Competency Validation helps students understand precisely what makes them competent in a specific skill.

Scenarios give real-life examples so students understand the application and importance of critical thinking skills.

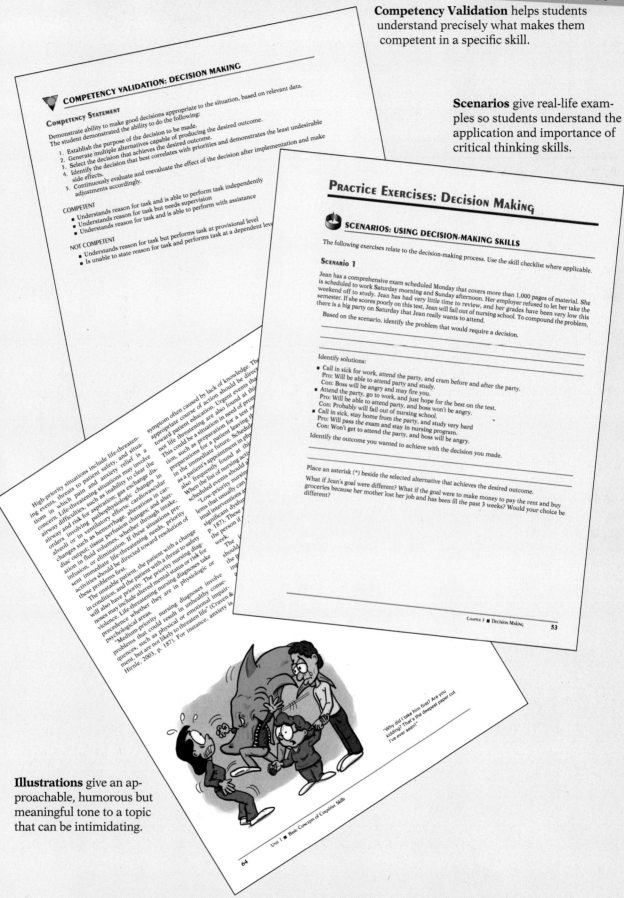

COMPETENCY VALIDATION: DECISION MAKING

Competency Statement

Demonstrate ability to make good decisions appropriate to the situation, based on relevant data.
The student demonstrated the ability to do the following:

1. Establish the purpose of the decision to be made.
2. Generate multiple alternatives capable of producing the desired outcome.
3. Select the decision that achieves the desired outcome.
4. Identify the decision that best correlates with priorities and demonstrates the least undesirable side effects.
5. Continuously evaluate and reevaluate the effect of the decision after implementation and make adjustments accordingly.

COMPETENT
- Understands reason for task and is able to perform task independently
- Understands reason for task but needs supervision
- Understands reason for task and is able to perform with assistance

NOT COMPETENT
- Understands reason for task but performs task at provisional level
- Is unable to state reason for task and performs task at a dependent level

PRACTICE EXERCISES: DECISION MAKING

SCENARIOS: USING DECISION-MAKING SKILLS

The following exercises relate to the decision-making process. Use the skill checklist where applicable.

SCENARIO 1

Jean has a comprehensive exam scheduled Monday that covers more than 1,000 pages of material. She is scheduled to work Saturday morning and Sunday afternoon. Her employer refused to let her take the weekend off to study. Jean has had very little time to review, and her grades have been very low this semester. If she scores poorly on this test, Jean will fail out of nursing school. To compound the problem, there is a big party on Saturday that Jean really wants to attend.

Based on the scenario, identify the problem that would require a decision.

_____

Identify solutions:
- Call in sick for work, attend the party, and cram before and after the party.
  Pro: Will be able to attend party and study.
  Con: Boss will be angry and may fire you.
- Attend the party, go to work, and just hope for the best on the test.
  Pro: Will be able to attend party, and boss won't be angry.
  Con: Probably will fail out of nursing school.
- Call in sick, stay home from the party, and study very hard
  Pro: Will pass the exam and stay in nursing program.
  Con: Won't get to attend the party, and boss will be angry.

Identify the outcome you wanted to achieve with the decision you made.

_____

Place an asterisk (*) beside the selected alternative that achieves the desired outcome.

What if Jean's goal were different? What if the goal were to make money to pay the rent and buy groceries because her mother lost her job and has been ill the past 3 weeks? Would your choice be different?

_____

CHAPTER 3 ■ Decision Making   53

High-priority situations include life-threatening events, threats to patient safety, and situations in which pain and anxiety relief is a concern. Life-threatening situations may involve airway difficulties, such as inability to clear the airway and risk for aspiration; gas exchange disorders or in ventilatory efforts; cardiovascular changes such as hemorrhage, alterations in cardiac output; tissue perfusion changes; and alteration in fluid volumes, or elimination. If these situations present immediate life-threatening needs, priority activities should be directed toward resolution of these problems first.

The unstable patient, the patient with a change in condition, and the patient with a threat to safety will also have priority. The priority nursing diagnoses may include altered mental status or risk for violence, whether they are in physiologic or psychological areas.

"Medium-priority nursing diagnoses involve problems that could result in unhealthy consequences that could result in unhealthy consequences, such as physical or emotional impairment, but are not likely to threaten life" (Craven & Hirnle, 2003, p. 187). For instance, anxiety is

symptom often caused by lack of knowledge. The appropriate course of action should be directed toward patient education. Urgent events that are not life threatening are also found at this level. This could be a situation in need of preparations for a patient leaving the immediate future. Scheduling t as a patient's appointment in ph also frequently found at this When the list of nursing acti scheduled events should a

"Low-priority nursing lems that usually can imal interventions a significant dysfun p. 187). These the person if week.

The should the in

Illustrations give an approachable, humorous but meaningful tone to a topic that can be intimidating.

"Why did I take him first? Are you kidding? That's the deepest paper cut I've ever seen!"

UNIT 1 ■ Basic Concepts of Cognitive Skills

64

Objectives alert students to the important points that are discussed in each chapter.

Key Points summarize main concepts from the chapters.

CRITICAL THINKING in NURSING: A COGNITIVE SKILLS WORKBOOK

SAUNDRA K. LIPE, RN, MSN

Rend Lake College
Ina, Illinois

SHARON BEASLEY, RN, MSN, PHD

Rend Lake College
Ina, Illinois

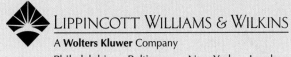

LIPPINCOTT WILLIAMS & WILKINS
A **Wolters Kluwer** Company

Philadelphia • Baltimore • New York • London
Buenos Aires • Hong Kong • Sydney • Tokyo

Acquisitions Editor: Quincy McDonald
Managing Editor: Joseph Morita
Editorial Assistant: Marie Rim
Senior Production Manager: Helen Ewan
Managing Editor / Production: Erika Kors
Design Coordinator: Brett MacNaughton
Cover Designer: Melissa Walter
Interior Designer: Melissa Olson
Illustrator: Matt Andrews
Senior Manufacturing Coordinator: Michael Carcel
Manufacturing Manager: William Alberti
Indexer: Ellen S. Brennan
Compositor: Circle Graphics
Printer: Quebecor Dubuque

9 8 7 6 5

Library of Congress Cataloging-in-Publication Data

Lipe, Saundra K.
   Critical thinking in nursing: A cognitive skills workbook / Saundra K. Lipe, Sharon Beasley.
     p. ; cm.
   Includes bibliographical references and index.
   ISBN 13: 978-0-7817-4042-5
   ISBN 10: 0-7817-4042-8 (alk. paper)
    1. Nursing. 2. Cognition. 3. Critical thinking. I. Beasley, Sharon. II. Title.
   [DNLM: 1. Cognition. 2. Nursing Process. 3. Thinking. WY 100 L764c 2004]
  RT84.5.L565 2004
  610.73—dc22

                            2003058864

Care has been taken to confirm the accuracy of the information presented and to describe generally accepted practices. However, the authors, editors, and publisher are not responsible for errors or omissions or for any consequences from application of the information in this book and make no warranty, express or implied, with respect to the content of the publication.

The authors, editors, and publisher have exerted every effort to ensure that drug selection and dosage set forth in this text are in accordance with the current recommendations and practice at the time of publication. However, in view of ongoing research, changes in government regulations, and the constant flow of information relating to drug therapy and drug reactions, the reader is urged to check the package insert for each drug for any change in indications and dosage and for added warnings and precautions This is particularly important when the recommended agent is a new or infrequently employed drug.

Some drugs and medical devices presented in this publication have Food and Drug Administration (FDA) clearance for limited use in restricted research settings. It is the responsibility of the health care provider to ascertain the FDA status of each drug or device planned for use in his or her clinical practice.

Reviewers

ILENE BORZE, RN, MS, CEN
Professor
Gateway Community College
Phoenix, Arizona

PAULA H. BRYANT, RN, MSN
Associate Professor of Nursing
Middle Georgia College
Cochran, Georgia

JEANIE BURT, MA, RN
Assistant Professor
Harding University College of Nursing
Searcy, Arkansas

PEGGY ELLIS, PhD, RNCS, ANP
Clinical Associate Professor
Barnes College of Nursing, University of Missouri
St. Louis, Missouri

PAT GRACI, MSN, RN
Associate Professor
Western Connecticut State University
Danbury, Connecticut

PENNY HEASLIP, BScN, MEd, RN
Nursing Department Chairperson
University of the Cariboo
Kamloops, British Columbia

CHRISTINE HICKS, BSc, MSc, PhD
Lecturer, Department of Medicine
St. George Clinical School
Sydney, Australia

NANCY HINZMAN, MSN, RNC
Associate Professor
College of Mount Saint Joseph
Cincinnati, Ohio

MAGGIE KEIL, RN, MNE
Assistant Professor
Victor Valley College
Novato, California

BRENDA MICHEL, MS, RN
Professor
Lincoln Land Community College
Springfield, Illinois

BRENDA MORRIS, EDD, RN
Clinical Associate Professor
Arizona State University
Tempe, Arizona

LAUREN E. O'HARE, MS, EdD
Assistant Professor
Wagner College
Staten Island, New York

PEGGY PRZYBYCIEN, RNMS
Associate Professor
Onondaga Community College
Syracuse, New York

BARBARA B. REES, RN, DSN
Chair, Health Sciences Division and
Professor of Nursing
Floyd College
Rome, Georgia

BETTY E. RICHARDS, RN, MSN
Professor
Middle Georgia College
Cochran, Georgia

ESTHER SALINAS, RN, MSN, MS ED
Associate Professor
Del Mar College
Corpus Christi, Texas

SANDRA SCHULER, RN, MS
Professor
Montgomery College
Takoma Park, Maryland

ALITA K. SELLERS, PhD
Professor
West Virginia University Parkersburg
Parkersburg, West Virginia

SANDRA P. SMALL, RN, MScN
Associate Professor
School of Nursing, Memorial University of
Newfoundland
St. Johns, Canada

JOANN THOMAS, MN, ARNP, CNAA, BC
Director of Nursing/Allied Health
Fort Scott Community College
Fort Scott, Kansas

RANDONNA TIMS, RN, MS
Faculty
Tulsa Community College
Tulsa, Oklahoma

SHARON J. WALTERS, RN, MSN
Assistant Professor
University of Arkansas
Fayetteville, Arkansas

PAT WINBERG, RN, MSN
Faculty
Penn Valley Community College
Kansas City, Missouri

PREFACE

Critical Thinking in Nursing is designed to present the cognitive skills required of the professional nurse. In order to enhance the understanding and application of these skills, they are presented in a competency-based, clinically oriented format. The goal of this textbook is to teach nurses how to think critically while applying the skills necessary to practice nursing in a competent manner.

CHAPTER ORGANIZATION

The chapters are arranged in an order that reflects the progressive application of concepts. *Critical thinking* is the basic construct, and is incorporated in all the processes; it is addressed in the first chapter. The second chapter introduces the generic *problem solving* process, discussing concepts related to solving both nursing, and non-nursing problems. Effective problem solving involves critical thinking. It also usually requires making a decision. *Decision making* is explored next, and is presented as a step in the problem-solving process. During the course of a day, the nurse must make many decisions, often while under a time constraint and while juggling multiple demands. A working understanding of priority setting is essential in today's health care environment. *Priority setting* is part of the decision making process, and is discussed in Chapter 4.

All these concepts are meshed in the process of problem solving particular to the nursing profession, which is known as the *nursing process*. This process is systematic, and involves the following steps: assessment, analysis, outcome identification, planning, implementation, and evaluation. The nursing process is the topic of Chapter 5.

Delegation allows increased productivity through the effective use of resources. Nurses must learn to transfer responsibility for performing specific tasks, while retaining accountability for the quality of the performance. Chapter 6 presents delegation principles that can be learned by applying the nursing process.

The remaining chapters deal with the application of cognitive skills in processing clinical data. Unlike the nursing process, which is usually performed in set steps, nurses use cognitive skills as

they are needed. These skills are further developed in Chapters 7 through 11: *Communication; Patient Teaching; Applying Clinical Reasoning to Various Practice Settings; Ethical Decision Making; and Applying Nursing Judgment in Clinical Settings.*

CHAPTER FORMAT

All of the chapters are arranged in a consistent format. In the beginning of each chapter, basic theory is interspersed with examples. Active learning exercises follow this theory. To reinforce the concepts, the authors recommend routinely incorporating the practice exercises into the study of the chapter. Next, cognitive skills, which are accompanied by competency statements, are presented in a checklist format. The checklist allows novice nurses to develop their critical thinking while using a concrete format to which they are accustomed.

The skill sheets were developed to guide the new nurse in safe nursing practice. Key elements in each step of the nursing process are identified. The tool can be applied to a specific task, an individual patient, or to the skill mix and care delivery needs of an entire work assignment.

The skill checklists can be used in several ways. Instructors may use the scenarios provided with all of the skill checklists to practice the process discussed in the chapter. Instructors may also provide their own scenarios to complete the process. These may be performed in a laboratory setting. For example, to add realism to the process of learning to telephone a physician, students may be required to place calls to an instructor who is role-playing a physician. The instructor can then evaluate the student by using the checklist as a tool. This practice will help internalize the processes, so that the students will feel comfortable applying them to clinical settings in the management of patient care. Finally, instructors can use some of the checklists for evaluation in the clinical setting.

AUDIENCE

The target group for this book is students in the second semester of nursing courses. Chapters 1 through 5 can be used by LPN/LVN students to develop critical thinking skills. The returning LPN/LVN student who is making a transition to the RN role, as well as the generic nursing student, can use this book to develop skills needed to process information, manage care, and make nursing judgments. Designed for students engaged in independent study or traditional classrooms, this book provides content, exercises, and strategies to enhance the thinking skills of the novice nurse. The goal is to make these concepts clear, concise, and applicable to the practice setting.

Acknowledgments

Many people have been very supportive and helpful in making this book a reality. Our deepest appreciation goes to the nursing students at Rend Lake College for giving us the inspiration to create the book. We gratefully acknowledge our colleagues and friends for their assistance and contributions to the exercises in Chapters 9, 10, and 11. They generously shared their knowledge, experiences, and ideas with us. These people include: Mary Kuhl, RN, PhD; Trish Bennett-Minor, RN, MSN; Bonnie Tolbert, RN, MSEd; Barbara Crouse, RN, MSN; Dorothy Donoho, RN (Saundra's mom); Maggie Peters, RN, BSN; Pricella Edwards, RN, BSN; Rhonda Edwards, RN, BSN; Virginia Telford, RN, MSN; Lynn Lenker, RN, MSN; Mike Adamson, RN, BSN; and Dale Allen, MSES.

Special thanks go to the staff at Lippincott Williams & Wilkins, including Marilee LeBon, Editor, whose caring attention and positive reinforcement made the project easier; Ilze Rader, former Executive Editor, for believing in the project; and Joe Morita for fitting the bits and pieces together. We are ever grateful to our design coordinator, Brett Mac-Naughton, through whose efforts we have achieved the visual effects we had hoped for, and to our managing editor, Erika Kors, for her efforts in ensuring that the final product was of the utmost quality. It was also a pleasure to work with Matt Andrews, whose wonderful job with the humorous illustrations enhances the text.

Finally, thanks to the reviewers for sharing their time and expertise, which helped to improve the quality and broaden the perspective encompassed in the work. All of these contributions have provided an opportunity for our personal and professional growth. We'd like to express our thanks and appreciation to all who have been involved in so many different ways.

SAUNDRA K. LIPE
SHARON BEASLEY

CONTENTS

UNIT ONE

BASIC CONCEPTS OF COGNITIVE SKILLS

CHAPTER 1

Critical Thinking

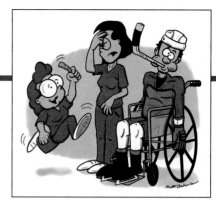

1. Define critical thinking.

2. Differentiate among critical thinking, problem solving, and decision making.

3. Describe the characteristics of a critical thinker.

4. Explain the intellectual standards used in second-order thinking (critical thinking).

5. Delineate the process involved in critical thinking.

The role of the nurse has shifted from one of "hand-maiden" to one of an autonomous partner in health care delivery. The impact of technological expansion and the increased acuity level of patients, combined with consumer demand for accountability and responsibility, have fueled this change. Currently, novice nurses must possess cognitive skills that require critical thinking. The nurse uses critical thinking to solve problems, make decisions, and establish priorities in the clinical setting. The framework for solving patient problems is called the nursing process. Critical thinking is inherent to *the nursing process.*

DEFINITION

Critical thinking is an essential skill in the administration of safe, competent nursing care. Critical thinking may be defined as "the process of purposeful, self regulatory judgment. The process gives reasoned consideration to evidence, contexts, conceptualizations, methods, and criteria" (American Philosophical Association, 1990, p. 2).

Ennis describes critical thinking as "reasonable, reflective thinking that is focused on deciding what to believe or do" (Nosich, 2001, p. 2).

Critical thinking is goal directed; it is thinking with a purpose. Critical thinking also involves questioning. These questions include: *Why? Who? What if? When? Where?* Data are collected and organized within the critical thinking process. Pertinent data are separated from irrelevant data. Related data are clustered together to encourage the recognition of patterns. These clusters of data are then analyzed, and successful solutions to problems are identified.

RELATIONSHIP TO PROBLEM SOLVING AND DECISION MAKING

The practice of nursing involves setting priorities, making decisions, and solving problems. If these activities were approached in a haphazard fashion, patient outcomes would suffer. The purpose of this book is to outline a systematic process that can be used to perform these activities.

Frequently, terms such as *critical thinking, problem solving,* and *decision making* are used interchangeably in nursing literature, resulting in confusion for the reader. Although these processes are related, they are also distinct and can be studied individually.

Problem solving is a systematic approach, resulting in the formation of solutions. It involves the identification of the root problem through analysis. The nursing process is a type of problem solving used in developing a plan of care for each patient. The nursing process can be applied to solve problems relating to issues that affect patients as well as staff, such as cost containment, productivity, and quality of care.

Decision making involves choosing from among options. It is a step in the problem-solving process. However, not all decisions are the result of a problem. Therefore, the term *decision making* is not synonymous with problem solving. Priority setting is included in the decision-making process. Because of the complex nature of these processes, decision making and priority setting are discussed in separate chapters of this book.

Critical thinking is a style of thinking that is necessary for success with all the other processes. It represents the rational thought process that underlies problem solving and decision making.

- Comes to well-reasoned conclusions and solutions, testing them against relevant criteria and standards.
- Thinks open-mindedly within alternative systems of thought, recognizing, and assessing, as need be, their assumptions, implications, and practical consequences.
- Communicates effectively with others in figuring out solutions to complex problems.

Critical thinking is, in short, self-directed, self-disciplined, self-monitored, and self-corrective thinking.

INTELLECTUAL STANDARDS IN THINKING

Thinking occurs spontaneously in daily life without consideration of the process. This nonanalytical thinking can be filled with biased, preconceived notions and incorrect information. Second-order thinking, as identified by Paul and Elder, raises the level of thought process so that the parts of a situation are consciously reviewed. This involves assessing each aspect and restructuring thinking to focus on central issues. "Critical thinkers routinely take their thinking apart" (Paul & Elder, 2001a, p. 52).

Standards are essential to increasing the quality of thinking. Increased skill in the application

THE CRITICAL THINKER

The critical thinker has many typical characteristics. This individual is an independent thinker who is not influenced by the people who state, "We have always done it that way." Critical thinkers question conventions and habits, basing decisions on sound reasoning. They recognize biases and assumptions, and they possess an open mind. Critical thinkers are observant and able to organize and prioritize data. Good judgment, intuition, and past experiences are all used by the critical thinker to develop solutions and analyze actions.

Nurses can cultivate critical thinking by questioning and by seeking knowledge. Paul and Elder (2001c, p. 1) state:

A well-cultivated thinker:

- Raises vital questions and problems, formulating them clearly and precisely.
- Gathers and assesses relevant information, and can effectively interpret it.

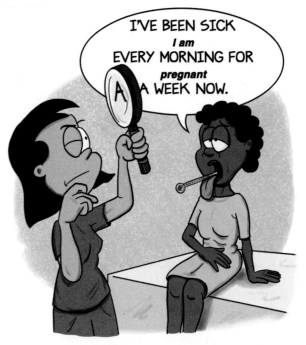

Read between the lines.

of standards improves reasoning. This leads to clearer, more precise thinking with less personal bias. Therefore, critical thinkers should check their thinking according to standards.

Paul and Elder (2001b) identified these standards as:

- Clarity
- Accuracy
- Precision
- Relevance
- Depth
- Breadth
- Logic
- Significance
- Fairness

Important questions the critical thinker should ask to reinforce each standard are listed in Table 1-1.

The standards of critical thinking are certainly applicable to nursing. A well-disciplined critical thinker attempts to be clear and precise, to verify and clarify data, and to sort out and discard unnecessary information. These are important actions for the nurse. After gathering enough data to make fair assumptions that are free of personal bias, the nurse can use the data to make sound judgments related to patient care. The critical thinking process is also essential in giving directions to staff and communicating information clearly in complex nursing situations.

CLARITY

Can u elaborate give an example?

Thinking clearly is central to understanding. If a concept is clear in one medium of communication, but the thought cannot be transferred into one of the other media, (e.g., thinking to written word or written word to verbalized communication), the concept needs better definition. Reasoning is essential to all forms of communication—reading, writing, speaking, listening, and collaborative learning. For example, if the reader of this text cannot

TABLE 1-1	QUESTIONS TO REINFORCE EACH STANDARD OF CRITICAL THINKING
STANDARD	**QUESTIONS**
Clarity	Could you elaborate further? Could you give me an example? Could you illustrate what you mean?
Accuracy	How could we check on that? How could we find out if that is true? How could we verify or test that?
Precision	Could you be more specific? Could you give me more details? Could you be more exact?
Relevance	How does that relate to the problem? How does that bear on the question? How does that help us with the issue?
Depth	What factors make this a difficult problem? What are some of the complexities of this question? What are some of the difficulties we need to deal with?
Breadth	Do we need to look at this from another perspective? Do we need to consider another point of view? Do we need to look at this in other ways?
Logic	Does all this make sense together? Does your first paragraph fit in with your last? Does what you say follow from the evidence?
Significance	Is this the most important problem to consider? Is this the central idea to focus on? Which of these facts are most important?
Fairness ·	Are my selfish desires keeping me from being fair to others? Am I sympathetically entering the viewpoints of others? Am I putting views I oppose in their strongest form?

Used with permission from Paul, R., & Elder, L. (2001). *Mini-guide: How to study and learn.* Dillon Beach, CA: Foundation for Critical Thinking.

explain the concept of critical thinking to a classmate, then her or his thinking lacks clarity.

ACCURACY

The need for accuracy in health care is self-evident. Amputating the wrong limb, administering incorrect medications, and performing treatments on the wrong patient are all examples of front-page news involving inaccuracy. Accuracy in the interpretation of evidence and data are critical to the outcome of nursing care. The critical thinker obtains information from reliable sources.

PRECISION

Nurses experience many demands in the delivery of health care. In an effort to meet these demands, the nurse may fail to meet the critical need of being exact. Precise reflection of thoughts takes time. Errors in patient care can occur when the nurse takes shortcuts. For example, the nurse who fails to identify patients before medication administration has sacrificed precision.

Nosich (2001, p. 137) advised nursing students to use the following measures for developing precision:

- Anticipate where others will need details to follow your reasoning.
- When you report what other people say, or the results of an experiment, or a procedure, try to say it exactly.
- Look up details in the text.
- When you take detailed notes, do so in outline form.
- Keep going from the general to the specific and from the specific to the general: What is a specific instance of this generality?
- How does this detail fit into the whole picture?
- Get feedback on where you need to be more specific, more exact.
- Ask fellow students where they need you to supply more detail.

RELEVANCE

All data pertinent to the situation or concept should be collected. Then, nonpertinent or insignificant data can be deleted. The mind can become cluttered with irrelevant facts; therefore, the individual needs to figure out what is most important and stay focused. Suppose, for example, that the nurse is as-

sessing a patient with a diagnosis of congestive heart failure. While checking for peripheral edema, the nurse notes an old tattoo on the patient's ankle. This is most likely trivial information not related to the assessment. The nurse should not allow it to interfere with his or her thought processes at this time. There are enough important facts to remember while performing the assessment.

DEPTH

Dealing with a very complex issue in a superficial way does not address the underlying cause of the problem. Being able to perceive the complexities of a situation and to visualize the relationship among various aspects is important. For example, if diabetic patient is admitted with a blood sugar level of 500 to 600 mg/dL, the health care team will quickly treat the blood sugar elevation to get it under control. However, if the problem that caused the elevated blood sugar is not treated, the patient will return with more problems later. The mind works in a similar fashion. Controlling the way information is processed produces better outcomes. The critical thinker must explore deeply enough to get beyond the surface issues.

BREADTH

Breadth concerns thinking about a situation from several different points of view. At times, people are so adamant about their own point of view that they cannot see the complexities involved in the problem. The critical thinker gathers more information and gives reasoned consideration to other points of view. Differing points of view occur frequently in health care settings. For example, consider the following circumstances surrounding a patient who has been placed on a ventilator. Her son, who lives 3,000 miles away, would like the ventilatory assistance to continue. He states, "I'm not ready to give up on Mom." However, the patient's daughter has been the primary caregiver. She feels her mother has suffered enough. The nurse must consider both points of view before taking action.

LOGIC

When using logic, one seeks to discover whether things make sense. To arrive at an accurate conclusion, assumptions must be valid. The conclusion must be based on the evidence. Nursing procedures must be performed in a logical order. For

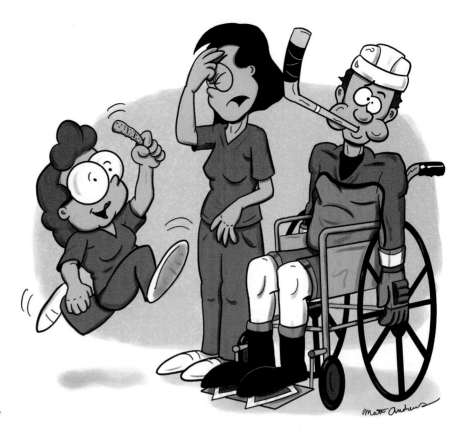

"Good news! I found a Band-Aid!"

example, if procedures involving sterile technique are not done in a certain order, asepsis will be compromised.

Significance

Significance is a measure of whether information is critical rather than peripheral or trivial in a given situation. For instance, for a patient just returning from the postanesthesia care unit (PACU), vital signs would be critical information. If the nurse leaves the room to obtain a blanket for a family member before taking vital signs, an error in significance has occurred.

Fairness

Fairness pertains to being open to new ideas or information. Other viewpoints should be given adequate consideration. Consider the following example: A nursing unit has always charted in three different places. The new nurse suggests the use of a flow sheet to streamline the data entry and save time. The regular staff refuse to consider the idea because "that's just not the way we do it here." This refusal to consider new ideas demonstrates unfair thinking.

PROCESS OF CRITICAL THINKING

Critical thinking is not a step-by-step process. The order in which the thinker proceeds depends on the nature of the situation. However, there are aspects the individual must consider in order to think critically. These areas are identified in Figure 1-1.

We Think For a Purpose

Critical thinking should be purposeful. Undirected thought is not critical thought. The thinker must identify the purpose of the thought and should check periodically during the process to ensure that he or she is still on target. Data that pertain to the issue being studied should be collected and organized. It is important that all pertinent data be collected; therefore, the critical thinker tries to discover what data might be missing. For example, a high school student might use critical thinking when considering a career in nursing. After collecting data concerning educational requirements, desired skills, and the job market for nurses, the student looks over the collected information and discovers that data on ability are missing.

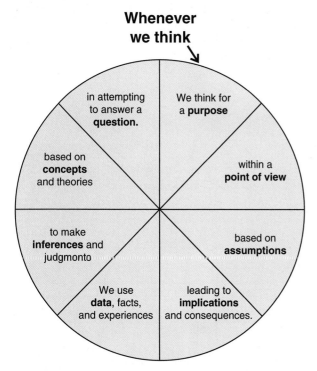

Whenever we think

- We think for a **purpose**
- within a **point of view**
- based on **assumptions**
- leading to **implications** and consequences.
- We use **data**, facts, and experiences
- to make **inferences** and judgmonto
- based on **concepts** and theories
- in attempting to answer a **question.**

FIGURE 1-1

Universal structures of thought. Adapted from Paul, R., & Elder, L. (2001). *Critical thinking: Tools for taking charge of your learning and your life.* Upper Saddle River, NJ: Prentice Hall.

Consequently, the student accesses computer software that analyzes the abilities required for a nursing career. By using critical thinking skills, the student has identified missing data. He or she then proceeds to obtain the needed information.

Within a Point of View

Critical thinkers seek out other points of view. For maximum benefit, the opinions of others must be evaluated fairly. Everyone has assumptions and biases. To minimize the negative impact of preconceived notions, the opinions of others should be sought. The thinker should listen carefully with an open mind. In the previous scenario, the student seeking to learn more about nursing as a career could discuss nursing with current practitioners.

Based on Assumptions

Every decision is influenced by assumptions. Critical thinkers must examine assumptions and assess their validity and accuracy. For example, a student may assume that newly graduated nurses work from 9:00 AM to 5:00 PM on week-

days or spend most of the shift on the phone, as depicted in a television program. If a career decision is based on these questionable assumptions, dissatisfaction can occur when the truth is discovered.

Consider the following scenario that demonstrates the presence of assumptions: A woman who appears to be in her late thirties was admitted to the same-day treatment area for an epidural injection to treat intractable back pain. The patient is of medium weight, wearing false eyelashes and clothing that would be more appropriate for an adolescent. The patient has a history of hepatitis C. She is very friendly with all the staff, even those she has never met. She repeatedly uses "Honey" and "Dear" when addressing staff members. The patient complains continuously of severe back pain. Her visitor is wearing a blazer, heavy eye makeup, tight leather pants, and a lot of costume jewelry. The patient and visitor are laughing and talking loudly. Based on this limited information, answer the following questions:

1. How do you think the patient got hepatitis C?
2. Who do you think the visitor is?
3. Will the patient and visitor share any medication upon discharge?
4. How often does the patient come for epidural injections?

Some people would assume that the patient is an intravenous drug user who contracted hepatitis from substance abuse and is seeking drugs and attention. In reality, the patient is younger than she appears. She has a history of cancer of the uterus and ovaries. She also has a history of chemotherapy, multiple surgeries, and blood transfusions, from which she contracted the hepatitis. She wears false eyelashes because her natural lashes grew back very thin after chemotherapy. She also has a history of a fall, resulting in lumbar disk damage and back pain. The visitor is her younger sister, who came to visit her after attending rehearsal for a play, without changing out of her costume. Inaccurate assumptions can result in faulty reasoning with undesirable consequences.

Leading to Implications and Consequences

All reasoning has implications and consequences. It is vital to consider the results of chosen strategies early in the process. Inconsistencies in the thinking process should also be identified. For example, in the previous scenario, if the nurse assumes the patient is seeking drugs and allows a personal bias to influence decision making, the nurse may limit pain medication. As a direct result of this personal bias, patient care would be negatively affected. Faulty reasoning may result from using flawed logic or imposing personal bias.

We Use Data, Facts, and Experiences

Related information should be clustered. This involves putting related information together. To cluster information, it is necessary to identify signs, symptoms, and trends. The information should be sorted into normal data and data that deviate from normal standards. The nurse obtains data during a patient assessment and notes deviations from normal. The data are then clustered to identify problems and trends. For example, consider a patient admitted for appendicitis who presented with an elevated white blood cell count, elevated temperature, and rebound tenderness in the right lower quadrant. This trend in data is consistent with the medical diagnosis.

To Make Inferences and Judgments

All reasoning contains interpretations from which conclusions are drawn and data are given meaning. Critical thinkers infer only what the evidence implies. Instincts should always be checked. If it doesn't feel right, it probably isn't. For example, consider a patient who demonstrates moderate changes in vital signs, with a decrease in urinary output and pale skin. Using nursing instincts and available data, the nurse infers that the patient has active blood loss, despite absence of obvious bleeding. The inference and judgment are appropriate for the data. The nurse must give meaning to all the data, or poor judgment can result.

Based on Concepts and Theories

Data should be compared with theories of nursing practice. This helps ensure that thinking is accurate. To verify the thinking, more information should be gathered. The present situation should be compared with past experience or theory information learned in class. A sound knowledge base founded in the classroom can help the learner to validate information and ensure that it is correct. Strategies should be selected that reflect that transfer of theory knowledge to the practice setting. Evidence-based practice requires the use of research-based interventions to ensure appropri-

ate and consistent quality care. Nursing Interventions Classification (NIC) includes a full range of interventions that are research based. Therefore, selecting from the NIC list for an intervention to apply to the practice setting will ensure an appropriate research-based choice.

In Attempting to Answer a Question

All reasoning leads somewhere. As data are collected, the critical thinker should be able to identify key concepts and explain them clearly. If thinking has proceeded in a logical fashion, the thinker will be able to verbalize relevant, accurate explanations for the cause-and-effect relationship. For example, if a patient demonstrates symptoms of depression, the nurse needs to consider the cause. A patient may exhibit similar symptoms whether the depression is a result of life events or is endogenous. However, treatment and nursing interventions vary, depending on the underlying pathology. Therefore, the cause-and-effect relationship must be considered, not just the symptoms.

SKILLS OF CRITICAL THINKING

Certain skills are important for effective critical thinking (Box 1-1). These mental abilities contribute to clear, rational thought. Nurses use critical thinking skills daily to analyze and interpret patient care situations. As with most skills, proficiency in critical thinking increases with practice.

The cognitive skills used to analyze and interpret data through critical thinking are applied within a framework called the *nursing process*. This process provides a structure for applying critical thinking to nursing tasks and managing patient care. These cognitive skills direct the nurse to focus on the outcome assessment. The six essential cognitive skills described here will be applied to the nursing process framework and demonstrated further in Chapter 5, Nursing Process Applications.

Box 1-1 Skills of Critical Thinking

Interpretation
Analysis
Evaluation
Inference
Explanation
Self-regulation

INTERPRETATION

The skill of interpretation includes the ability to understand and explain the meaning of information or an event. It requires knowledge of theory and its subsequent application. For instance, the nurse uses theory knowledge to interpret a patient's lab results. The nurse must also look at the significance of the event. For example, consider a nurse who observes a patient attempting to strike a staff member. Using interpretive skills and the patient's diagnosis, the nurse would consider the possible causes and significance of the action.

ANALYSIS

Nurses are practicing analysis when they investigate a course of action based on objective and subjective data. Various measures may be considered to solve a problem. The nurse should consider the advantages, disadvantages, and consequences of all possibilities. The analysis of assessment data provides direction in determining the problems the nurse can treat independently and the problems that require collaboration. It also helps to identify patient care that needs to be referred.

EVALUATION

The process of evaluation is the assessment of the information obtained. The nurse must consider the source of the information. Is the source reliable? Is the information credible? What are the chances that bias could be involved? Is the information relevant to the current problem? In the previous example, suppose family members of the combative patient state that they have never witnessed this behavior before. The nurse must apply the questions listed above to this new information. The nurse must also apply this skill to assess whether the desired outcome for the patient was achieved.

INFERENCE

Critical thinkers who are skilled at inference can make correct conclusions based on available information. Their decisions are based on sound reasoning. Again, in the case of the combative patient, the nurse would gather lab results, baseline data from the chart, information from old charts, and a history of the onset of symptoms. The nurse would

also consult with the patient and the family concerning the behavior. From these data, the nurse might conclude that the patient is suffering from an electrolyte imbalance. In this case, the nurse has used several reliable sources to come to a conclusion. The nursing diagnoses on the patient's plan of care are based on these conclusions. The nurse applies this skill of clinical reasoning while monitoring the patient's changes in health status.

EXPLANATION

Another important critical thinking skill is the ability to explain one's conclusions. The nurse should be able to provide sound rationales for answers. The ability to explain the reasoning process itself is also beneficial. This involves describing the events that lead to a particular conclusion.

SELF-REGULATION

Self-regulation involves monitoring one's own thinking. The individual should reflect on the process leading to his or her conclusion. Did I perform the thinking process appropriately? Did I obtain all the pertinent facts? Am I making any incorrect assumptions? While monitoring thinking, the individual should self-correct the thinking process as needed. The skill of evaluation is used to assess the accuracy and validity of information obtained. Self-regulation involves the recognition and correction of errors in one's thought process. Self-regulation occurs in response to self-evaluation of thinking.

PITFALLS IN CRITICAL THINKING

Many errors in thinking can be seen as pitfalls to the critical thinking process. Errors in the critical thinking process may result in illogical or biased thinking. The disciplined thinker recognizes and avoids these pitfalls.

Illogical Process

Critical thinking fails as a process when logic is not used. A common fallacy can arise from using a circular argument (e.g., it is true because it is so). There is no step that proves the assumptions. For example, a nurse might write the nursing diagnosis "Ineffective coping: Individual related to

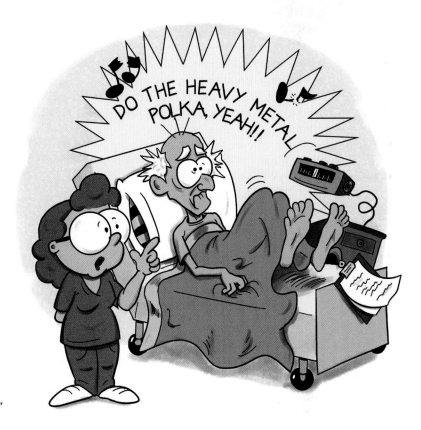

"I should have known that **Heavy Metal Memories** wouldn't relax you that much."

poor coping skills as evidenced by inability to cope." This does not define the problem; it simply makes a circle.

The logic of the conclusion must be examined. Is the conclusion based on true assumptions? Does it follow logically? For example, Mary claims that all of the students in her nursing fundamentals class are cheating. Robert states that at least one student is not cheating because he is not cheating. Robert cannot then conclude that no students cheat. This has not been proved by the assumptions.

A common pitfall resulting in illogical thinking is called *appeal to tradition*. This is the argument that "we have always done it this way." Creativity is stifled, and new strategies are ignored. Critical thinking results in the careful consideration of various options and the solicitation of input from others.

Errors in logic also occur when the thinker makes hasty generalizations without considering all the evidence. The critical thinker does not jump to conclusions.

Bias

Everyone has biases. Critical thinkers examine their biases and do not allow them to compromise the integrity of the thinking process. Biases can in-

terfere with quality patient care. For example, Jane feels that patients with alcoholism could stop drinking if they wanted to badly enough. She feels that these patients are manipulative. When the patient with alcoholism complains of anxiety, Jane may dismiss this as attention seeking and thereby miss the signs of delirium tremens.

Closed-mindedness

Another deterrent to critical thinking is a tendency to be closed-minded. The close-minded individual ignores alternative points of view. Input from important sources such as experts, patients, and significant others is ignored. This results in limited options and the decreased use of innovative ideas.

SUMMARY

The practice of nursing includes solving problems, making decisions, and setting priorities. Clarity of thought is essential to all of these. The importance of critical thinking cannot be overemphasized. Critical thinking differs from random thinking in that it is goal directed and purposeful. The purpose of critical thinking is often the solution of a problem.

- Critical thinking is an essential skill in the administration of safe, competent nursing care.
- Critical thinking is goal directed. It involves the clustering and analysis of data to solve problems systematically.
- Critical thinking is inherent to problem solving and decision making.
- The critical thinker is unbiased, open-minded, and observant. The critical thinker possesses good judgment and intuition and the abilities to use analytical reasoning and to communicate effectively.
- The standards of critical thinking are clarity, accuracy, precision, relevance, depth, breadth, logic, significance, and fairness.
- In the process of thinking, we think for a purpose, within a point of view, based on assumptions leading to implications and consequences; we use data, facts, and experiences to make inferences and judgments, based on concepts and theories, in attempting to answer a question.
- Nurses use critical thinking skills daily for interpretation, analysis, evaluation, inference, explanation, and self-regulation in delivering patient care.
- Errors in thinking are pitfalls to the critical thinking process.

REFERENCES

Alfaro-LeFevre, R. (1999). *Critical thinking in nursing.* Philadelphia: W.B. Saunders.

Alfaro-LeFevre, R. (2001). Thinking critically about your assignments. *Nurse Educator, 26*(1), 15–16.

American Philosophical Association (1990). *Critical thinking: A statement of expert consensus for purposes of educational assessment and instruction, recommendations prepared for the Committee on Pre-college Philosophy.* ERIC Doc. No. ED 315-423.

Davies, R., & McDermott, D. (1996). *Mind opening training games.* New York: McGraw-Hill.

Facione, N. C., & Facione, P. A. (1996). Externalizing the critical thinking in knowledge development and critical thinking. *Nursing Outlook, 44*(3), 129–136.

Jacobs, P. M., Ott, B., Sullivan, B., Ulrich, Y., & Short, L. (1997). An approach to defining and operationalizing critical thinking. *Journal of Nursing Education, 36*(1), 19–22.

Marquis, B. L., & Huston, C. J. (2003). *Leadership roles and management functions in nursing.* Philadelphia: Lippincott Williams & Wilkins.

McCoy, C. W. (2002). *Why didn't I think of that: Think the unthinkable and achieve creative greatness.* Upper Saddle River, NJ: Prentice Hall.

Nosich, G. (2001). *Learning to think things through.* Upper Saddle River, NJ: Prentice Hall.

Paul, R. (1995). *Critical thinking: How to prepare students for a rapidly changing world.* Dillon Beach, CA: Foundation for Critical Thinking.

Paul, R., & Elder, L. (2001a). *Critical thinking: Tools for taking charge of your learning and your life.* Upper Saddle River, NJ: Prentice Hall.

Paul, R., & Elder, L. (2001b). *Mini-guide: How to study and learn.* Dillon Beach, CA: Foundation for Critical Thinking.

Paul, R., & Elder, L. (2001c). *Miniature guide to critical thinking: Concepts and tools.* Dillon Beach, CA: Foundation for Critical Thinking.

Rubenfeld, M. G., & Scheffer, B. K. (1999). *Critical thinking in nursing.* Philadelphia: Lippincott Williams & Wilkins.

Sedlak, C. A. (1997). Critical thinking of beginning baccalaureate nursing students during the first clinical nursing course. *Journal of Nursing Education, 36*(1), 11–18.

STUDENT WORKSHEETS

 ## SKILL SHEET: CRITICAL THINKING

PURPOSE

To demonstrate the transition to a higher-level thinking process that is necessary to perform competently in the role of a professional nurse.

Objectives

1. Place data in logical order to sequence events.
2. Demonstrate deliberate strategies that reflect a transfer of theory knowledge to the practice setting.
3. Analyze situations for similarities with previous experiences.
4. Identify the cause-and-effect relationship.
5. Adapt knowledge and skill gained in previous situations to present the problem.
6. Demonstrate the ability to apply sound reasoning to nursing practice.

 ## COMPETENCY VALIDATION: CRITICAL THINKING

COMPETENCY STATEMENT

1. The student will demonstrate a logical systematic thought process in analyzing and synthesizing data.
2. The student will demonstrate skill in evaluation and self-correction for her or his own thinking.

The student demonstrated the ability to do the following:

1. Identify purpose.
2. Assess data.
3. Utilize all appropriate resources to gather information.
4. Search for missing data.
5. Delete nonpertinent facts.
6. Seek and evaluate other points of view.
7. Recognize assumptions.
8. Assess validity and accuracy of assumptions.
9. Identify inconsistencies in thinking.
10. Examine bias.
11. Form a cluster with the data.
12. Identify signs, symptoms, and trends.
13. Sort signs and symptoms into normal data and those that deviate from normal standards.
14. Demonstrate an ability to recognize similarities and differences between situations.
15. Identify significant factors in the data.
16. Establish priorities based on urgency and need.
17. List valid conclusions based on evidence.
18. Select strategies that reflect transfer of theory knowledge to the practice setting.
19. Demonstrate logical thought processes to sequence events.
20. Explain key concepts.
21. Confirm the relationship between cause and effect.
22. Review and modify thinking as needed.

COMPETENT

- Understands reason for task and is able to perform task independently
- Understands reason for task but needs supervision
- Understands reason for task and is able to perform with assistance

NOT COMPETENT

- Understands reason for task but performs task at provisional level
- Is unable to state reason for task and performs task at a dependent level

 ## SKILL CHECKLIST: CRITICAL THINKING

CRITICAL THINKING	SATISFACTORY	UNSATISFACTORY	NI/COMMENTS
Identify the purpose.			
Identify all pertinent data.			
Collect significant and relevant data in an organized manner.			
Search for missing data.			
Seek other points of view.			
Evaluate opinions of others fairly.			
Recognize assumptions.			
Assess validity and accuracy of assumptions.			
Identify inconsistencies in thinking.			
Examine any bias.			
Cluster related information.			
Identify signs, symptoms, and trends.			
Sort the signs and symptoms into normal data and those that deviate from normal standards.			
Infer only what the evidence says.			
Recognize similarities and differences between situations.			
Select strategies that reflect transfer of theory knowledge to the practice setting.			
Explain key concepts.			
Verbalize relevant accurate explanations for the cause-and-effect relationship.			
Review and modify thinking as needed.			

SCENARIO TO ACCOMPANY STUDENT WORKSHEETS

During the assessment, Mr. Fellows relates a history of sudden onset of chest pain rated at 10 on a 1 to 10 scale, unrelieved by rest, which started while he was mowing the lawn. He describes the pain as "crushing, like a truck ran over my chest." His blood pressure is 200/110 mm Hg, temperature is 98.0°F (36.7°C); pulse is 106 beats/min; and respirations are 24 breaths/min. The pulse is irregular and thready, and the respirations are slightly dyspneic. The cardiac monitor reveals atrial fibrillation. During the assessment, his wife confides to the nurse that Mr. Fellows was treated 3 years ago for alcohol dependence. Currently, he is complaining of nausea and indigestion. His skin is pale and diaphoretic. He is restless and anxious. His wife is sitting at the bedside very tearful and emotional.

Apply the Critical Thinking Skill Sheet to the scenario. Work your way through the process, identifying important aspects:

Identify the purpose of critical thinking during the data collection.
List where you might find pertinent data.
Identify what the nurse can do to collect significant data in an organized manner.
Where would the nurse seek information to identify missing data?
What other points of view should the novice nurse seek in order to verify conclusions?
How can the nurse evaluate the opinions of others fairly?
Recognize assumptions.
Continue to apply the skill sheet to this patient scenario.

SITUATION	WHAT POSSIBLE INFERENCE CAN BE MADE?	WHAT ASSUMPTION LED TO THE INFERENCE?
The physician informed the patient that the lab data results are positive for cancer and that the disease has spread to the liver. The patient is very upset and crying.	The diagnosis of cancer caused the patient to feel sad.	All patients who learn they have a life-threatening disease are sad.
The physician told the patient that his WBC (white blood cell count) was abnormal and that it indicated an infection.		
The patient rang the call light for pain medication. The nurse had gone to lunch, and a delay resulted in the patient experiencing extreme pain for an extended time.		
The hospital is operated by a managed care company that frequently short-staffs the patient care areas. As a result of the working conditions, many of the nurses have quit. The result of increased short-staffing is poor patient care and overworked nurses.		
The patient was admitted to the nursing unit at the beginning of the 12-hour shift. The nursing staff had nine primary care patients to attend to. The nurse assigned to the patient was so busy that she failed to write a plan of care for the patient. The nurse failed to monitor the intravenous fluids and urinary output. As a result of the nurse's neglect, the patient went into cardiac failure due to the fluid overload.		

See the Answer Key in Appendix A for sample answers for this exercise.

PRACTICE EXERCISES: Critical Thinking

 ## SCENARIO: THINKING CRITICALLY

Think critically about the following question: In what area of nursing would you prefer to work upon graduation?

You have been given the purpose of critical thought. Work your way through the process, identifying important aspects.

- Identify the data you think would be pertinent to this decision.
- Collect and organize the data.
- List where you might find data regarding whether this would be a good choice for you.

Answers will vary with student experience.

 ## SCENARIO: USING SKILLS OF CRITICAL THINKING

Situation: Frank Fellow, a 72-year-old patient admitted for acute confusion presented in the emergency department (ED) with a history of hypertension (high blood pressure), diabetes mellitus, type 1 (insulin-dependent) diabetes, and arthritis. He lives in a single-family home with his wife.

The patient is slightly confused and has an unsteady gait. He frequently forgets to use his walker and fails to call for assistance from the nursing staff when ambulating to the bathroom.

Based on this scenario, discuss your interpretation, analysis, evaluation, inference, and explanation and how you would use these to resolve a situation related to the patient's safety.

Interpretation: Clarify what the behavior means.

_____

_____

_____

_____

_____

_____

_____

Analysis: During the assessment, what questions should the nurse ask to determine the best plan of care?

_____

_____

_____

_____

_____

_____

_____

_____

Evaluation: What outcomes do you expect to achieve with your patient today?

_____

_____

_____

_____

_____

_____

Inference: What conclusion (explanation for behavior) could the nurse make, based on the analysis?

_____

_____

_____

_____

_____

_____

_____

Explanation: During implementation, how can the nurse justify the actions being initiated?

_____

_____

_____

_____

_____

_____

Self-regulation: What issues should the nurse reexamine to correct or improve the nursing care?

_____

_____

_____

_____

_____

_____

_____

See the Answer Key in Appendix A for sample answers for this exercise.

QUIZ

Please take 5 minutes to complete this short quiz. Work as quickly as you can, making sure you attempt to answer all questions.

1. If a doctor gave you three pills and told you to take one every half hour, how long would they last?
2. Divide 30 by one half. Add 10. What is the answer?
3. If you had only one match and entered a dark room where there was an oil lamp, an oil heater, and some kindling wood, which would you light first?
4. Take two apples from three apples. What do you have?
5. Some months have 30 days, some have 31; how many months have 28 days?
6. A man builds a house with four sides, a rectangular structure with each wall having a southern exposure. A bear comes wandering by one day. What color is the bear?
7. How many animals of each species did Moses take on the ark?
8. I went to bed at 8:00 in the evening and wound up the alarm clock to get me up at 9:00 in the morning. How many hours of sleep did this allow me?

Adapted from Davies, R., & McDermott, D. (1996). *45 Activities for developing a learning organization*. Aldershot, UK: Gower Publishing Limited.

See the Answer Key in Appendix A for answers to this exercise.

CHAPTER 2

Problem Solving

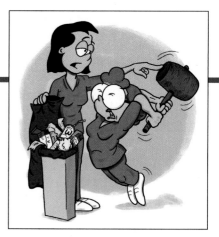

OBJECTIVES

1. Define problem solving.

2. Identify the relationship of critical thinking to the problem-solving process.

3. Compare problem solving and decision making.

4. Describe the difference between the nursing process and problem solving.

5. List the steps involved in problem solving.

6. Describe the five-star problem solving method.

7. List possible errors in the problem-solving process.

As defined in Chapter 1, critical thinking is the process of purposeful, self-regulatory judgment. Critical thinking enables an individual to solve problems and make decisions; therefore, problem solving and decision making are practical applications of critical thinking skills. Problem solving is a systematic process, leading to the achievement of outcomes. The ability to solve problems effectively contributes to the delivery of safe, competent nursing care. Decision making, which is imbedded in the problem solving process, will be further explained in Chapter 3, Decision Making.

DEFINITION

Webster defines a problem as "a question raised for inquiry, consideration, discussion, decision, or solution" and as something "difficult to solve or decide." (Webster's, 1993, p. 1807). For the purpose of this text, a problem will be defined as the gap between "what is" and "what should be." The gap exists as a result of a deficit or an excess of something. To be classified as a problem, this deficit or surplus must be significant enough to the problem solver to warrant further investigation.

Various problems are present in everyday situations. On any given day, a nurse may encounter problems related to patients, coworkers, mechanical breakdowns, or personal issues. Problems are an inescapable part of life.

Problem solving involves identifying the problem and making choices that direct the course toward the desired outcome. Effective problem-solving skills are essential to the delivery of competent nursing care.

NURSING PROCESS

The nursing process differs from generic problem solving in that it is patient centered. "Nursing process is considered to be a specialized form of systematic inquiry or problem solving process used in drawing conclusions about the patient's problems and the corresponding nursing actions to solve problems" (Saucier, Stevens, & Williams, 2002, p. 246). Table 2-1 compares the nursing process to the problem-solving process and the scientific method of problem solving.

Problem solving is a generic process that can be applied to any problem. It is not unique to the nursing field. In this chapter, problem solving is presented in a nursing process format, but problem solving encompasses more areas than just the nursing process. The problem-solving process places emphasis on judgment, priorities, and decision making. It encourages clinical judgment and accountability. Therefore, the problem-solving process is the foundation of the nursing process, but the terms cannot be used interchangeably.

DECISION MAKING

Decision making and problem solving are frequently viewed as synonymous processes. In reality, there is a difference between the two. Decision making is a choice between options. Making a decision is a step in the problem-solving process. Although these processes do overlap, not all decision making is the result of a problem. For example, a decision is to be made when the checker at the grocery store asks, "Do you want paper or plastic?" or when an individual chooses which television program to watch. Therefore, a decision may be made without a preexisting problem.

STEPS IN THE PROBLEM-SOLVING PROCESS

ASSESSMENT

The problem-solving process begins with assessment. First, the existence of a problem must be recognized. The effective problem solver is alert to problems. Related data should be collected, compiled, and organized at this time. For example, during shift report, the nurse observes a postoperative patient grimacing and holding his chest. Immediately, the nurse begins to collect data, including vital signs, physical assessment, pain assessment, history of discomfort, and physician's orders. These data lead to the definition of the problem.

Analysis

After recognizing the problem's existence, the problem solver enters the analysis phase. In the process of analysis, the problem should be identified and defined clearly and precisely. If the nurse focuses only on solving the symptoms of the problem, the original problem will still exist. Problem solving involves asking questions such as "Why?" "What is the problem?" and "Why do you think this is a problem?"

Once the problem has been identified, the problem solver needs to determine the priority of the problem. Some problems require immediate solutions, whereas other decisions can be delayed. This subject is covered more thoroughly in Chapter 4, Priority Setting.

TABLE 2-1	Comparison of the Scientific Method, Problem-Solving Process, and Nursing Process	
SCIENTIFIC METHOD	**PROBLEM-SOLVING PROCESS**	**NURSING PROCESS**
1. Define problem.	1. Encounter problem.	1. Assess
2. Collect data.	2. Collect data.	2. Diagnosis (Analysis)
3. Formulate hypothesis.	3. Analyze data to specify problem.	3. Outcome identification
4. Design plan to test hypothesis.	4. Determine plan of action to resolve problem.	4. Plan
5. Test hypothesis.	5. Execute action plan.	5. Implement
6. Interpret results.	6. Evaluate plan for effectiveness in problem resolution.	6. Evaluate
7. Evaluate for study conclusion or revision.		

Adapted from Harrington, N., & Terry, C. L. (2003). *LPN to RN transitions* (p. 185). Philadelphia: Lippincott-Williams & Wilkins.

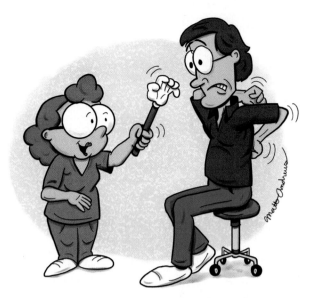

"Poison ivy on the back? I've got just the thing!"

At this point, the problem solver should develop a list of all possible strategies. This is a critical step in the problem-solving process. If the solutions or alternatives identified do not provide the means to solve the problem, there is little chance of achieving the desired outcome. The problem solver should always focus on a range of solutions before selecting the best one. For example, a staff nurse knows that a patient is being discharged in a few days. This nurse has been informed that the patient will need to continue injections of subcutaneous heparin following discharge. In planning the necessary education, the nurse might consider several strategies:

- Contacting the patient education department for collaboration
- Showing a video demonstrating the technique
- Delegating the education to an assistant
- Using a demonstration–return demonstration method of instruction

Of course additional strategies exist. Creativity is a critical element in generating options or solutions. In developing a list of all possible problem-solving strategies, the nurse should not be limited to always using the same methods. People who exercise creativity are more flexible and independent in their thinking and, therefore, are able to conceptualize new and innovative approaches to a problem. Questioning current practice allows for the opportunity to promote change. However, the effective problem solver has also thoroughly re-

searched available data concerning the problem. In nursing, evidence-based practice is validated with research and best-practice models. When solutions exist that have been researched and proved effective, it is a waste of time to experiment with something creative, which might delay solving the problem.

OUTCOME IDENTIFICATION

Another important aspect of problem solving is having a clear, concise idea of the desired destination. The decisions made should lead the problem solver in the correct direction. In the earlier example of discharge teaching, the nurse might identify the desired outcome as, "The patient will demonstrate correct self-administration of subcutaneous heparin within 72 hours." This outcome is measurable and gives the nurse direction in organizing patient education. The nurse should reject strategies that do not lead to this outcome.

With invalid strategies eliminated, the problem solver should consider the potential effect of each remaining strategy. Positive and negative outcomes must be determined (Table 2-2). Unexpected results can be an unwelcome surprise at the end of the process if this step is ignored. The next step is

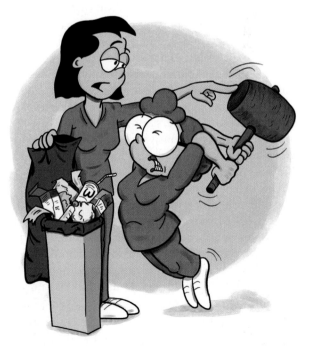

"You know, maybe there's a better way to empty the trash."

TABLE 2-2 Examples of Positive and Negative Outcomes for Potential Choices

METHOD	POSITIVE EFFECTS	NEGATIVE EFFECTS
Collaborate with patient education department	May learn more quickly because experienced educator can teach to specific learning style	Education may be delayed owing to busy department
Video	May be easy for learner to visualize process as presented in step-by-step format	May not learn owing to inability to ask questions during video Doesn't work well with kinesthetic learners who need to handle equipment
Delegate to an assistant	Gives nurse time to perform other higher-priority interventions	May decrease understanding because assistant is not properly trained May not be able to delegate to this assistant because of state nurse practice act or institutional policy
Demonstration–return demonstration	Instruction can be individualized with one-on-one instruction, which allows adequate time for questions Education can be designed to meet the patient's individual learning needs	May not have time to provide education Nurse may be interrupted frequently

to predict the likelihood of each outcome occurring. Negative consequences that occur rarely may not be as much of a concern.

Plan

During the planning phase, the nurse should select the alternative that has the best chance of success and the least undesirable outcome. A final decision on which plan to use should not be made prematurely, because this decision may eliminate all alternative courses of action. Principles of the scientific method should be used in selecting the desired alternative. The scientific method involves analyzing each alternative or hypotheses as a possible solution. See Table 2-1 for the steps used in the scientific method.

Once the alternative is selected, the nurse develops and consults a list of resources. This includes all sources of information regarding the problem. Examples of appropriate resources include the patient, the patient's chart, nursing textbooks, medication books, policy and procedure books, and individuals with expertise in this area. Planning in the nursing process involves establishing a plan of care for the patient. The plan of care is developed with strategies to resolve the patient's problems.

Next, the nurse must identify actions that will produce the desired outcome and assign each action a priority in order to prepare a time schedule. Finally, the nurse must make decisions regarding assignment of these actions.

Implementation

After the planning phase, the chosen solution should be implemented. If actions have been delegated to personnel, clear and thorough directions must be given. In addition to delegation, this may require performing nursing actions to achieve the established goals.

Evaluation

Evaluation is a necessary step in the problem-solving process. Changes may occur in the problem that necessitate immediate revisions. Therefore, the nurse should monitor the response to the strategy and modify ineffective actions. For example, if the nurse administers acetaminophen for pain relief and it is not effective, an alternative may be preferable. The nurse should always compare the results obtained with the desired outcome. The care plan may need revision because of weaknesses in the plan, changes in the patient's condition, or a redefinition of the problem. Evaluation in the nursing process is the assessment of

Box 2-1 TEMPLATE FOR PROBLEM SOLVING

To be an effective problem solver:

1. Figure out, and regularly rearticulate, your goals, purposes, and needs. Recognize problems as emergent obstacles to reaching your goals, achieving your purposes, and satisfying your needs.
2. Whenever possible, take problems one by one. State the problem as clearly and precisely as you can.
3. Study the problem to make clear the "kind" of problem you are dealing with. Figure out, for example, what sorts of things you are going to have to do to solve it. Distinguish problems over which you have some control from problems over which you have no control. Set aside the problems over which you have no control. Concentrate your efforts on those problems you can potentially solve.
4. Figure out the information you need and actively seek that information.
5. Carefully analyze and interpret the information you collect, drawing what reasonable inferences you can.
6. Figure out your options for action. What can you do in the short term? In the long term? Recognize explicitly your limitations as far as money, time, and power.
7. Evaluate your options, taking into account their advantages and disadvantages in the situation you are in.
8. Adopt a strategic approach to the problem and follow through on that strategy. This may involve direct action or a carefully thought-through, wait-and-see strategy.
9. When you act, monitor the implications of your action as they begin to emerge. Be ready at a moment's notice to revise your strategy if the situation requires it. Be prepared to shift your strategy or your analysis or statement of the problem, or all three, as more information about the problem becomes available to you.

Adapted from Paul, R., & Elder, L. (2001a). *Mini-guide: Critical thinking* (p. 16). Dillon Beach, CA: Foundation for Critical Thinking.

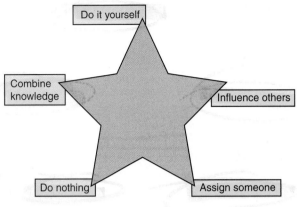

FIGURE 2-1

Five star solution wheel and problem-solving strategies.

the information to determine the patient's progress toward the desired outcome. Box 2-1 provides a summary of advice for effective problem solving.

PROBLEM-SOLVING STRATEGIES

Many strategies may be used to assist in problem solving. The five-star solution wheel lists these strategies (Figure 2-1):

Do it yourself
Influence others
Assign someone
Do nothing
Combine knowledge

Do It Yourself

The problem solver might intervene to solve the problem if he or she determines that expending time and energy will make a positive difference in resolving the problem. Time is a valuable resource. The problem solver should evaluate his or her capabilities and expertise and determine whether this is the preferred option.

Influence Others

The problem solver may decide that he or she does not have ownership of the problem. At times, it is wise to allow the person owning the problem to solve it. For example, a nurse manager notes that the conflict between two employees has resulted in increased tension on the unit. The nurse manager could bring the employees together to discuss their issues. Interpersonal skills might be used to assist in conflict resolution, but, essentially, the employees would be allowed to work out their own solution.

Assign Someone

Effective, efficient nursing care may involve assigning responsibilities and tasks to others. Delegation is the "transferring to a competent individual the authority to perform a selected nursing task in a selected situation" (National Council of State Boards of Nursing, 1995, p. 2). The goal is to achieve quality patient outcomes. Factors influencing delegation are covered in Chapter 6, Delegation.

Do Nothing

Often a problem will subside on its own without the need to waste valuable resources in an effort to fix it. The problem solver should recognize when a problem has the potential to resolve by itself and should consider making a conscious effort not to intervene. Even when the decision is to "do nothing," the facts should be documented if patients are involved.

Combine Knowledge

Consultation and collaboration with an expert nurse facilitates a higher-quality decision or choice. Collaborating or consulting with an expert or more learned person in the specialty area will help ensure that the correct problem has been identified and clearly defined. Other sources of input might include patient interviews, physicians, nursing rounds, and conferences. Talking through the situation often helps put the problem into perspective. Any one or a combination of these techniques can be used to facilitate problem solving.

PITFALLS IN PROBLEM SOLVING

There can be several reasons for ineffective problem solving. These include:

- Failure to clearly identify the real problem
- Failure to eliminate preconceived ideas in the identification of solutions
- Failure to communicate
- Failure to follow up
- Failure to use appropriate resources

Failure to Clearly Identify the Real Problem

One common pitfall in the problem-solving process is the failure to identify the problem correctly. This pitfall includes dealing with symptoms instead of the problem, secondary problems instead of the main problem, or problems that the problem solver does not "own."

Treating symptoms may provide temporary relief, but if the underlying problem is not resolved, it will resurface. Consider the following example: Urinalysis results have been placed on a patient's chart indicating that the patient has a urinary tract infection (UTI). Neither the nurse nor the physicians have noted the lab work. The nurse observes that the patient has an elevated temperature. The nurse does not investigate further, but

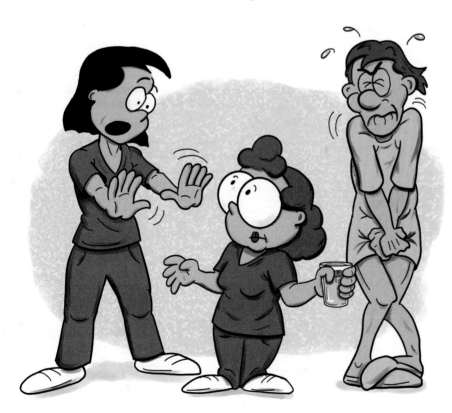

"Trust me! The patient's problem isn't lack of fluids!"

administers acetaminophen. The temperature may temporarily decrease, but the patient still has the UTI.

Attempting to resolve secondary issues may bring about change, but the original problem still exists. For example, a student with low reading skills enrolls in nursing school. The student experiences difficulty with the coursework in one class and is placed on academic probation. The student identifies the problem as failure in that course. In attempting to solve the problem, the student changes study habits by increasing the amount of time devoted to the course. Because this results in decreased time for other courses, the student experiences difficulty completing reading assignments. The grades in other courses begin to drop. The student has not identified the underlying problem.

Problem solvers also experience difficulty in attempting to resolve problems over which they have no control. For example, suppose your 21-year-old son has chosen a partner you dislike. If the problem is the partner, you do not own the problem. You cannot change the partner; you can only change your reaction to the partner. Therefore, if you incorrectly identify actions of the partner as the problem, frustration and ineffective problem-solving attempts will follow. Consider another example: a nurse is upset over the older equipment used at her place of employment. She spends the whole shift complaining about the equipment. This accomplishes nothing because she has no control over the decision to purchase equipment.

Failure to Eliminate Preconceived Ideas in Identification of Solutions

High-quality decisions require consideration of all possible solutions. At times, problem solvers are reluctant to try new, creative solutions. They may be fearful of looking foolish. Conformity to a group may discourage creative thinking. A tradition of relying on one solution is difficult to change. The problem solver may also have personal bias against some solutions. For example, a critical care nurse is caring for an elderly patient with a myocardial infarction. The patient is begging to see her 5-year-old grandson who lives with her. The old rule was: Children must be 12 years old to visit in the intensive care unit. In this case, the decision is up to the nurse in charge of the patient's care. This nurse strongly believes that children should never be allowed in the unit under any circumstance.

It is imperative to remember that rarely does a problem have only one solution. To discover the best solution, all possible solutions should be considered.

Failure to Communicate

Communication is very important in the problem-solving process. Assessments, strategies, and outcomes should be communicated for continuity of care. Collaboration, consulting, and delegation all require effective communication. Failure to communicate often results in inefficient problem solving. For example, during change of shift report, failure to report progress toward expected outcomes with patient teaching may result in premature discharge.

Failure to Follow Up

Great plans often go wrong because no one monitored the progress and outcomes following implementation. Without follow-up, untoward events can affect the progress. As changes, delays, or unexpected events develop, the problem solver must intervene to direct the situation toward the desired outcome.

Failure to Use Appropriate Resources

People have a tendency to use the same solutions that worked in the past. In today's changing health care arena, it is essential to initiate change, question current practice, and challenge the status quo. In questioning current practice, an awareness of appropriate resources to validate our decisions is necessary. Some of the resources available for use in this process include nursing textbooks, facility policy, procedure manuals, Standards of Care, and experienced colleagues.

SUMMARY

Problem solving is a systematic process. The nurse should approach problems using a scientific method instead of dealing with them in a haphazard manner. Strategies for effective problem solving exist, and skills in implementation of these strategies improve with use. Therefore, nurses should practice problem-solving skills in a systematic manner. The application of problem solving in nursing is called the *nursing process*. This process is further discussed in Chapter 5, Nursing Process Applications.

KEY POINTS

- Problem solving is a systematic process leading to the achievement of outcomes.
- Problem solving is a generic process based on the scientific method, which is applicable to all fields.
- Assessment involves identification of the problem.
- During outcome identification, the nurse establishes the desired goal and explores potential effects of each strategy.
- During the planning phase, the nurse should select the alternative with the best chance of success that has the least risk. After the planning phase, the selected alternative is implemented.
- Evaluation of results is essential to determine whether the desired outcome has been reached.
- Strategies for problem solving include: do it yourself, influence others, assign someone else, do nothing, and combine knowledge.
- Ineffective problem solving may result from the failure to identify the real problem, eliminate preconceived ideas, communicate, follow-up, or use appropriate resources.

REFERENCES

Davies, R., & McDermott, D. (1996). *Mind opening training games.* New York: McGraw-Hill.

Eitington, J. (1996). *The winning trainer: Winning ways to involve people in learning.* Houston: Gulf.

Garofalo-Ford, J. (1979). *Applied decision making for nurses.* St. Louis: Mosby.

Harrington, N., & Terry, C. (2003). *LPN to RN transitions.* Philadelphia: Lippincott-Williams & Wilkins.

Huber, D. (2000). *Leadership and nursing care management.* Philadelphia: W.B. Saunders.

National Council of State Boards of Nursing (NCSBN). (1995). *Delegation: Concepts and decision-making process.* Chicago: Author.

Paul, R., & Elder, L. (2001a). *Mini-guide: Critical thinking.* Dillon Beach, CA: Foundation for Critical Thinking.

Paul, R., & Elder, L. (2001b). *Critical thinking: Tools for taking charge of your learning and your life.* Upper Saddle River, NJ: Prentice Hall.

Tappen, R. (1995). *Nursing leadership and management: Concepts and practices.* Philadelphia: F.A. Davis.

Saucier, B. L., Stevens, K. R., & Williams, G. B. (2002). Critical thinking outcomes of computer-assisted instruction versus written nursing process. *Nursing and HealthCare Perspectives, 21*(5), 240–246.

Webster's third new international dictionary (1993). Springfield, MA: Merriam-Webster.

Student Worksheets

 ## SKILL SHEET: PROBLEM SOLVING

Purpose

1. Increase the student's ability to use the collected data for problem or need identification.
2. Develop the student's skill in applying the decision-making steps to problem solving.
3. Enable the student to participate in evaluating the effectiveness of the selected solutions for problems.

Objective

To apply an organized process that facilitates appropriate judgment and reasoning skill in the solution of problems.

Steps: Problem Solving

ASSESSMENT

1. Recognize the existence of the problem.
2. Collect, compile, and organize data.

ANALYSIS

1. Define the problem clearly and precisely.
2. Focus on controllable problems.
3. Establish priorities.
4. Develop a list of all possible strategies that could resolve the problem.

OUTCOME IDENTIFICATION

1. Establish the desired outcome.
2. Consider the potential effect of each strategy.
3. Predict the likelihood of each outcome occurring.

PLAN

1. Utilize principles and rationale of scientific method in selection of desired alternative.
2. Choose the alternative that has the best chance of success and the least undesirable outcome.
3. Develop a list of resources.
4. Prepare a list of desired actions.
5. Prepare a time schedule.
6. Delineate assignments for people.

IMPLEMENTATION

1. Implement the solution.
2. Give clear directions to involved personnel.

EVALUATION

1. Monitor the response to the strategy and modify ineffective actions.
2. Compare the desired outcomes with the results to determine the effectiveness of the plan.
3. Revise the plan as needed.

 COMPETENCY VALIDATION: PROBLEM SOLVING

COMPETENCY STATEMENT

The student identifies and defines problems, develops strategies, and selects appropriate solutions to produce desired outcomes.

The student demonstrated the ability to do the following:

1. Describe the problem clearly and precisely.
2. Focus on controllable problems.
3. Identify strategies that are plausible.
4. Use scientific principles and rationale to develop alternative courses of action.

COMPETENT

- Understands reason for task and is able to perform task independently
- Understands reason for task but needs supervision
- Understands reason for task and is able to perform with assistance

NOT COMPETENT

- Understands reason for task but performs task at provisional level
- Is unable to state reason for task and performs task at a dependent level

SKILL CHECKLIST: PROBLEM SOLVING

PROBLEM SOLVING	SATISFACTORY	UNSATISFACTORY	NI/COMMENTS
ASSESSMENT			
1. Recognize that a problem exists.			
2. Collect, compile, and organize data.			
ANALYSIS			
1. Define the problem clearly and precisely.			
2. Focus on controllable problems.			
3. Establish priorities.			
4. Develop a list of all possible strategies that could resolve the problem.			
OUTCOME IDENTIFICATION			
1. Establish desired outcome.			
2. Consider the potential effect of each strategy.			
3. Predict the likelihood of each outcome occurring.			
PLAN			
1. Use principles of scientific reasoning in selection of method.			
2. Choose the alternative that has the best chance of success and the least undesirable outcome.			
3. Develop a list of resources.			
4. Prepare a list of desired actions.			
5. Prepare a time schedule.			
6. Delineate assignments for people.			
IMPLEMENTATION			
1. Implement the solution.			
2. Give clear directions to involved personnel.			
EVALUATION			
1. Monitor the response to the strategy and modify ineffective actions.			
2. Compare the desired outcomes with the results to determine effectiveness of the plan.			
3. Revise the plan as needed.			

SCENARIO TO ACCOMPANY STUDENT WORKSHEETS

Frank Fellow is a 72-year-old man who was admitted to the step-down unit from intensive coronary care 24 hours after cardioversion. Patient education is to include self-administration of heparin, 5,000 units subcutaneously twice a day. The patient has a visual impairment and is experiencing difficulty drawing the correct dosage of medication from the vial. He can administer the injection independently.

During the evening while you are teaching the patient and his wife, the patient complains of left-sided chest pain rated at 5 on a 0 to 10 scale. He is moderately short of breath. Upon hearing his complaints of shortness of breath, his spouse becomes frantic and tearful.

1. Underline the problems in the scenario.

_____

_____

_____

_____

2. Identify the alternatives. What should the nurse do?

_____

_____

_____

_____

_____

_____

See the Answer Key in Appendix A for sample answers for this exercise.

PRACTICE EXERCISES: PROBLEM SOLVING

 SCENARIOS: IDENTIFYING PROBLEM-SOLVING METHODS

Practice the following scenarios using the problem-solving checklist.

SCENARIO 1

The nurse prepares medication for one of the patients in Room 102. After administering the medication, the nurse realizes the meds were given to the wrong patient. The nurse immediately reports the incident to the physician. Following this action, the nurse returns to the patient's room and informs and assesses the patient. The nurse completes an occurrence report and continues to monitor the patient for adverse reactions.

What problem-solving method was used?

Do it yourself. ~~and~~ The nurse is kind of doing everything ~~but~~
~~I think~~

What other problem-solving methods could have been included?

Combine knowledge.

SCENARIO 2

Betty arrives for work and discovers that the other RN scheduled for her unit has called in sick. There are no replacements available. Betty completes a list of patient needs and gives assignments to the remaining staff, including an LPN and two UAPs. Betty retains the patient needs that require RN-level interventions.

What problem-solving method was used?

What other problem-solving methods could have been included?

Scenario 3

Mary Rodriguez has been diagnosed with breast cancer. Her insurance company has refused reimbursement for an expensive, experimental medical procedure. Marcus Jones, Mary's case manager, forms a committee to discuss fundraisers.

What problem-solving method was used?

_____

_____

_____

What other problem-solving methods could have been included?

_____

_____

SCENARIOS: DETECTING ERRORS IN THE PROBLEM-SOLVING PROCESS

Scenario 4

Jane's family always stressed punctuality. Jane believes in arriving 15 minutes before scheduled start of events. As Jane prepares for her first clinical rotation, she can't find her stethoscope. Jane races around the house searching. She walks by the stethoscope several times, but does not see it. She is very upset and unable to focus on her environment. Jane identified the problems as failure to place the stethoscope in a convenient place. She vowed always to have her stethoscope in her car.

What error in the problem-solving process is Jane making?

_____

_____

_____

What is the actual problem?

_____

_____

_____

Scenario 5

Don Smith is a 67-year-old patient on a medical floor admitted with pneumonia. He calls the nurse's station to complain of indigestion. His nurse obtains his mediation administration record (MAR) and administers the Mylanta ordered as needed (PRN). The nurse continues with the med pass. Upon returning to Mr. Smith's room an hour later, the nurse notes that Mr. Smith is pale and diaphoretic and that he is clutching his chest.

What error in the problem-solving process is the nurse making?

failure to clearly identify real problem.

What would be a strategy to remedy this error?

Find out what problem is, and be sure. Perform a thorough assessment.

Scenario 6

Dante is the charge nurse on a busy medical floor. He has been informed by administration that his unit has failed to document adequately the weights of patients with congestive heart failure. Dante creates a new procedure for this documentation. He posts copies explaining the change in the break room. An in-service is conducted at 2:00 PM that day to explain further the importance of following the procedure. Dante assumes that the procedure is being followed. At the end of 3 months, Dante is surprised when his supervisor reveals the statistics. There was increased compliance in the week following the in-service, but within a few weeks, documentation had slipped to even lower levels than previously noted.

What error in the problem-solving process is Dante making?

What would be a strategy to remedy this error?

See the Answer Key in Appendix A for sample answers for this exercise.

FUN EXERCISES

> **Fun Exercises: Problem Solving**
> **Check Your I.Q. (Imagination quotient)**
>
> Interpret the following:
>
> 1. Sand — *Sand box*
>
> 2. MAN / BOARD
>
> 3. STAND / I — *I understand*
>
> 4. |R|E|A|D|I|N|G|
>
> 5. WEAR / LONG
>
> 6. R / ROAD / A / D
>
> 7. CYCLE / CYCLE / CYCLE
>
> 8. T / O / W / N
>
> 9. LE   VEL
>
> 10. KNEE / LIGHT — *Knee on light*
>
> 11. DEATH/LIFE
>
> 12. ECNALG
>
> 13. O / M.D. / Ph.D. / D.D.S.
>
> 14. ii ii / O O — *Circles under the eyes*
>
> 15. DICE / DICE — *parr a dice*
>
> 16. CHAIR
>
> 17. T / O / U / C / H
>
> 18. GROUND / FEET / FEET / FEET / FEET / FEET / FEET
>
> 19. MIND / MATTER
>
> 20. HE'S/HIMSELF
>
> 21. GEGS / GGSE / EGSG
>
> 22. ✗–○✗

Adapted from Eitington, J. (1996). *The winning trainer: Winning ways to involve people in learning* (p. 17). Houston, TX: Gulf.

See the Answer Key in Appendix A for answers for this exercise.

DEMONSTRATION OF THE PROBLEM-SOLVING PROCESS

You are a nursing student enrolled in a required course. The instructor randomly divides the class into groups. Each group is to submit a paper analyzing educational offerings available online. All group members will receive the same grade.

Your group members have delayed starting on the project. The paper is due in 1 week. Outline the steps you would take to solve the problem:

ASSESSMENT

_____

_____

_____

_____

_____

ANALYSIS

_____

_____

_____

_____

_____

OUTCOME IDENTIFICATION

_____

_____

_____

_____

_____

STRATEGY	NEGATIVE EFFECT	POSITIVE EFFECT
Do paper self		
Divide evenly, hope for best		
Complain to instructor		
Threaten team members		
Schedule group meeting to discuss progress		

PLAN

_____

_____

_____

_____

_____

IMPLEMENTATION

_____

_____

_____

_____

_____

EVALUATION

_____

_____

_____

_____

_____

CHAPTER 3

DECISION MAKING

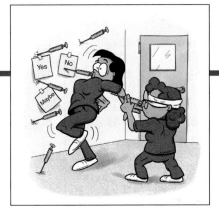

OBJECTIVES

1. Define decision making.

2. Identify the difference between problem solving and decision making.

3. List the steps involved in decision making.

4. Describe how desirability, probability, and risk affect the analysis of the solutions being considered.

5. Identify errors in decision making and state actions to correct these errors.

Decision making is the process of choosing among alternatives. Emphasis on cost-effective health care requires the nurse to possess astute decision-making skills. Critical thinking is inherent in the process of rational, purposeful decision making. Therefore, critical thinking skills are vital to nursing practice.

This chapter focuses on the application of sound decision-making principles as they relate to nursing situations. Regular practice is necessary to make quality decisions. Exercises to assist in the development of decision-making skills are included at the end of this chapter.

DEFINITION

Ellis and Hartley (2000, p. 111) define decision making for nurses as "a systematic cognitive process in which you identify alternatives, evaluate those alternatives, come to a conclusion, and select an option." For the purpose of this text, *decision making* is a purposeful, goal-directed effort applied in a systematic way to make a choice among alternatives. It is "action to achieve a foreseen result, which is preceded by reflection and judgment to appraise the situation, and by a thoughtful, deliberate choice of what should be done" (Orem, 1971, p. 31). It is important to remember that a decision has consequences. Ignoring a problem is a decision. Deciding not to act is also a decision. Therefore, accountability and responsibility for the outcome are key elements.

DIFFERENTIATING DECISION MAKING FROM PROBLEM SOLVING

Problem solving and decision making are sometimes viewed as synonymous terms. However, the concepts are different. Problem solving involves assessment and analysis of a problem. This leads to the formulation and implementation of solutions. Decision making involves choosing between options. It is a critical step in the problem-solving process. However, not all necessary decisions are related to problems. For example, choosing what to eat for breakfast is a decision. Normally, there is no need to proceed through the entire problem-solving process to make this decision. It is a matter of preference. Therefore, decision making is a vital step in problem solving, but it is not the same process.

FACTORS INFLUENCING DECISION MAKING

Decisions are influenced by many factors, including emotions, values, perceptions, and the current social climate. It is very difficult to make sound decisions while experiencing extreme emotions. The values of the decision maker enter into the process. Values are affected by cultural factors, religious beliefs, spirituality, and past experiences. Furthermore, values often differ from person to person. Some people, for example, measure their self-worth by their salary or the amount of money in their bank account; others measure self-worth by their contributions to society or by their number of friends.

Perception is also a significant factor affecting decisions. Perception involves biases and personal interpretation of the situation. What makes something attractive to one person may not be perceived as appealing by another individual.

Human beings have the unique capacity for self-awareness, imagination, conscious control, and interdependent will. These qualities provide us with the tools necessary to make choices.

CHARACTERISTICS OF AN EFFECTIVE DECISION MAKER

Effective decision makers tend to possess certain skills. These skills can be learned and, with practice, can be integrated into the decision process.

People who approach decisions with self-confidence and a degree of assertiveness are generally more effective. A proactive approach is also beneficial. Proactive individuals have examined their values and make decisions based on them. This differs from the approach of reactive people, who allow circumstances, conditions, and the environment to control their responses. People with a reactive stance do not feel control over their decisions.

With some decisions, flexibility is helpful. Even though every attempt is made to select the best option, sometimes a perfect solution does not exist. The decision maker may have to give the most attractive solution a limited trial. During this period, the decision maker will increase his or her knowledge about the advantages and disadvantages of the chosen answer.

A knowledgeable decision maker understands that all decisions have consequences, but also understands that no one always makes the right decision. The ability to accept responsibility for the consequences of one's decision making is essential. For example, a nurse might make a poor decision resulting in undesirable consequences for the patient but must accept responsibility for the action chosen.

A final important trait for a decision maker is the ability to focus. Priority decisions should be considered first. Some individuals become overwhelmed when making inconsequential decisions and delay action on high-priority decisions. The critical thinker should first concentrate on important decisions and then focus on controllable factors. The focal point should be issues in which a difference can be made and situations that can be changed.

DECISION MAKING IN NURSING

In addition to personal choices, nurses make decisions in many areas of their practice, including clinical, ethical, and group decisions and decisions involving the delegation of duties. Making competent, sound decisions in nursing practice is one of the most critical processes a nurse must learn in developing professional skill.

Clinical decisions are generally related to patient care. Today, nurses direct, control, and manage multiple resources in the health care setting. Nursing decisions are judged by the quality of care and by competency issues. The complexity of clinical practice often makes clinical decisions difficult or unclear. Repeatedly practicing decision making by reviewing the process step by step will increase one's ability to make sound decisions.

Delegation is an example of a useful decision-making process found in nursing practice. It involves differentiating the skills of professional and technical staff and assessing the acuity level of patients. These factors are considered along with the amount of time and resources that are available. A decision concerning what should be delegated is

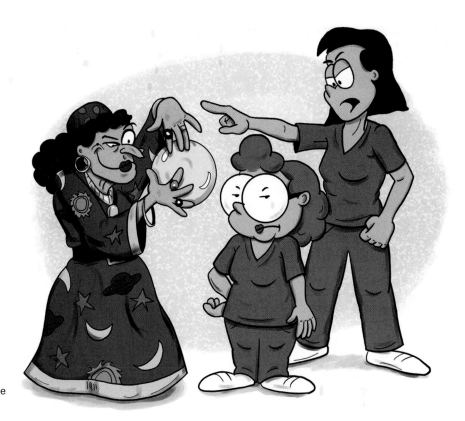

"I don't care what her accuracy percentage is! You have to make your own decisions!"

then made. (See Chapter 6, Delegation, for more information on the process of delegation.)

Ethical decisions are often very difficult. Moral issues such as cloning and euthanasia may be involved. All of the available options may have negative or undesirable consequences. Chapter 10, Ethical Decision Making, describes ethical decision making in more detail.

Nurses must also make decisions as a member of a group. Working with interdisciplinary treatment teams and other institutional committees is frequently included as a nursing responsibility. When dealing with groups, people should value the individual differences of the group members. The talents of each member should be used to the advantage of the group. For instance, a member who is good with details may be assigned to take notes. Group dynamics are enhanced when the participants are skilled listeners. Individuals in the group should listen to the viewpoints of others with the goal of understanding them. At times, group members will have opposing views. Options to solve this impasse should be considered. Sometimes a compromise is possible. Alternatively, the participants may agree to disagree about the issue.

listen not enforcing ideas

Approaches to Participative Decision Making

When group members are allowed to participate in decision making, various approaches can be used. Occasionally, a group is formed to deal with a single problem or issue. After the problem is resolved, the group is disbanded. This is generally known as a *task force*.

A *quality circle* is another method of group decision making. Quality circles are groups of people with common concerns. These individuals work together and discuss everyday job issues.

Another example of group participation is *brainstorming*. During these sessions, group members are encouraged to identify as many alternative solutions as possible. Creativity is encouraged.

In *nominal group technique*, the supervisor selects seven to ten individuals. A problem is presented, and each group member writes a possible solution. All solutions are written on a board or flip chart. Then, each group member ranks the list of solutions. The alternative with the most favorable response is identified as the first alternative.

The *Delphi method* does not involve bringing a group of people together; however, a group makes the decision. Personnel are approached individually and given a list of possible solutions. These individuals are asked to rank the solutions. The solution with the highest ranking is selected as the first alternative.

Group decisions can also be made by *consensus*. This process involves a decision by participants to accept the group's solution. Original proposals are revised until they are acceptable to the entire group.

Another accepted method of group decision making is *majority rule*. Group decisions are made by voting for the best solution. The solution with the most votes is adopted by the group.

Each method of group decision making has its advantages and disadvantages. See Table 3-1 for a comparison of these factors. Because nurses are involved in many types of decisions, increased ability in this area is a desired skill.

Decision-Making Tools

Fortunately, tools are available to assist the nurse in making decisions. For example, the decision-making grid at the end of this chapter prompts nurses to follow certain steps as they make a decision.

Decision trees are also useful decision-making devices. These include clinical pathways and algorithms. *Clinical pathways* are standardized plans set in a time frame. They are an adaptation of a nursing care plan. An *algorithm* is a systematic guide to decision making. The nurse works down a "tree," answering questions specific to the current decision. If the answer is yes, the reader proceeds down one side of the tree. If the answer is no, the nurse is directed down the other side of the tree. A sample algorithm and clinical pathway can be seen in Figures 3-1 and 3-2, respectively.

Another tool that can be used to facilitate decisions is a cost–benefit analysis, which involves preparing a column of advantages and a column of disadvantages, listed side by side. This process is repeated for each possible solution. Often, putting thoughts on paper helps to clarify the issue.

PROCESS OF DECISION MAKING

To maintain consistency throughout the text, the decision-making process described below is presented in a nursing process format. The steps for

TABLE 3-1	Advantages and Disadvantages of Group Decision-Making Approaches	
TYPE OF PROCESS	**ADVANTAGES**	**DISADVANTAGES**
Task force	▪ Uses the expertise of appointed members.	▪ Members with dominant personalities may influence the group. ▪ May leave members dissatisfied because the group dissolves after making recommendation.
Quality circle	▪ Uses the expertise of volunteer members who share a common concern.	▪ Time consuming. ▪ Because of voluntary membership, may not get the best input. ▪ Productivity relies on the ability of the group to work together effectively.
Brainstorming	▪ Generates a large number of creative approaches.	▪ Because focus is on generating a number of solutions, quality may be lacking. ▪ Process can be stifled by premature critique of solutions posed.
Nominal group technique	▪ Allows for consideration of a large number of alternatives. ▪ Group members are not pressured toward a particular solution.	▪ Time consuming. ▪ Requires advance planning. ▪ Members may not realize much satisfaction in the process.
Delphi method	▪ Generates many alternatives. ▪ Can involve a large number of participants because they do not have to come together. ▪ Because participants do not meet together, one cannot influence another.	▪ Requires much time from start to finish. ▪ Requires advance planning. ▪ Participants may have a low sense of accomplishment.

Adapted from Ellis, J. R., & Hartley, C. L. (2000). *Managing nursing care* (p. 123). Philadelphia: Lippincott Williams & Wilkins.

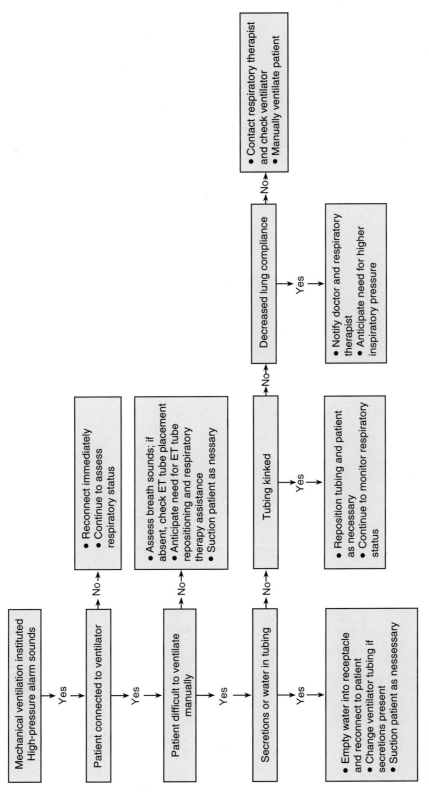

FIGURE 3-1

Decision tree: troubleshooting high-pressure ventilator alarms. Alarms are used to monitor changes in rate, rhythm, and pressure and to help ensure ventilator safety. Types of alarms vary from one machine to another. If an alarm sounds, assess the situation and take appropriate nursing actions immediately. This decision tree shows the troubleshooting process for a high-pressure ventilator alarm. Adapted from Smith-Huddleston, S., & Ferguson, S. G. (1997). *Critical care and emergency nursing*. Springhouse, PA: Springhouse Corp.

Text within the figure:

- Mechanical ventilation instituted / High-pressure alarm sounds
  - Yes → Patient connected to ventilator
    - No → • Reconnect immediately / • Continue to assess respiratory status
    - Yes → Patient difficult to ventilate manually
      - No → • Assess breath sounds; if absent, check ET tube placement / • Anticipate need for ET tube repositioning and respiratory therapy assistance / • Suction patient as nessary
      - Yes → Secretions or water in tubing
        - No → Tubing kinked
          - No → Decreased lung compliance
            - Yes → • Notify doctor and respiratory therapist / • Anticipate need for higher inspiratory pressure
            - No → • Contact respiratory therapist and check ventilator / • Manually ventilate patient
          - Yes → • Reposition tubing and patient as necessary / • Continue to monitor respiratory status
        - Yes → • Empty water into receptacle and reconnect to patient / • Change ventilator tubing if secretions present / • Suction patient as nessessary

Clinical Pathway: Colon Resection Without Colostomy

	Patient Visit	Presurgery Day 1	O.R. Day	Postop Day 1
Assessments	History and physical with breast, rectal, and pelvic exam Nursing assessment	Nursing admission assessment	Nursing admission assessment on TBA patients in holding area. Review of systems assessment	Review of systems assessment*
Consults	Social service consult Physical therapy consult	Notify referring physician of impending admission		
Labs and diagnostics	Complete blood count (CBC) Coagulation profile ECG Chest X-ray (CXR) Chem profile CT ABD w/wo contrast CT pelvis Urinalysis Barium enema & flex sigmoidoscopy/colonoscopy Biopsy report	Type and screen for patients with hemoglobin (Hgb) <10	Type and screen for patients in holding area with Hgb <10	CBC
Interventions	Many or all of the above labs/diagnostics will have already been done. Check all results and fax to the surgeon's office.	Admit by 8 a.m. Check for bowel prep orders Bowel prep Antiembolism stockings Incentive spirometry Ankle exercises I.V. access Routine vital signs (VS) Pneumatic inflation boots	Shave and prep in O.R. Nasogastric (NG) tube maint.* Intake and output (I/O)* VS per routine* Catheter care* Incentive spirometry* Ankle exercises I.V. site care Head of bed (HOB) 30º* Safety measures* Wound care* Mouth care*	NG tube maintenance* I/O* VS per routine* Catheter care* Incentive spirometry* Ankle exercises* I.V. site care* HOB 30º* Safety measures* Wound care* Mouth care* Antiembolism stockings*
I.V.s		I.V. fluids, D_5 1/2NSS	I.V. fluids, D_5 LR	I.V. fluids, D_5 LR
Medication	Prescribe GoLYTELY/Nulytely 10a–2p Neomycin @2p, 3p, and 10p Erythromycin @ 2p, 3p, and 10p	GoLYTELY/Nulytely 10a–2p Erythromycin @ 2p, 3p, and 10p Neomycin @2p, 3p, and 10p	Preop antibiotics (ABX) in holding area Postop ABX x 2 doses PCA (basal rate 0.5 mg) S.C. heparin	PCA (basal rate 0.5 mg) S.C. heparin
Diet/GI	Clears presurgery day NPO after midnight	Clears presurgery day NPO after midnight	NPO/NG tube	NPO/NG tube
Activity			4 hours after surgery, ambulate with abdominal binder D/C pneumatic inflation boots once patient ambulates	Ambulate t.i.d. with abdominal binder May shower Physical therapy b.i.d.
Key: *NSG activities V=Variance N= No var.	1. 2. 3. V V V Ⓝ N N	1. 2. 3. V V V Ⓝ Ⓝ Ⓝ	1. 2. 3. V V V Ⓝ Ⓝ Ⓝ	1. 2. 3. V V V Ⓝ Ⓝ Ⓝ
Signatures:	1. _C. Mollon, RN_ 2. _____ 3. _____	1. _C. Mollon, RN_ 2. _CC. Roy, RN_ 3. _CC. Roy, RN_	1. _L. Singer, RN_ 2. _J.Smith,RN_ 3. _P. Joseph, RN_	1. _L. Singer, RN_ 2. _J.Smith,RN_ 3. _P. Joseph. RN_

FIGURE 3-2A

Following a clinical pathway. Adapted from *Mastering Documentation* (1999). Springhouse, PA: Springhouse.

Clinical Pathway: Colon Resection Without Colostomy (continued)

	Postop Day 2	Postop Day 3	Postop Day 4	Postop Day 5
Assessments	Review of systems assessment*	Review of systems assessment*	Review of systems assessment*	Review of systems assessment*
Consults		Dietary consult		Oncology consult if indicated (or to be done as outpatient
Labs and diagnostics	Electrolyte 7 (EL–7) CXR	CBC EL–7	Pathology results on chart	CBC EL–7
Interventions	D/C NG tube if possible* (per guidelines) I/O* VS per routine* D/C catheter* Ambulating* Incentive spirometry* Ankle exercises* I.V. site care* HOB 30º* Safety measures* Wound care* Mouth care* Antiembolism stockings	I/O* VS per routine* Incentive spirometry* Ankle exercises* I.V. site care* Safety measures* Wound care* Antiembolism stockings	I/O* VS per routine* Incentive spirometry* Ankle exercises* I.V. site care* Safety measures* Wound care* Antiembolism stockings	Consider staple removal Replace with Steri–Strips Assess that patient has met d/c criteria*
I.V.s	I.V. fluids, D_5 1/2NSS + MVI	I.V.– Heplock	Heplock	D/C Heplock
Medication	PCA (5 mg basal rate)	D/C PCA P.O. analgesia Resume routine home meds	P.O. analgesia	P.O. analgesia
Diet/GI	D/C NG tube per guidelines: (Clamp tube at 8 a.m. if no N/V and residual <200 mL, D/C tube @ 12 noon) (Check with doctor first)	Clears if pt. has BM/flatus Advance to postop diet if tolerating clears (at least one tray of clears)	House	House
Activity	Ambulate q.i.d. with abdominal binder* May shower Physical therapy b.i.d.	Ambulate q.i.d. with abdominal binder* May shower Physical therapy b.i.d.	Ambulate q.i.d. with abdominal binder* May shower Physical therapy b.i.d.	
Teaching	Reinforce preop teaching* Patient and family education p.r.n. re: family screening*	Reinforce preop teaching* Patient and family education p.r.n. re: family screening* Begin D/C teaching*	Reinforce preop teaching* Patient and family education p.r.n.* D/C teaching re: reportable s/s, F/U and wound care*	Review all D/C instructions and Rx including follow–up and appointments: with surgeon within 3 weeks, with oncologist within 1 month if indicated*
Key: *NSG activities V=Variance N= No var. Signatures:	1. 2. 3. V V V Ⓝ Ⓝ Ⓝ 1. A. McCarthy, RN 2. **R. Moyer, RN** 3. P.Drake, RN	1. 2. 3. V V V Ⓝ Ⓝ Ⓝ 1. A. McCarthy, RN 2. **R. Moyer, RN** 3. P.Drake, RN	1. 2. 3. V V V Ⓝ Ⓝ Ⓝ 1. L. Singer, RN 2. J.Smith,RN 3. P. Joseph, RN	1. 2. 3. V V V Ⓝ Ⓝ Ⓝ 1. L. Singer, RN 2. J.Smith,RN 3. P. Joseph, RN

FIGURE 3-2B

making a decision mirror the nursing process as they proceed from the assessment of the problem all the way through to the evaluation of results.

ASSESSMENT

Decision making starts with an assessment phase, during which appropriate information is gathered. For example, a problem may surface in the form of a complaint. Data regarding the complaint should be obtained. If a choice relates to the delivery of a nursing service, appropriate resources should be consulted. These resources may include reference books, institutional policy and procedure manuals, the American Nurses Association (ANA) Standards of Care, and the state Board of Nursing regulations governing practice. Experienced colleagues are another valuable resource in the work setting. Pertinent facts should be organized to clarify the issue. Say, for example, that a family complains to the nurse that their mother cannot sleep. The nurse gathers appropriate information regarding the complaint from several sources, including the patient, the family, and nursing personnel, and reviews the patient's chart for contributing factors. After collecting the information, the nurse identifies the source of the problem as the level of noise and activity in the nurse's station during the night. The nurse consults the policy and procedure manual for guidelines on room transfers and confers with the nursing supervisor.

ANALYSIS

During the analysis phase, the decision maker determines the necessity of making a decision. In some cases, the situation will resolve itself; there may be no benefit in making a choice.

If a choice must be made, however, the decision maker should generate multiple alternatives, which in turn should be analyzed and ranked, based on desirability, probability, and personal risk. Desirability includes factors that make the option more attractive at the time. It is highly influenced by personal values, bias, and patient preference. Consider whether the option fits with one's religious views, values, and personal beliefs. There may be other issues affecting desirability, such as lack of equipment, lack of available staff, lack of time, or lack of clinical competency with the procedure. Probability is the likelihood the alternative will achieve the desired outcome. An ideal alternative is one that is highly likely to lead to the desired outcome with few undesirable effects. The amount of risk involved with each alternative should be considered. In the field of nursing, decisions are made under conditions of uncertainty and change. A decision has a risk because it brings about change. It is important to explore emotional and social risk as well as physical risk. Risk to both patient and staff should also be considered. For example, consider a patient who is complaining of pain rated as 9 on a 1 to 10 scale. The respiratory rate is 10 breaths/min, and the patient is moaning in pain. The only pain prescription on the medication administration record (MAR) is a narcotic analgesic that suppresses the respirations. Alternatives include administering the medication, holding the medication, or calling the physician to obtain a new prescription.

The nurse evaluates these options based on desirability, probability, and personal risk. The analysis might reveal that the risk for negative consequences of administering the ordered pain medication outweighs the desirability of pain control until the physician can be consulted for a different medication order.

OUTCOME IDENTIFICATION

It is always necessary to identify the desired destination clearly. The first step in a journey is to decide where you want to end up. The expected outcome is a guide in choosing the direction of your decisions. Often, people sacrifice what is really important so that they can achieve a goal that doesn't really matter. This reflects a failure to keep the ultimate destination in sight. Consider the following illustration from *Alice's Adventures in Wonderland* by Lewis Carroll.

One day Alice came to a fork in the road and saw a Cheshire cat in a tree. "Would you tell me please, which road I ought to go from here?" asked Alice. "That depends a good deal on where you want to go," said the cat. "I don't care where," said Alice. "Then it doesn't matter which way you go," said the cat (as cited in Tappan, Weiss, & Whitehead, 2001, p. 79).

In another example related to nursing practice, a nurse begins diabetic education without identifying that the goal for the patient is to self-administer insulin. Without knowing the final destination, the nurse might use all the available teaching time before providing injection instruction.

With clearly stated outcomes, success becomes measurable. A poor-quality decision is a more likely result when the objective or goal is not clearly defined or when the goal is inconsistent with the values of the individual affected.

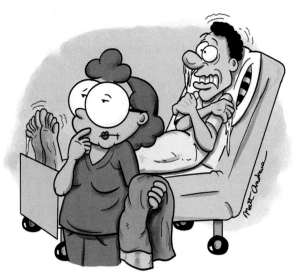

"Hmm... would the patient be warmer with this blanket or with the white one?"

In nursing practice, the appropriate nursing diagnosis must first be identified. Next, the desired outcome is selected from those identified in the Nursing Outcomes Classification (NOC) (Johnson, Maas, & Moorhead, 2000). (This process is further explained in Chapter 5, Nursing Process Applications.) After the desired outcome is recognized, each alternative must be compared. A cost–benefit analysis can be used to examine positive and negative aspects. The following scenario is an example of cost–benefit analysis:

A terminal patient has a large mass in the left lung. It has been determined that there is no cure available. Palliative measures being considered include the use of medications for pain control or the use of chemotherapy and radiation to reduce the size of the tumor. The nurse discussed the palliative treatment, including pain management, only with the patient. Positive aspects include increased quality time with family and friends, less financial expense, and promoting death with dignity. However, breathing difficulty would increase over time, and physical mobility and the ability to perform activities of daily living would gradually diminish. The increasing doses of pain medication would cause altered mentation as well as physiologic side effects, such as dry mouth, constipation, and drowsiness.

On the other hand, chemotherapy and radiation would reduce the size of the tumor. This would enhance respiratory efforts, maintain mobility, and decrease the pain. However, the chemotherapy would result in nausea, vomiting, and immune system suppression, necessitating isolation from family and friends. Multiple blood transfusions would be needed to treat the side effects of the therapy. These treatments would create huge medical bills.

The positive and negative aspects of both treatment modalities should be examined and compared before making a decision with the aim of producing the desired outcome.

PLAN

During the planning stage, the decision maker should choose the best option or combination of options that correlates with the priority while achieving the desired outcome. Allowing others to determine the solution does not foster growth in decision-making skills. Also, choices that would solve only the symptoms of the problem should not be selected. Until the real problem is identified, decision-making efforts will be counterproductive. By staying focused on the outcome, the decision maker remains focused on the real problem.

IMPLEMENTATION

During the implementation phase, nursing care is initiated that is appropriate to the alternatives selected by the patient.

EVALUATION

The results of the decision should always be evaluated. Questions should be asked and the responses monitored. Did the solution generate the desired outcome? Did the benefits outweigh the risks?

Consider again the terminally ill patient in the previous example, weighing the risks and benefits of various treatments. After analyzing the options, pain management only is selected and implemented. During the evaluation phase, the outcomes are monitored to determine that the best choice was selected. Figure 3-3 presents a schematic example of the evaluation process.

ERRORS IN DECISION MAKING

Failure to make a good decision can occur even after careful deliberation and consideration of all the facts. Reasons for failure may include bias, a narrow focus, or impatience (Box 3-1).

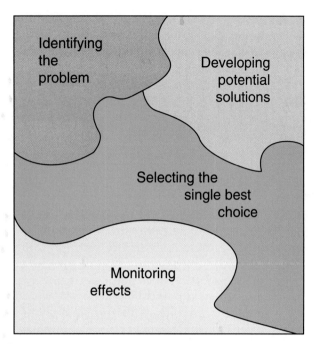

FIGURE 3-3
Evaluation process.

Bias

Bias can surface at various times during the decision-making process. Some people will place excessive emphasis on the first data received. They reject later information that does not support their first impression. Issues of prejudice could also surface. Some people tend to be closed-minded in their decision making. They are not open to con-

---

Box 3-1 Potential Errors in Decision Making

BIAS

Placing excess emphasis on first data received
Avoiding information that is contrary to one's opinion
Selecting alternatives to maintain status quo
Being predisposed toward a single solution
Stating the problem in a way to support one's choices
Making decisions to support past choices

FAILURE TO CONSIDER THE TOTAL SITUATION

Using inaccurate data
Problem was not clearly defined
Failure to prioritize or rank the problems in order of importance
Unrealistic goals

IMPATIENCE

Failure to identify multiple solutions
Incorrect implementation
Failure to use appropriate resources

---

sidering the opinions of others. These individuals typically avoid information that is contrary to their opinion. Therefore, data are excluded from the decision-making process.

Problems with decision making can also occur at the time that alternatives are selected. Some people resist change and thus favor alternatives that maintain the status quo. A similar problem happens when a person becomes attached to a single solution, choosing this familiar alternative even if it does not fit the situation. It is also possible to choose an option and then to restate the problem in a way that supports the choice. This represents a failure to identify the original problem. Decisions can be made that serve the purpose of supporting past choices. These can all lead to bias contaminating the decision-making process. Consider, for example, the case of a nurse who believes that substance abuse is caused by lack of will power and that individuals who are dependent on illicit drugs simply lack the desire to stop. Failure to examine her or his own thought processes for clarity and openness can cause a bias when this nurse delivers care to a patient admitted for substance abuse.

Failure to Consider the Total Situation

Failure to consider the total situation can also cause errors in decision making. The decision could be based on inaccurate data. For example, a nurse may assume that the new unlicensed assistive personnel (UAP) can obtain blood sugar readings and delegates this task. The UAP might not use the equipment properly. Consequently, the nurse would be making an error in the decision-making process if treatment decisions were made based on an incorrect reading.

Sometimes, the decision-maker does not clearly define the problem. This may lead to solving symptoms instead of the problem. For example, a 13-year-old patient, small for his age, weighing 79 pounds, is admitted with insulin-dependent diabetes mellitus. Even though there are three bedrooms in his home, he sleeps on the living room floor. His sister sleeps on the sofa, and the foster parents sleep in a bedroom. The family receives money to provide care for both children. Their food menu consists primarily of fast-food hamburgers, french fries, and macaroni with cheese and is lacking fruits or vegetables. Treating the blood sugar and teaching about the etiology of diabetes would resolve symptoms, not the problem.

Directing the care toward changing the environment and teaching dietary modifications would be more effective in problem resolution.

Decision-making failures can also be related to unrealistic goals. For example, it would be unrealistic to write a care plan goal expecting the patient with severe contractures to return to unassisted ambulation.

Finally, failure to rank the problems in order of importance can cause the decision-making process to break down. If the patient is experiencing difficulty breathing, this is a high-priority situation, and decisions must be made immediately. It does not matter at this point if the patient's room is cluttered. Ignoring the patient's serious problem and focusing on one that is trivial could result in undesirable consequences.

Impatience

The decision-making process can fail to function properly because of impatience. Most problems have more than one solution. If the decision maker chooses the first one that comes to mind, it might not be the optimum solution. For example, racing from room to room doing a little here and a little there results in a loss of productivity instead of a time saving. The outcome of haphazard management is frequently the consumption of large amounts of time, energy, and resources.

In an effort to proceed quickly, the nurse may fail to use appropriate resources. For instance, consider a situation in which a procedure that is unfamiliar to the nurse has been ordered. If the nurse fails to consult experts or to refer to appropriate texts to learn the procedure, a poor decision could result. Eagerness to finish a procedure quickly may lead to incorrect implementation. For example, when taking a blood pressure measurement on a very large patient, the nurse might use a normal-sized adult cuff to save the time involved in finding the large cuff. The decisions based on this reading would be incorrect. The decision-making process would have failed.

To reach a quality decision, decision makers should consciously evaluate the quality of their thinking for accuracy and clarity. Using the decision-making skill checklist provided at the end of this chapter will assist in this procedure.

SUMMARY

Decision-making is a purposeful, goal-directed system designed to help individuals select among alternatives. It is an important step in the problem-solving process. Nurses must know how to make wise decisions in their practice; they must know how to choose alternatives that achieve the desired outcome with an acceptable amount of risk. The best way to accomplish this level of competent decision making is to use a systematic approach.

IMPORTANT

KEY POINTS

- Decision making is a purposeful, goal-directed effort applied in a systematic way to make a choice among alternatives.
- Decision making is a step in the problem-solving process.
- Various factors influence decision making, including emotions, values, perceptions, and social climate.
- Effective decision makers are self-confident, proactive, flexible, focused, and accountable for their actions.
- Nurses must be skilled at making decisions in a group setting. Approaches to group decision making include task forces, quality circles, brainstorming, nominal group technique, the Delphi method, consensus, and majority rule.
- The first step of the decision-making process involves gathering appropriate information. Multiple alternatives should be generated and considered; identified alternatives are then ranked, based on desirability, probability, and personal risk.
- In making a decision, the desired outcome should be clearly stated. The decision maker

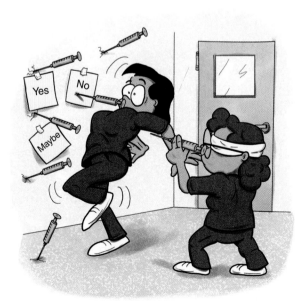

should choose the option that best achieves the outcome with an acceptable amount of risk.

- The selected alternative should be monitored for achievement of the desired outcome.
- Errors in the decision-making process include bias, failure to consider the entire situation, and impatience.

REFERENCES

Covey, S. (1989). *The 7 habits of highly effective people.* New York: Simon and Schuster.

Ellis, J. R., & Hartley, C. L. (2000). *Managing and co-ordinating nursing care.* Philadelphia: Lippincott Williams & Wilkins.

Huber, D. (2000). *Leadership and nursing care management.* Philadelphia: W.B. Saunders.

Johnson, M., Maas, M., & Moorhead, S. (2000). *Nursing outcomes classifications (NOC).* St. Louis: Mosby.

Jones, R., and Beck, S. (1996). *Decision making in nursing.* Albany, NY: Delmar.

National Council of State Boards of Nursing (NCSBN). (1995). *Delegation: Concepts and decision-making process.* Chicago: Author.

Marquis, B. L., & Huston, C. J. (2003). *Leadership roles and management functions in nursing.* Philadelphia: Lippincott Williams & Wilkins.

Mastering Documentation (1999). Springhouse, PA: Springhouse.

McCloskey, J. C., & Bulechek, G. M. (2000). *Nursing interventions classification (NIC).* St. Louis: Mosby.

Orem, D. (1971). *Nursing concepts of practice.* New York: McGraw-Hill.

Smith-Huddleston, S., & Ferguson, S. G. (1997). *Critical care and emergency nursing* (pp. 52–53). Springhouse, PA: Springhouse.

Tappen, R. M. (1995). *Nursing leadership and management.* Philadelphia: F.A. Davis.

Tappen, R. M., Weiss, S. A., & Whitehead, D. (2001). *Essentials of nursing leadership and management.* Philadelphia: F.A. Davis.

Yoder-Wise, P. S. (1999). *Leading and managing in nursing.* St. Louis: Mosby.

Student Worksheets

SKILL SHEET: DECISION MAKING

Purpose

To facilitate the student's development in making appropriate decisions in an organized manner based on relevant data. To increase the effectiveness of decision-making skills to solve problems.

Objective

To apply an organized process that facilitates appropriate judgment and reasoning skill in making decisions.

Steps: Decision Making

ASSESSMENT

1. Gather information.
2. Clarify the issue.
3. Sort and organize to identify pertinent facts and related issues.
4. Integrate existing knowledge.
5. Validate the available information.

ANALYSIS

1. Use critical thinking skills to interpret the data.
2. Determine the necessity for a decision to be made.
3. Establish the purpose of the decision and what needs to be determined.
4. Integrate existing knowledge related to previous experiences with similar situations.
5. Examine own value system and its effect on decisions.

OUTCOME IDENTIFICATION

Identify desired outcome of decision.

PLAN

1. Generate multiple alternatives that are capable of producing the desired outcome.
2. Analyze and rank alternatives based on desirability, probability, and personal risk.
3. Compare each alternative in terms of priorities.
4. Choose the option that best correlates with priorities and demonstrates the least undesirable side effects.

IMPLEMENTATION

Initiate the decision.

EVALUATION

1. Determine whether the decision resolves the priority area of the situation.
2. Establish whether the desired outcome was achieved.
3. Take responsibility for decisions.
4. Evaluate and reevaluate effect of decision after implementation and make adjustments accordingly.

COMPETENCY VALIDATION: DECISION MAKING

COMPETENCY STATEMENT

Demonstrate ability to make good decisions appropriate to the situation, based on relevant data.
The student demonstrated the ability to do the following:

1. Establish the purpose of the decision to be made.
2. Generate multiple alternatives capable of producing the desired outcome.
3. Select the decision that achieves the desired outcome.
4. Identify the decision that best correlates with priorities and demonstrates the least undesirable side effects.
5. Continuously evaluate and reevaluate the effect of the decision after implementation and make adjustments accordingly.

COMPETENT

- Understands reason for task and is able to perform task independently
- Understands reason for task but needs supervision
- Understands reason for task and is able to perform with assistance

NOT COMPETENT

- Understands reason for task but performs task at provisional level
- Is unable to state reason for task and performs task at a dependent level

SKILL CHECKLIST: DECISION MAKING

DECISION MAKING	SATISFACTORY	UNSATISFACTORY	NI/COMMENTS
ASSESSMENT			
1. Gather information.			
2. Clarify the issue.			
3. Sort and organize to identify pertinent facts and related issues.			
4. Integrate existing knowledge.			
5. Validate the available information.			
ANALYSIS			
1. Interpret the data.			
2. Determine the necessity for a decision to be made.			
3. Establish the purpose of the decision.			
4. Integrate existing knowledge related to previous experience with similar situations.			
5. Examine own value system and its effect on decisions.			
OUTCOME IDENTIFICATION			
1. Identify desired outcome of decision.			
PLAN			
1. Generate multiple alternatives that are capable of producing the desired outcome.			
2. Analyze and rank alternatives based on desirability, probability, and personal risk.			
3. Compare each alternative in terms of priorities.			
4. Choose the option that best correlates with priorities and demonstrates the least undesirable side effects.			
IMPLEMENTATION			
1. Initiate the decision.			
EVALUATION			
1. Determine whether the decision resolves the priority area of the situation.			
2. Establish whether the desired outcome was achieved.			
3. Take responsibility for decisions.			
4. Evaluate and reevaluate effect of decision and make adjustments accordingly.			

SCENARIO TO ACCOMPANY STUDENT WORKSHEETS

Refer to the patient in the Skill Sheet Scenario in Chapter 2, Problem Solving. Frank Fellow is a 72-year-old man who was admitted to the step-down nursing unit after myocardial infarction and cardioversion. Education for self-administration of heparin is continued. He can administer the injection independently. He continues to have difficulty drawing the correct dose of medication because of poor visual acuity.

What should the nurse do?

_____

_____

_____

_____

_____

See the Answer Key in Appendix A for sample answers for this exercise.

PRACTICE EXERCISES: DECISION MAKING

 ## SCENARIOS: USING DECISION-MAKING SKILLS

The following exercises relate to the decision-making process. Use the skill checklist where applicable.

SCENARIO 1

Jean has a comprehensive exam scheduled Monday that covers more than 1,000 pages of material. She is scheduled to work Saturday morning and Sunday afternoon. Her employer refused to let her take the weekend off to study. Jean has had very little time to review, and her grades have been very low this semester. If she scores poorly on this test, Jean will fail out of nursing school. To compound the problem, there is a big party on Saturday that Jean really wants to attend.

Based on the scenario, identify the problem that would require a decision.

_____

_____

_____

Identify solutions:

- Call in sick for work, attend the party, and cram before and after the party.
  Pro: Will be able to attend party and study.
  Con: Boss will be angry and may fire you.
- Attend the party, go to work, and just hope for the best on the test.
  Pro: Will be able to attend party, and boss won't be angry.
  Con: Probably will fail out of nursing school.
- Call in sick, stay home from the party, and study very hard
  Pro: Will pass the exam and stay in nursing program.
  Con: Won't get to attend the party, and boss will be angry.

Identify the outcome you wanted to achieve with the decision you made.

_____

_____

Place an asterisk (*) beside the selected alternative that achieves the desired outcome.

What if Jean's goal were different? What if the goal were to make money to pay the rent and buy groceries because her mother lost her job and has been ill the past 3 weeks? Would your choice be different?

Scenario 2

Linda has just returned to school and has been out of the study habit for 7 years. She has found it very difficult to get back into the habit of studying.

Based on the scenario, identify the problem that would require a decision.

_____

_____

Identify two solutions:

- Study when she first gets home, without stopping for supper and chores until studying is done.
  Pro: Will get studying done while not being so tired from housework.
  Con: Will be hungry and in a messy house.
- Leave studying until after supper and chores are done.
  Pro: Anxiety will be decreased about messy house and husband being hungry.
  Con: Will be too tired to study, stressed from being tired and not being finished with studying.
- Ask husband to do supper and help with the chores.
  Pro: Will get studying done.
  Con: Will have distractions with husband cooking; will feel inadequate for not being all things to all people.

Identify the outcome you wanted to achieve with the decision you made.

_____

_____

Place an asterisk (*) beside the selected alternative that achieves the desired outcome.

Scenario 3

Joel is working as an unlicensed assistive personnel (UAP). He wants to be a nurse but can't decide if he should attend nursing school in the fall. He and his partner have discussed their bills; he would have little time for working to assist with household expenses. He is also concerned about having enough time to study and participate in family events.

Identify a problem that required you to make a decision.

_____

_____

Identify solutions:

- Go to school and work part-time too.
  Pro: Will get an education for a better job and eventually make more money.
  Con: Will be stressed, interrupt family routine, and make grades lower than desired owing to job and family demands.
- Go to school and quit job.
  Pro: Will get an education for a better job and have fewer disruptions with family. Also, will have more time to study.
  Con: Will have less money to spend while going to school.

- Don't start school, and keep working as a UAP.
  Pro: Life will be uninterrupted.
  Con: Will have a job with poor pay and little chance for advancement.

Identify the outcome you wanted to achieve with the decision you made.

_____

_____

Place an asterisk (*) beside the selected alternative that achieves the desired outcome.

Scenario 4

Michelle submitted a request for a personal day off. The request was denied. She really needed the day off to go to her son's Christmas program.

Based on the scenario, identify a problem that would require a decision.

_____

_____

Identify solutions:

- Call in sick for that day.
  Pro: Will be able to attend son's program.
  Con: May be suspended for requesting time off and then calling in sick.
- Trade shifts with someone else.
  Pro: Will be able to attend son's program.
  Con: Will have to work on day off to replace regular shift.
- Go to work and miss program.
  Pro: Boss won't be angry.
  Con: Son will be upset because Mom missed the Christmas program.

Identify the outcome you wanted to achieve with the decision you made.

_____

_____

Place an asterisk (*) beside the option that correlates with the priorities and demonstrates the least undesirable side effects.

Scenario 5

A 66-year-old female patient had a right fractured hip and went to surgery for a right hip pinning procedure. The patient has an order for Vicodin tablets, 1 every 4 hours as needed for complaints of pain. It has been 3½ hours since her last pain medication. Physical therapists just finished range-of-motion exercises, and the patient will be getting up in the chair soon. She requested another pain pill now before she gets up in chair.

Identify a problem that requires you to make a decision.

_____

_____

Identify solutions:

- Give the pain pill early this time.
  Pro: Patient will be pain free and more likely to comply with therapy.
  Con: Face being chastised for not following the doctor's orders and risking possible legal issues.
- Call the doctor and report the pain.
  Pro: Be absolutely within legal limits.
  Con: Doctor will be interrupted and probably angry.
- Ask the patient to wait the 30 minutes.
  Pro: Nurse will not have to decide.
  Con: Patient who is already in pain will have a procedure that will increase her pain (violation of the Patient Care Partnership).
- Give pain medications as written and get the patient up in chair without it.
  Pro: Nurse will not have to decide.
  Con: Patient's pain will be increased.

Identify the outcome you want to achieve.

_____

_____

Place an asterisk (*) beside the selected alternative that achieves the desired outcome.

Scenario 6

A 33-year-old male patient is sitting in a chair beside the bed. He is alert and oriented. He was admitted for pneumonia and is receiving intravenous (IV) antibiotics that are expected to continue for 2 more days. The patient reports to the nurse that IV fluid is leaking around the needle, and the treatment has to be discontinued. You are trying to determine whether it is necessary to reinsert the needle.

Identify a problem that requires you to make a decision.

_____

_____

Identify solutions:

- Restart the IV.
  Pro: Patient will continue to get IV fluids and antibiotics.
  Con: Temporary discomfort of the needle stick.
- Leave the needle out.
  Pro: Patient can move more freely without discomfort.
  Con: Patient will not get the antibiotics needed for treatment of his disease.
- Ignore the situation and let someone else deal with it.
  Pro: Nurse will not be bothered with the procedure.
  Con: Fluids will continue to leak, and patient will not get needed treatment.

Identify the outcome you wanted to achieve with the decision you made.

_____

_____

Place an asterisk (*) beside the option that correlates with priorities and demonstrates the least undesirable side effects.

SCENARIO 7

An 83-year-old woman was admitted with a fractured hip yesterday evening and was taken to surgery for a repair on admission. She was admitted to your nursing unit at 1:30 AM. When you came on at 7:00 AM, she was drowsy and tired. The admitting orders are to get her up three times a day. You are trying to decide whether to let her sleep this morning because of her late return to the floor.

Identify a problem that required you to make a decision.

_____

_____

Identify solutions:

■ Get her up per doctor's order.
  Pro: Promotes mobility, and early mobility reduces chance for blood clots.
  Con: She may still be under the effect of anesthetic and injure herself.
■ Leave her in bed until this afternoon.
  Pro: Patient can better assist in the transfer and minimize risk for injury. Also promotes rest.
  Con: Bed rest increases risk for skin breakdown and promotes blood clots.

Identify the outcome you want to achieve with the decision you make.

_____∅____Bloodclots_____

_____

Place an asterisk (*) beside the option that correlates with priorities and demonstrates the least undesirable side effects.

See the Answer Key in Appendix A for sample answers for this exercise

PERSONAL EXPERIENCE

Write a brief scenario describing a patient you treated.

_____

_____

_____

_____

_____

_____

_____

_____

Identify a problem that required you to make a decision.

_____

_____

Identify two or more alternatives to resolve the problem.

_____

_____

_____

_____

Describe the consequences of each alternative (pros and cons).

_____

_____

_____

_____

_____

_____

_____

Place an asterisk (*) beside the option that correlates with priorities and demonstrates the least undesirable side effects.

Identify the outcome you wanted to achieve with the decision you made.

_____

_____

Answers will vary with student experience.

CHAPTER 4

Priority Setting

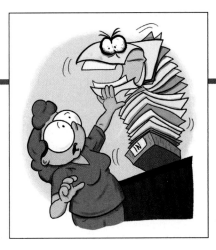

Priority setting is a complex step in the decision-making process. It is used to rank patient needs, determine the order of nursing activities, and manage resources. With a multitude of demands on their time, nurses need to be aware of priority-setting principles before making choices. Critical thinking supplies the logic within this process.

DEFINITION

A *priority* is something that is more important than anything else at a given time. On a busy nursing unit, priorities may include patient, team, or organizational needs. The values of the patients, their families, doctors, and other members of the health care team may be in opposition. For this reason, setting priorities is unique to each patient or situation. However, there are principles of pri-

ority setting that assist in arranging activities based on urgency, importance, significance, or preference. Use of these principles enhances competent nursing care.

TIME MANAGEMENT

Time management is an important skill for all busy people, including nursing students. Nursing students must make decisions regarding what information should be studied, which assignment should be studied first, how much time can be spent with family and friends, whether time permits a job while attending school, and how much leisure time is available. Juggling these responsibilities successfully requires a plan. Without a plan, a person spends the day simply "putting out fires." In other words, problems are merely handled as they occur, without considering relevance or significance. This can lead to spending excessive time on inconsequential problems. Lack of time also diminishes the ability to delegate. Consequently, the individual may experience more problems than one person can solve. Finally, preventive measures are largely ignored if action is delayed until a problem exists. This strategy creates new problems, which could have been prevented with an adequate plan. The effective problem solver is proactive instead of reactive. Box 4-1 depicts a plan of action for managing time on a busy nursing unit.

The formulation of a plan requires decisions about priorities. Steven Covey (1989) describes management as "putting first things first." To accomplish this, he recommends making a list of expected activities. These activities tend to fall into one of three categories: "must do," "should do," or "nice to do." "Must do" activities are a high priority. This category includes pressing problems and deadline-driven issues. In a student role, "must do" could be a large written assignment due tomorrow. "Should do" activities include preventive measures, certain interruptions, and homework that is not deadline driven but would be beneficial. For example, the student who recopies notes in a more readable, organized fashion is taking measures to prevent loss of information. While studying, the student receives a phone call from a creditor, interrupting the recopying process. This is a "should do" situation. Another example of "should do" tasks is the nongraded exercises at the end of the chapter. "Should do" tasks are of medium priority. "Nice to do" tasks are those that are aesthetic or pleasurable but are of low priority. An example would be going to the theater to see a show portraying a patient with a disease that is being studied in class.

People often tend to perform "nice to do" tasks first. These tasks are more enjoyable and less complex. Workers can become so immersed in "nice to do" tasks that they never finish important tasks. "Must do" tasks may be put off if they are more difficult or unpleasant. At times, individuals will concentrate only on tasks in which they are proficient. This strategy may result in ignoring activities that are of higher priority.

Once priorities are set, a time frame should be developed. Some people start with a time analysis. They may reflect on, or keep track of, how their time is spent. This activity reveals the person's current level of organization. It can lead to improvement in organizing time. The principles of time management can be summarized in one statement: "Organize and execute around priorities." (Covey, 1989, p. 149) Time management procedures are outlined in Box 4-2.

PRIORITIZING PATIENT NEEDS

An important component in determining nursing care priorities is defining patient needs. Once defined, these needs can be prioritized using Maslow's Hierarchy of Needs. This theory of motivation, developed by Abraham Maslow, is based on human needs. Maslow identified five levels of needs and arranged them in a pyramid form. Physiologic needs, including sleep, food, and water, are the lowest level of needs and are located at the base of the pyramid. Above physiologic needs on the pyramid are psychological needs, including safety and security, and love and belonging. The remaining levels of needs comprise higher-level or "meta-needs," including self-esteem and self-actualization. In Maslow's model, the basic needs found at the

---

Box 4-1 ORGANIZING THE WORKDAY

1. Gather data from available sources:
   - Shift report
   - Nursing Kardex
   - Review of patient's chart
   - Medication administration record (MAR)
   - Review of diagnostic test results
   - Collaboration with other health team members
   - Brief assessment of assigned patients
2. Examine the data.
3. Establish a plan for delivery of care.
4. Implement the plan.
5. Delegate if necessary to accomplish all tasks.
6. Attend to the most immediate concerns first.
7. Organize your work based on priorities.
8. Review and revise the plan as situations change.

Box 4-2 TIME MANAGEMENT PROCEDURES

Identify tasks, obligations, and activities.
Write them down.
Identify which must be completed in specified time frames.
Prioritize according to importance.
Work on the most important first.
Cross off tasks as they have been accomplished (a very satisfying activity).
Delegate tasks that do not require your expertise.
Do not accept assignments that you are not capable of completing.
Avoid the need to be perfect.
Control interruptions.
Evaluate how effectively time was used.

---

base of the pyramid must be at least partially met before the individual can concentrate on meta-needs. For example, if a person is starving, self-esteem is not a pressing issue.

Nurses can use Maslow's Hierarchy of Needs to prioritize patient needs. This list of needs assists the nurse in selecting nursing diagnoses and determining the priority of the diagnoses. Maslow's system of prioritizing patient need is particularly effective when physiologic needs are compared with psychological needs. Consider the following example: A 47-year-old patient had a right modified radical mastectomy performed yesterday. While reviewing the plan of care, the nurse notes that all of the following nursing diagnoses are appropriate. Which diagnosis would the nurse select as the highest priority?

Disturbed body image
Anxiety
Deficient fluid volume
Ineffective coping

Physiologic needs always take precedence. Deficient fluid volume is a physiologic need and therefore the priority. The exception to this rule would be if the psychosocial problem interferes with the patient's ability to participate in the physiologic care. For example, imagine that the same patient needs to learn how to dress the wound for home management. Discharge is planned as soon as this is accomplished. The patient's inability to cope is demonstrated by her refusal to look at the incision and participate in the dressing change. In this case, the nurse should address ineffective coping first. Refer to Figure 4-1 and Table 4-1 for a de-

scription of Maslow's Hierarchy of Needs with a corresponding list of nursing diagnoses.

One of the disadvantages of relying only on Maslow's Hierarchy of Needs is that numerous physiologic needs are placed on the same level. For this reason, many nurses rely on the refinement of Maslow's model developed by Kalish. This model adds another level to clarify the priorities in physiologic needs, ranking some nursing activities at the physiologic level. Kalish identified the most basic level needs as food, air, water, temperature regulation, elimination, rest, and pain avoidance. The second level of physiologic needs includes sex, activity, exploration, manipulation, and novelty. For example, Kalish's model supports giving priority to hydration over providing activity. Current patient circumstances and goals must be taken into consideration when prioritizing needs, but Kalish's model serves as a useful guide (Figure 4-2).

PRIORITIZING NURSING DIAGNOSES

Occasionally, it is not possible to prioritize nursing diagnoses simply by differentiating physical and psychological needs. The Craven and Hirnle (2003) model is useful in these cases. Craven and Hirnle developed theories about priorities that are somewhat similar to Covey's. Their model organizes priorities into three categories: high, medium, and low priority. Prioritizing nursing diagnoses in this manner leads to determining the priority of nursing activities.

The diagram below depicts Maslow's hierarchy of needs. You can use this system when determining priorities for patient care. Shown at left is the ascending hierarchy of human needs; the definitions at right explain the five need categories.

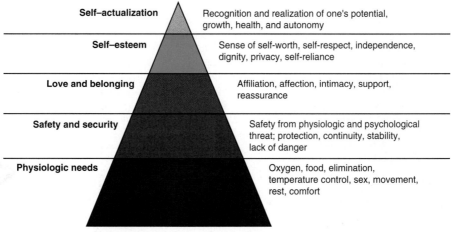

Self–actualization — Recognition and realization of one's potential, growth, health, and autonomy

Self–esteem — Sense of self-worth, self-respect, independence, dignity, privacy, self-reliance

Love and belonging — Affiliation, affection, intimacy, support, reassurance

Safety and security — Safety from physiologic and psychological threat; protection, continuity, stability, lack of danger

Physiologic needs — Oxygen, food, elimination, temperature control, sex, movement, rest, comfort

FIGURE 4-1

Nursing diagnoses and Maslow's Hierarchy of Needs. Adapted from Sparks, S. M., & Taylor, C. M. (1998). *Nursing diagnosis reference manual.* Springhouse, PA: Springhouse.

SELF-ACTUALIZATION	SELF-ESTEEM	LOVE AND BELONGING	SAFETY AND SECURITY	PHYSIOLOGIC NEEDS
Development, risk for delayed	Adjustment, impaired	Anxiety	Autonomic dys-reflexia	Activity intolerance
Disturbed energy field	Coping, defensive	Caregiver role strain	Autonomic dys-reflexia, risk for	Activity intolerance, risk for
Growth and development, delayed	Coping, in-effective	Caregiver role strain, risk for	Communication, impaired verbal	Airway clearance, ineffective
Health-seeking behaviors	Coping, in-effective community	Compromised family coping	Death anxiety	Aspiration, risk for
Spiritual distress	Decisional con-flict (specify)	Failure to thrive, adult	Deficient knowl-edge (specify)	Bed mobility, impaired
Spiritual well-being, readiness tor enhanced	Deficient diversional activity	Family processes, interrupted	Disuse syn-drome, risk for	Body temperature, risk for imbalanced
Therapeutic regimen management, effective	Denial, in-effective	Loneliness, risk for	Falls, risk for	Breastfeeding, effective
	Disturbed body image	Parent-infant attachment, risk for impaired	Fear	Breastfeeding, ineffective
	Disturbed personal identity	Parental role conflict	Grieving, anti-cipatory	Breastfeeding, interrupted
	Family pro-cesses, dys-functional: Alcoholism	Parenting, impaired	Grieving, dys-functional	Breathing pattern, ineffective
	Hopelessness	Parenting, impaired, risk for	Growth, risk for dispropor-tionate	Cardiac output, decreased
	Noncompliance (specify)	Readiness for enhanced family coping	Impaired home maintenance	Confusion, acute
	Post-trauma response	Relocation stress syndrome	Infection, risk for	Confusion, chronic
	Post-trauma response, risk for	Social inter-actions, impaired	Injury, risk for	Constipation
	Powerlessness	Social isolation	Injury, risk for perioperative positioning	Constipation, perceived
	Powerlessness, risk for		Latex allergy response	Deficient fluid volume
	Rape trauma syndrome		Latex allergy response, risk for	Deficient fluid volume, risk for
	Rape trauma syndrome: Compound reaction		Peripheral neurovascular dysfunction, risk for	Dentition, impaired
	Rape trauma syndrome: Silent reaction		Poisoning, risk for	Diarrhea
	Relocation stress syndrome, risk for		Sorrow, chronic	Disturbed sensory perception (specify) (visual, auditory, kinesthetic, gustatory, tactile, olfactory)
	Role perfor-mance, ineffective		Suffocation, risk for	Disturbed sleep pattern
	Self-esteem, chronic low		Therapeutic regimen man-agement, in-effective	Environmental interpretation syndrome, impaired
	Self-esteem disturbance		Therapeutic regimen man-agement, ineffective community	Excess fluid volume
			Therapeutic regimen management, ineffective family	Fatigue
				Fluid volume, imbalanced, risk for
				Gas exchange, impaired
				Hyperthermia
				Hypothermia
				Incontinence, bowel
				Incontinence, functional urinary
				Incontinence, reflex urinary
				Incontinence, risk for urinary
				Incontinence, stress urinary
				Incontinence, total urinary
				Incontinence, urge urinary
				Infant behavior, disorganized
				Infant behavior, readiness for enhanced organized
				Infant behavior, risk for disorganized
				Infant feeding pattern, ineffective
				Intracranial adaptive capacity, decreased
				Memory, impaired
				Nausea
				Nutrition, imbalanced: Less than body requirements
				Nutrition, imbalanced: More than body requirements
				Nutrition, imbalanced: Risk for more than body requirements
				Oral mucous membranes, impaired
				Pain, acute
				Pain, chronic
				Physical mobility, impaired
				Protection, ineffective
				Self-care deficit, bathing/hygiene

(continued)

TABLE 4-1	List of Nursing Diagnoses Categorized Using Maslow's Hierarchy (Continued)			
SELF-ACTUALIZATION	**SELF-ESTEEM**	**LOVE AND BELONGING**	**SAFETY AND SECURITY**	**PHYSIOLOGIC NEEDS**
	Self-esteem, situational low		Trauma, risk for Unilateral neglect	Self-care deficit, dressing/grooming
	Self-esteem, situational low, risk for			Self-care deficit, feeding
	Self-mutilation			Self-care deficit, toileting
	Self-mutilation, risk for			Sexual dysfunction
	Suicide, risk for			Sexuality patterns, ineffective
	Violence, risk for: Self-directed or other-directed			Skin integrity, impaired
				Skin integrity, impaired, risk for
				Sleep deprivation
				Surgical recovery, delayed
				Swallowing, impaired
				Thermoregulation, ineffective
				Thought processes, disturbed
				Tissue integrity, impaired
				Tissue perfusion, ineffective (specify) (renal, cerebral, cardiopulmonary, gastrointestinal, peripheral)
				Urinary elimination, impaired
				Ventilation, impaired spontaneous
				Ventilatory weaning response, dysfunctional
				Walking, impaired
				Wheelchair mobility, impaired
				Wheelchair transfer mobility, impaired

Adapted from Schuster, P. M. (2002). *Concept mapping: A critical-thinking approach to care planning* (pp. 159–160). Philadelphia: F.A. Davis.

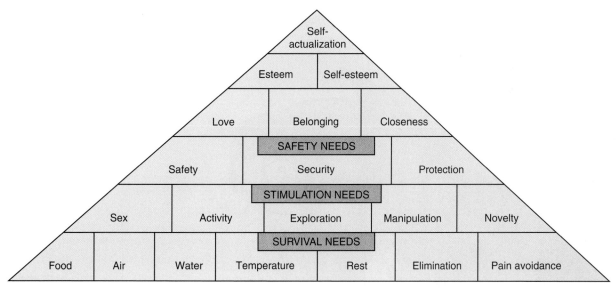

FIGURE 4-2

Kalish's expanded hierarchy. Adapted from Doenges, M. E., Moorhouse, M. F., & Burley, J. T. (2000). *Application of nursing process and nursing diagnosis: An interactive approach.* Philadelphia: F.A. Davis.

High-priority situations include life-threatening events, threats to patient safety, and situations in which pain and anxiety relief is a concern. Life-threatening situations may involve airway difficulties, such as inability to clear the airway and risk for aspiration; gas exchange disorders involving pathophysiologic changes in alveoli or in ventilatory efforts; cardiovascular changes such as hemorrhage, alterations in cardiac output; tissue perfusion changes; and alteration in fluid volumes, whether through intake, infusion, or elimination. If these situations present immediate life-threatening needs, priority activities should be directed toward resolution of these problems first.

The unstable patient, the patient with a change in condition, and the patient with a threat to safety will also have priority. The priority nursing diagnoses may include altered mental status or risk for violence. Life-threatening nursing diagnoses take precedence whether they are in physiologic or psychological areas.

"Medium-priority nursing diagnoses involve problems that could result in unhealthy consequences, such as physical or emotional impairment, but are not likely to threaten life" (Craven & Hirnle, 2003, p. 187). For instance, anxiety is a symptom often caused by lack of knowledge. The appropriate course of action should be directed toward patient education. Urgent events that are not life threatening are also found at this level. This could be a situation in need of prompt attention, such as preparation for a test or discharge preparations for a patient leaving the institution in the immediate future. Scheduled events, such as a patient's appointment in physical therapy, are also frequently found at this level of priority. When the list of nursing activities is prepared, pre-scheduled events should always be noted.

"Low-priority nursing diagnoses involve problems that usually can be resolved easily with minimal interventions and have little potential to cause significant dysfunction" (Craven & Hirnle, 2003, p. 187). These problems have no major effect on the person if not attended to this day or even this week.

The important principles discussed here should always be considered when deciding on the priority of an action. When the priority nursing diagnoses are selected, the nurse has a list of activities. When scheduling time, the nurse must keep these priorities in mind. Examples of high-, medium-, and low-priority diagnoses can be seen in Box 4-3.

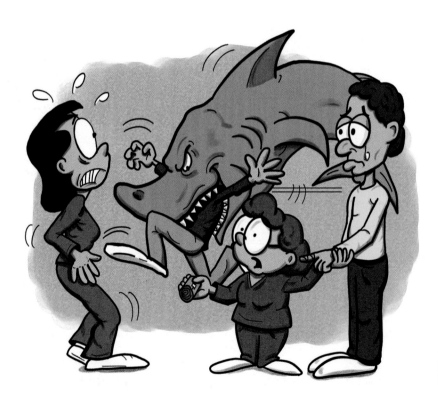

"Why did I take him first? Are you kidding? That's the deepest paper cut I've ever seen!"

PRIORITY ACTIVITIES

Realistically, there are other factors than those previously discussed that influence the scheduling of activities. The availability of resources in terms of material and staff is a concern. Urgent or scheduled activities may be a priority even if they are not life threatening. Rubenfeld and Scheffer (1999) developed a model that considers these issues.

Rubenfeld and Scheffer (1999) discuss four levels of priority: life-threatening issues, safety, patient priorities, and nursing priorities. At the first priority level are life-threatening issues such as airway, breathing, and circulation (ABCs). However, the nurse should also beware of using ABCs to establish priorities when the situation does not imply a problem in this area.

The second level concerns safety issues. Safety involves protecting the patient from injury during activities and includes areas such as fall prevention, safety devices, and seizure precautions. Safety also involves providing nursing care within the Scope of Practice and maintaining professional competence. As an example, the American Nurses Association Standards of Practice identify the expected level of performance and practice, which includes "doing no harm" and protecting the health and safety of the patient. This entails recognizing a changed or unstable patient status so that appropriate interventions can be initiated. In the case of changing patient status, the registered nurse (RN) would call the physician, whereas the licensed practical nurse (LPN) would notify the RN. When the patient has a changing, unstable condition, nursing activities related to this condition assume more importance. For instance, if a patient is confused and also un-

stable, there are two safety issues. Under the circumstances, the confusion would be a lesser priority than the unstable status.

Once life-threatening and safety issues have been taken into account, the nurse can consider the patient's priorities in scheduling activities. To the extent that his or her condition will allow, the patient should be consulted in planning activities. Health care providers are legally required to involve patients in health care decisions. For example, the Patient Care Partnership allows consumers to be active in their own health care. It embraces informed and shared decision making. The Joint Commission on Accreditation of Healthcare Organizations (JCAHO) standards mandate that outcomes be based on activities that are patient and family oriented. Therefore, the patient's beliefs regarding the level of importance must be considered in planning. This allows the plan of care to be carried out more efficiently. For instance, if a doctor orders a procedure, an early step in the process is to obtain informed consent. The nurse needs to consider this when planning activities related to the procedure. It might be a waste of time to gather the equipment first. If the patient refuses, the procedure will not be performed. Therefore, it is logical to obtain consent before gathering equipment.

Finally, establishing nursing priorities includes forming a composite of all of the patient's strengths and health concerns; moral and ethical decisions; issues regarding time, resources and setting; and Maslow's Hierarchy of Needs. A composite of all the patient's strengths and health concerns involves physical, emotional, mental, and spiritual aspects. Personal expectations related to beliefs and values and earlier experiences with health and illness also bear on patient decisions. This priority level also includes health promotion and illness prevention. These are essential elements needed to improve quality of life. A health risk appraisal will facilitate risk reduction interventions tailored to each individual's needs. For example, during the admission assessment, a 72-year-old patient showed a history of falling, unsteady gait, and impaired mobility. These are all indicators of a patient at risk for injury. The facility has a policy that a patient demonstrating three risk indicators for fall criteria must be placed on a "high-risk fall prevention" protocol. Interventions designed to reduce the risk for falls are therefore initiated.

The Rubenfeld and Scheffer model (1999) is well suited to nursing care delivery situations involving outpatient care, long-term care, and community-based settings. It encourages consulting the patients for their preferences (see Figure 4-3).

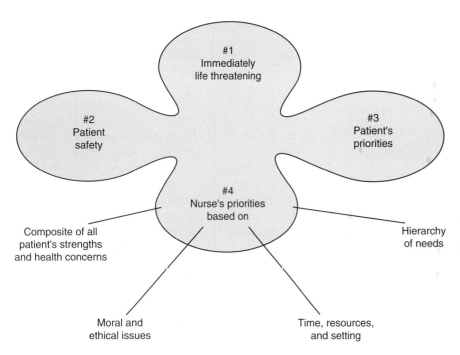

FIGURE 4-3

Guidelines for determining priorities. Adapted from Rubenfeld, M. G., & Scheffer, B. K. (1999). *Critical thinking in nursing: An interactive approach.* Philadelphia: Lippincott Williams & Wilkins.

Multitasking

Setting priorities is not a linear activity, because several needs or concerns are frequently addressed simultaneously. The nurse does not work on one priority, finish it, and then work on the second priority. The ability to multitask is important in time management. Learning to take charge and make efficient use of time is the key to time management. However, it is critical that the nurse recognize exactly what the top priority is, in order to ensure high-quality nursing care for all the patients under his or her care.

In applying information from the models, the nurse may want to prepare a daily "to do" list of activities. This is an efficient time management tool that emphasizes priorities. Organizing work increases productivity. Zerweth and Claborn (2000) have developed a useful tool for time management (Box 4-4).

Making a to do list facilitates the nurse's ability to complete several tasks at once. Routine nursing activities should be noted as well as patient-specific activities. This list should be developed early in the shift. During report, the nurse can identify the patient who is most seriously ill. This patient will likely require the most time and will also be at greatest risk for a change in status. The nurse must be alert for these status changes. Early intervention is essential to the delivery of high-quality care and will certainly produce a more effective use of time.

When scheduling activities, it is best to plan time for charting after the performance of the activity. This will help to ensure an accurate description of events. The priority-setting checklist included at the end of this chapter identifies the essential steps of time management. Students can use this checklist as a guide, or it can be used in

Box 4-4	**Daily Nursing To Do List**	
A. Immediate Activities		
A-1	Check intravenous line	
A-2	Assess chest tube	
A-3	Suction endotracheal tube	
B. Scheduled Items		
B-1	9:00 AM	Dressing change
B-2	10:00 AM	Medications
B-3	12:00 PM	Scheduled diagnostic test
B-4	2:00 PM	Medications
B-5	3:00 PM	Change of shift report
C. When Time Allows		
C-1	Diabetic teaching	
C-2	Social service consultation	
D. If Time Is Available		
D-1	See new videos in tape library	
D-2	Reorganize reference material on unit	

Adapted from Zerwekh, J., & Claborn, J. C. (2000). *Nursing today: Transition and trends* (p. 219). Philadelphia: W.B. Saunders.

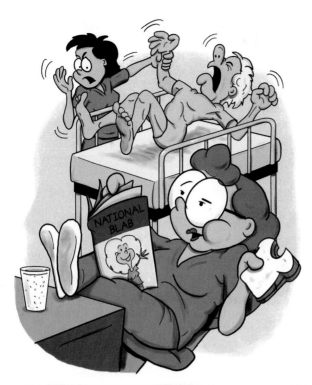

"Geez, I'll be there in a minute! Lunch **is** the most important meal of the day, you know. . ."

the lab setting accompanied by a scenario. Repeated practice is essential to the development of time management skills.

PRIORITIZING WITHIN THE NURSING PROCESS

Nursing care is complicated. Situational variables may affect decisions. Therefore, practical knowledge of several models may be necessary. In the prioritizing procedure, the nurse may need to use concepts from more than one source of guidance. This may include using Maslow's Hierarchy of Needs for prioritizing the nursing diagnosis and Rubenfeld and Scheffer's (1999) tool for ranking the importance of nursing activities. These can be tied together using the nursing process format.

ASSESSMENT

Assessment always takes precedence when prioritizing time. An assessment is used to collect data about the assigned patient and his or her health problems. This includes obtaining a health history,

performing a physical exam, evaluating lab and diagnostic results, talking to the patient, making observations, and collaborating with colleagues. The data are then sorted into clusters and validated with the patient. Patient problems are identified by sorting the defining characteristics into health-related situations. These defining characteristics are the "observable cues/inferences that cluster as manifestations of an actual or wellness nursing diagnosis." (NANDA, 2001, p. 245) The cues or inferences are the patient's response in a given condition. Each group of these data is referred to as a *cluster,* and conclusions drawn from a cluster lead to the nursing diagnosis. Clusters that support actual problems include existing data. Clusters of data for potential problems include related factors that point to a possible problem. Cue clusters bring together data on a potential problem in a way that gives meaning to them. Often, the same data looked at individually do not point toward the same conclusions. For example, refer to the following data cluster:

- The patient is 73 years old, has a fifth-grade education, and lives with her 55-year-old developmentally disabled son.
- The patient has recently been diagnosed with heart failure.
- The patient will probably need a digitalis preparation and ongoing diuretic therapy.

As the patient's data are collected, they should be compared with normal values. This will assist in the identification of patterns related to the disease process or patient need. The nurse can examine this information in relation to the cause and effect of the disease process. The nurse should never implement before assessing. However, in situations involving an urgent problem, performing only a partial assessment may be necessary. After implementation of interventions, a complete assessment can be performed. The following is an example of the assessment process: The patient was admitted for dehydration and needs a central line for fluid replacement. Vital signs upon arrival on the unit at 2:00 PM were temperature, 99°F (37.2°C); pulse, 102 beats/min; respirations, 24 breaths/min; and blood pressure, 90/60 mm Hg. These vital signs are consistent with previous recordings in the emergency room. The nurse finishes the patient report at 3:30 PM. The physician will be on the unit at 4:00 PM to place the central line. Which nursing activity has highest priority?

- Ensure that consent form is signed.
- Take the vital signs.
- Perform a body system assessment.

- Ensure that central line equipment is on the unit.
- Assess urinary output.

Assessing includes collecting, verifying, and organizing. Ensuring that the consent form is signed is verification. Without a consent form, the procedure cannot be done. It is included with the assessment and therefore is the first priority.

Analysis

In the analysis phase, the nurse prepares a list of patient needs and a list of nursing diagnoses based on the identified needs. For example, the nursing diagnosis for the data cluster of the previously discussed 73-year-old patient is: Deficient knowledge related to disease process, precautions, and side effects of diuretic and digitalis therapy.

Outcome Identification

Goals and measurable outcomes provide a means to determine whether the nursing diagnoses are appropriate for the situation. Priorities are established to help the nurse achieve the desired outcome.

The list of patient needs should be examined using Maslow's Hierarchy of Needs to determine priorities. In establishing the priority of nursing diagnoses, the model developed by Craven and Hirnle should also be used. After the nursing diagnoses are prioritized, the nurse can identify patient goals and outcomes based on the Nursing Outcomes Classification (NOC).

Plan

During the planning phase, nursing activities appropriate for the specified nursing diagnoses are selected from the Nursing Interventions Classification (NIC). Interventions are treatments that nurses perform to achieve the specified outcome. The NIC designates activities to be carried out by the nurse in order to execute these interventions. The activities listed in the NIC are research based to ensure that the appropriate activities are chosen to treat the patient's problem. The specific activities are then documented in the patient's plan of care.

Rubenfeld and Scheffer's (1999) tool has demonstrated a high level of utility in prioritizing nursing actions. For example, a 16-year-old boy was transported to the emergency department by ambulance following a motor vehicle accident. Witnesses report his car slid on ice, and the vehicle became airborne, throwing the adolescent from his car. Initial assessment reveals that the patient has a patent airway, is responsive to painful stimuli, has laceration to his left thigh covered with a dressing, and has contusions to the left flank area. The following activities need to be placed in order of priority:

- Immobilize head and neck.
- Assess level of consciousness and neurologic deficits.
- Assess left thigh and apply clean pressure dressing.
- Call the parents for consent to treat.
- Insert an indwelling Foley catheter.

Maslow's Hierarchy of Needs is not useful in rank ordering of these nursing activities or other complex nursing situations. However, an analysis of the situation and review of Rubenfeld and Scheffer's (1999) tool reveals that the priorities should be placed in the above order. Immobilizing the head and neck ensures the airway; assessing the neurologic aspects for potential problems that could cause tissue death and assessing potential bleeding are patient safety issues. Emergency treatment without consent extends only to a life-threatening situation; therefore, the next intervention should be to call the parents to ensure proper consent (patient's priorities). Nurse's priorities are next and involve the insertion of the indwelling Foley. This model is helpful in considering the complexity of each patient situation.

Implementation

The nurse must remember that the established priorities, listed as activities, must be implemented. This involves performing those immediate actions necessary to prevent harm first; actions for problems that could result in unhealthy consequences or physical or emotional impairment second; and the lowest-priority actions third. Lowest-priority actions are directed toward needs that would not be affected if not attended to until a later date.

During the implementation phase, patient care is given. This care may be provided through dependent (physician oriented), independent (nurse oriented), or interdependent actions (collaborative actions). The nurse should identify problems that are not within the scope of nursing practice and refer them to the appropriate health care member.

The stated goals should be used as a framework to deliver nursing care. The expected outcomes should be reviewed before taking action. The nursing actions and the patient's response to the action must be documented as appropriate for the institution.

Evaluation

As always, the plan should be reevaluated as the patient status or the situation changes. This might require an adjustment or revision of the plan. The nurse should continue to assess the patient's progress toward the outcome criteria established in the plan of care. Continued monitoring for improvement or deterioration in status, recording, and reporting is essential to making judgments about goal attainment. When changes do occur, an adjustment or revision of planned priorities is required. For example, a 65-year-old patient admitted for a cerebrovascular accident (CVA) has developed improvement in gross motor movement and fine motor skills since admission. Now the plan of care is revised to include independent living skills necessary to prepare for discharge.

PITFALLS IN PRIORITY SETTING

Priority setting is a complex critical thinking skill. Failure to identify tasks that cannot be delayed without serious consequences can occur even after consideration of all the variables. Patients must be monitored continuously for changing circumstances; thus, priorities may change as the shift progresses. Reasons for ineffective identification of priorities may include:

- Inadequate assessment and evaluation of patient needs
- Failure to differentiate between priority and nonpriority tasks
- Acceptance of others' priorities without assessing all the variables
- Performance of tasks with a "first identified, first completed" approach
- Completion of the easiest task first

Inadequate Assessment and Evaluation of Client Needs

Effective planning increases awareness of the knowledge, materials, and resources necessary to complete tasks. Preparing a "to do" list is essential to identify the knowledge and skills necessary to complete the activities required. This can also help the nurse avoid being placed in a situation for which he or she is unprepared. Thorough assessment provides a collection of significant, relevant data. Failure to gather current information and accurate data or to consider the total situation can cause errors. Poorly defined problems result in faulty analysis, thus yielding an inaccurate selection of priorities. For example, Mr. Jones's previous partial thromboplastin time (PTT) was 66 and the heparin infusion was continued at the same rate while the nurse provided personal care and administered routine oral medications for his or her assigned patients. Mr. Jones's most recent PTT was 122. The nurse failed to monitor these new lab results, causing the patient to have a bleeding episode as a result of excess medication.

Failure To Differentiate Between Priority and Nonpriority Tasks

Consider the impact of a delay in care activities for the patient. In order to rank the importance of activities, it is essential to determine not only which tasks are required for each individual in the care assignment, but which tasks have deadlines, and which are prerequisites to other tasks. Random completion of tasks without attending to the most immediate needs first—for example, starting patient care for the patients in the room closest to the nurse's station—can create poor results in delivering care.

Acceptance of Others' Priorities Without Assessing All the Variables

Assessing all the variables in the assignment is essential to produce quality care.

Accepting, without question, the opinions of others when determining the most important task to be completed can produce poor results. For example, a night nurse reports that the most urgent activity in need of attention is bathing a patient scheduled for surgery in two hours, while another patient admitted during the night for a fractured hip with pain rated at 9 (on a 1-10 scale) is kept waiting for a pain injection. Another example would be that of a nurse who is ordered to do a specific task immediately because a patient's family is "upset," even though one of the nurse's other patients is in respiratory distress.

Performance of Tasks With a "First Identified, First Completed" Approach

Preparing a "to do" list is essential to identify those activities in the workload that are scheduled and time-sensitive. Frequent reordering of the list is also important. Failure to plan frequently produces a first identified, first completed approach. For example, a nurse receives an order for an insulin injection for a newly admitted diabetic patient with a fasting blood sugar of 664 mg/dL. Instead of proceeding with this, the nurse administers all the morning medications and assists with basic care for other assigned patients.

Completion of the Easiest Task First

The novice nurse frequently completes simple tasks first because they are the most satisfying and comfortable. Failure to perform tasks in order of priority can result in poor outcomes for patient care. An example of this would be administering personal care instead of performing the complex dressing change that might lead to quicker recognition of the signs of infection.

It can be readily seen that priority setting is a vital aspect of the nursing process. In nursing practice, priority setting is used to select the order of nursing diagnoses. Principles of rank ordering are also used to choose the most important nursing action or activity. This does not imply that activities are left undone, only that nurses must select an order in which to perform them.

SUMMARY

In today's health care arena, more is expected of employees, despite the reality of a decreased staff. As patient acuity has increased, there has not been a corresponding increase in workers. Nurses often complain about a lack of time to complete assigned tasks. To ensure patient safety and satisfaction, nurses must decide which needs take precedence over other needs at that particular time. Success in caring for patients with multiple problems and needs demands the ability to direct care based on priorities.

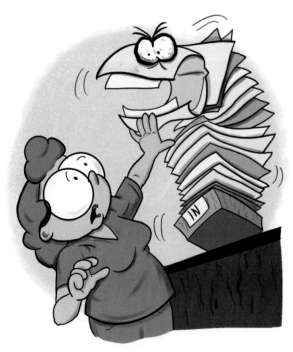
Don't let your priorities set you!

KEY POINTS

- Priority setting is an important step in the decision-making process. Critical thinking is inherent in the priority-setting process.
- Priority setting includes effective time management. To improve time management, tasks should be listed and categorized as "must do," "should do," or "nice to do."
- Patient needs must be identified to establish nursing care priorities.
- Maslow's Hierarchy of Needs can be used to establish patient priorities. Kalish's model provides a refinement of Maslow's theory by clarifying physiologic needs.
- To prioritize nursing diagnoses, Craven and Hirnle (2003) provide a model that organizes priorities into high, medium, and low priority.
- Rubenfeld and Scheffer (1999) divide nursing activities into four levels of priority: life-threatening issues, safety, patient priorities, and nursing priorities.
- Assessing always takes precedence when prioritizing time. In the assessment phase, data is sorted into clusters.
- A list of patient needs and corresponding nursing diagnoses is prepared in the analysis phase. Outcome identification helps determine which actions are priorities.
- In the planning phase, the nurse selects activities using the Nursing Intervention Classification (NIC) system. During implementation of the activities, care is directed by established goals and expected outcomes.
- Evaluation of care delivery should be performed to ensure quality.

REFERENCES

Alfaro-LeFevre, R. (1999). *Critical thinking in nursing.* Philadelphia: W.B. Saunders.

Burckhardt, J. A., Irwin, B. J., & Phillips-Arikian, V. (2001). *Kaplan NCLEX-RN.* New York: Simon & Schuster.

Castillo, S. L. (1999). *Strategies techniques and approaches to thinking.* Philadelphia: W.B. Saunders.

Covey, S. R. (1989). *The seven habits of highly effective people.* New York: Simon and Schuster.

Craven, R. F., & Hirnle, C. (2003). *Fundamentals of nursing: Human health and function* (4th ed.). Philadelphia: Lippincott Williams & Wilkins.

Doenges, M. E., Moorhouse, M. F., & Burley, J. T. (2000). *Application of nursing process and nursing diagnosis.* Philadelphia: F.A. Davis.

Ellis, J. R., & Hartley, C. L. (2000). *Managing and coordinating nursing care.* Philadelphia: Lippincott Williams & Wilkins.

Hendrickson, G., Doddato, T. M., & Kovner, C. (1990). How do nurses use their time? *Journal of Nursing Administration, 20* (3), 31–37.

North American Nursing Diagnosis Association (2001). *NANDA Nursing diagnosis: Definitions and classification (2001–2002).* Philadelphia: Author.

Orem, D. E. (1980). *Nursing concepts of practice.* St. Louis: McGraw-Hill.

Ringsven, M. K., & Bond, D. (1991). *Gerontology and leadership skills for nurses.* Boston: Delmar.

Rocchicciol, J. T., & Tilbury, M. S. (1998). *Clinical leadership in nursing.* Philadelphia: W.B. Saunders.

Rubenfeld, M. G., & Scheffer, B. K. (1999). *Critical thinking in nursing: An interactive approach.* Philadelphia: Lippincott Williams & Wilkins.

Schuster, P. M. (2002). *Concept mapping: A critical-thinking approach to care planning.* Philadelphia: F.A. Davis.

Sparks, S. M., & Taylor, C. M. (1998). *Nursing diagnosis reference manual.* Springhouse, PA: Springhouse.

Varcarolis, E. M. (2002). *Foundations of psychiatric mental health nursing: A clinical approach.* Philadelphia: W.B. Saunders.

Zerwekh, J., & Claborn, J. C. (2000). *Nursing today: Transition and trends.* Philadelphia: W.B. Saunders.

Student Worksheets

SKILL SHEET: PRIORITY SETTING

Purpose

To enable the student to determine the importance and urgency of the nursing diagnosis or performance of a nursing duty, based on the patient's situation and changing conditions.

Objectives

The student will demonstrate the ability to do the following:

1. Identify needs and tasks to be completed.
2. Analyze patient needs and tasks for their critical nature.
3. Identify the circumstance that takes precedence in position or is deemed most important among several items at this time.
4. Implement care based on priority ranking of problems.
5. Revise priorities as needs and situations change.

Steps: Priority Setting

ASSESSMENT*

1. Collect data from all available resources (e.g., review nursing history, perform physical examination, interview patient's family, and study the health record).
2. Sort, organize, and recognize deviations from the normal.
3. Validate the data with the patient.
4. Sort the clinical cues into related clusters.
5. Identify patterns in the data.
6. Relate the patterns to disease or need.

ANALYSIS

1. Examine the patterns to determine unmet needs as well as patient's strengths and health concerns.
2. Analyze all data for actual, potential, and collaborative problems.
3. Focus on actual or potential problems and needs.
4. Formulate diagnostic statement for identified needs.

OUTCOME IDENTIFICATION

1. Analyze needs and tasks for the critical or urgent nature of each.
2. Identify degree of threat to life or safety.
3. Rank priority of nursing diagnosis using Maslow's Hierarchy of Needs:
   - High priority: life-threatening issues that need immediate attention
   - Medium priority: problems that could result in unhealthy consequences such as physical or emotional impairment but that are not likely to threaten life
   - Low priority: problems that can be resolved easily with minimal intervention and that have little potential to cause significant dysfunction
4. Establish patient goals based on priorities identified.
5. Develop a list of patient outcomes based on NOC.

PLAN

1. Plan nursing interventions based on the identified priority nursing diagnosis.
2. Prioritize the interventions for each nursing diagnosis based on Rubenfeld and Scheffer's (1999) guidelines for setting priorities:
   A. Life-threatening problems always take precedence (i.e., issues that need immediate attention, such as changing or unstable status of the patient, preparation for test, and discharge from the facility that will occur shortly).
   B. Safety issues
   C. Patient's priorities (i.e., issues that are very important to the patient, including pain or anxiety)
   D. Nurse's priorities based on components of all patient's strengths and health concerns; moral and ethical issues; time, resources, and setting; and Maslow's Hierarchy of Needs
3. Write the nursing plan of care, selecting the nursing interventions most likely to relieve each problem.

IMPLEMENTATION

1. Perform tasks requiring immediate attention first.
2. Deal with high-priority problems that threaten life or safety first.
3. Intervene for medium-priority problems that are nonemergent or not life threatening next (i.e., problems that threaten health or coping ability).
4. Implement lowest-priority interventions, or deal with problems that do not directly relate to the specific illness or prognosis at this time (i.e., problems that have no major effect on the person if not attended to this day).
5. Identify problems not within the Scope of Nursing to treat and refer them to appropriate health care members.

EVALUATION

1. Continually evaluate and reevaluate problems after initial assessment to adjust ranking of problems.
2. Adjust plan of care based on current assessment of problems and needs.

*The steps of performance have been listed to show an appropriate sequence of completing the work; however, a different sequence of activities may be used during assessment.

 ## COMPETENCY VALIDATION: PRIORITY SETTING

COMPETENCY STATEMENT

To demonstrate the ability to rank order patient needs, nursing activities and manage resources based on importance and urgency.
The student demonstrated the ability to do the following:

1. List all tasks to be completed.
2. Identify degree of threat to life or safety.
3. Implement immediate actions necessary to prevent harm.
4. Implement actions that involved problems that could result in unhealthy consequences such as physical or emotional impairment, but are not likely to threaten life.
5. Implement actions that were of lowest priority, addressing problems that can be resolved easily with minimal interventions and have little potential to cause significant dysfunction.
6. Evaluate current data after initial assessment to adjust ranking of problems and plan of care as needed.

COMPETENT

- Understands reason for task and is able to perform task independently
- Understands reason for task but needs supervision
- Understands reason for task and is able to perform with assistance

NOT COMPETENT

- Understands reason for task but performs task at provisional level
- Is unable to state reason for task and performs task at a dependent level

SKILL CHECKLIST: PRIORITY SETTING

PRIORITIZING PROBLEMS	SATISFACTORY	UNSATISFACTORY	NI/COMMENTS
ASSESSMENT			
1. Collect data from available resources.			
2. Sort data into clusters.			
3. Validate the data with the patient.			
4. Identify patterns related to disease or need.			
ANALYSIS			
1. List unmet needs based on patterns.			
2. Identify nursing diagnosis based on problems or needs.			
3. List criteria that validate nursing diagnosis.			
OUTCOME IDENTIFICATION			
1. Analyze needs and tasks for their critical nature.			
2. Identify the priority based on Maslow's Hierarchy of Needs and nursing diagnosis based on NANDA.			
3. Establish patient goals based on priorities identified.			
4. Develop a list of patient outcomes based on NOC.			
PLAN			
1. Outline nursing interventions.			
2. List nursing interventions in order of priority based on Rubenfeld and Scheffer's (1999) guidelines.			
IMPLEMENTATION			
1. Implement immediate actions necessary to prevent harm first.			
2. Implement actions for problems that result in unhealthy consequences or physical or emotional impairment next.			
3. Implement lowest-priority actions, or deal with problems that do not directly relate to the specific illness or prognosis at that time, last.			
4. Use stated goals as a framework to deliver nursing care.			
5. Document nursing interventions and patient's response as appropriate.			
EVALUATION			
1. Reevaluate problems and needs as situation or patient status changes.			
2. Adjust plan of care as indicated.			

SCENARIO TO ACCOMPANY STUDENT WORKSHEETS

Grace Gelding, 73 years of age, was transferred to your nursing unit from the coronary care unit (CCU). Her medical diagnosis is heart failure of new onset, and the chart indicates that she is a full code.

Current orders include:

1. Digoxin, 0.125 mg orally per day
2. Furosemide, 40 mg orally per day
3. Serum electrolytes each morning
4. Oxygen, 2L per nasal cannula
5. Up in chair
6. Diet: soft; no added salt (NAS)

Physical assessment reveals skin cool, 1+ pitting edema in lower extremities. Lung sounds reveal fine crackles in bases bilaterally and an occasional dry, nonproductive cough. Her mentation is alert and oriented, and she complains about feeling tired easily. Vitals are as follows: temperature, 97.2°F (36.2°C); pulse, 74 beats/min; respirations, 24 breaths/min at rest; blood pressure, 142/78 mm Hg.

Discharge is scheduled as soon as assistance can be arranged in the home. She lives with a 55-year-old son who is developmentally disabled. Medications will include digoxin and furosemide, which are new prescriptions.

DATA CLUSTER	DATA CLUSTER
Patient is 73 years old, lives with 55-year-old developmentally disabled son	1+ pitting edema in lower extremities
Recent diagnosis of heart failure	Fine crackles in bases bilaterally
Anticipated need for digitalis preparation and ongoing diuretic therapy	Occasional dry, nonproductive cough
	Alert and oriented
	Respirations 24 breaths/min at rest

1. List the priority nursing diagnoses (review NANDA list and place in order of priority).

_____

_____

_____

_____

2. Identify interventions in order of priority to assess at the beginning of your shift.

_____

_____

_____

_____

See the Answer Key in Appendix A for sample answers for this exercise.

Practice Exercises: Priority Setting

SETTING PRIORITIES OF NURSING DIAGNOSES

Use Maslow's Hierarchy of Needs to identify the level of needs of the nursing diagnoses in column 1, and place the corresponding number in the blank space beside column 2.

1. Physiologic
2. Safety and security
3. Love and belonging
4. Self-esteem
5. Self-actualization

Column 1	Column 2
Activity intolerance	_____
Imbalanced nutrition: Less than body requirements	_____
Anxiety	_____
Social isolation	_____
Ineffective role performance	_____
Ineffective airway clearance	_____
Chronic confusion	_____
Impaired tissue integrity	_____
Constipation	_____
Acute pain	_____
Disturbed sleep pattern	_____
Deficient fluid volume	_____

See the Answer Key in Appendix A for answers to this exercise.

 ## SCENARIO: IDENTIFYING PRIORITY NURSING DIAGNOSES

Greg Smith, 35 years of age, was transferred to a medical unit for gastric evaluation after being in the intensive coronary care unit (ICCU), and a myocardial infarction has been ruled out. His condition appeared stable when suddenly he developed acute pain and bleeding. A diagnostic esophagogastroduodenoscopy (EGD) revealed gastric ulceration. He underwent emergency surgery. This is Greg's first hospital admission; he is divorced, with no family support system. Greg's boss has been making inquiries about his progress and is pressing the staff to tell him when Greg will be able to return to work. Greg has now returned to your unit after surgery, and you are developing his care plan.

You have developed the nursing diagnosis list in column 1. Identify the need addressed in column 2. For the purpose of this exercise, use Maslow's Hierarchy of Needs to set priorities:

1. Physiologic
2. Safety and security
3. Love and belonging
4. Self-esteem
5. Self-actualization

Column 1	Column 2
Situational low self-esteem related to fear of prolonged disability and threat to job	_____
Ineffective breathing pattern related to effects of anesthesia and history of smoking	_____
High risk for ineffective coping related to effects of acute illness, lack of support system	_____
High risk for infection related to hazards of invasive lines and contamination of peritoneum with gastric juices	_____
Acute pain related to surgical incision and irritation of gastric juice during bleed	_____

See the Answer Key in Appendix A for answers to this exercise.

SCENARIOS: PRIORITIZING NURSING ACTIVITIES

SCENARIO 1

You are making rounds after receiving the change-of-shift report. Allan Moore, 87 years of age, was admitted for pneumonia. Vitals were reported as follows: temperature, 99.8° F (37.7°C); pulse, 96 beats/min; respirations, 28 breaths/min; blood pressure, 150/90 mm Hg. The patient continues to be restless, complains of dyspnea, and is anxious. The oxygen saturation was 87% after he pulled his oxygen cannula off.

1. List the five top-priority nursing activities at this time.

> oxygen cannula.
> head of bed ↑
> calm him down. encourage to deep breath and cough.
> auscultate chest - listen for adventitious sounds. + liquid
> assess pulse quality
> check for edema.

SCENARIO 2

You continue your morning assessments when the patient in the next room complains of pain, rating it as 9 on a 1 to 10 scale. After you obtain an order for morphine, 2 to 4 mg intravenously as needed for severe pain, you enter the room and observe that the patient has pulled out the central line catheter.

1. What is your initial action at this time and why?

_____

_____

_____

_____

_____

Scenario 3

After morning break, the unit secretary informs you that a new admission from the emergency department (ED) is on the way to the nursing floor. A 50-year-old diabetic patient was admitted with a blood sugar level of 388. The ED nurse reported that insulin was given, but the chart does not include the time or dose given. Your initial assessment reveals the following: temperature, 99.8°F (37.7°C); pulse, 88 beats/min regular; respirations, 22 breaths/min; and blood pressure, 148/78 mm Hg. He is alert to person only, which the daughter states is unusual for him. His skin is warm and dry, and he is requesting a drink. His face is flushed, and he is moving around in bed continuously and pulling at the covers. He verbalizes an inability to eat this morning.

Orders include:

18 U Humulin Regular/38 U Novolin, intermediate-acting insulin (NPH), to be given subcutaneously (SC) every morning before breakfast
Rocephin, 1 gram intravenous piggyback (IVPB) every 24 hours
Ativan, 1 mg intramuscularly (IM) every 8 hours as needed (PRN)
Dressing change on foot ulcerations PRN
Culture and sensitivity tests on open wounds in right foot
Insulin to sliding scale per protocol

1. What is your first priority?

_____

_____

_____

_____

_____

Scenario 4

Sandra Walker, 68 years of age, was admitted for persistent abdominal pain and nausea during the past several weeks. Her history revealed that she stopped using sugar in her coffee to lose weight, with a resultant weight loss of 30 pounds during the past 4 months. Diagnostic testing reveals a colon lesion thought to be malignant, and the patient is scheduled for a colon resection in the morning. Sandra is very anxious after discussing the plan of care and refuses to sign a surgical consent form. Sandra tells the nurse that she is having severe abdominal pain and demands "a pain shot right now." The nurse notes that about 3 hours have passed since her last pain shot.

All of these nursing diagnoses are appropriate to this patient; which one is the priority at this time?

Deficient knowledge related to procedure
Anxiety related to procedure
— Acute pain related to the disease process
Risk for imbalanced nutrition related to disease

Based on this decision, select the priority nursing activity at this time.

— Administer intramuscular (IM) pain medication
Sit and talk with patient
Call the physician
Offer to call a family member

Scenario 5

Mary Jones is a 48-year-old insulin-dependent diabetic patient. She was admitted to the hospital for circulatory impairment to the lower extremity and an open draining wound on the right foot. The patient manages her own blood glucose monitor and insulin injections at home. Her orders include blood glucose monitoring before meals and at bedtime. Monitoring glucose and insulin are to be done by the morning nurse. All of the following need to be completed. In what order would you perform them?

_____ Complete assessment

_____ Teach patient about complications of diabetes and circulation

_____ Perform morning care and grooming

_____ Administer morning insulin injection

_____ Take vital signs

_____ Perform finger stick for blood glucose monitoring

_____ Assist with breakfast tray

Scenario 6

Randy Wheeler, 52 years old, was admitted with a diagnosis of cirrhosis related to chronic alcoholism. He is complaining of his abdomen being tight and distended, which is due to ascites. He also complains of shortness of breath and restlessness this morning. His morning vitals were as follows: temperature, 99.2°F (37.3°C); pulse, 102 beats/min; respirations, 36 breaths/min; and blood pressure, 138/96 mm Hg. The vital signs were consistent with previously recorded vitals. When the physician made rounds, he informed you that he would be back in 30 minutes to perform an abdominal paracentesis.

Which nursing activity is the priority? Identify in order of priority as numbers 1 through 5, with number 1 being top priority.

_____ Make sure the paracentesis equipment is available.

_____ Perform a body system assessment

_____ Ensure that the patient voids to empty the bladder.

_____ Take vital signs.

_____ Get patient signature on informed consent.

See the Answer Key in Appendix A for answers to this exercise.

TIME MANAGEMENT

Evaluating Use of Time

Review the following Daily Time Log. Under the comments, note what you would do differently to be more efficient and to provide better care. (Not every entry needs a comment.)

TIME	ACTIVITIES	EVALUATION OF TIME USE
7:00–7:30	Received shift report; checked medication administration record (MAR); delegated vitals for stable patients	
7:30–8:00	Shared "horror stories of yesterday" with nurse who had day off; checked labs	
8:00–8:30	Assessed patients, served meal trays, helped nursing assistant (NA), cleaned up spills on carpet	
8:30–9:00	Evaluated Mrs. Green's shortness of breath; finished picking up trays; started treatments	
9:00–9:30	Started medications pass; took two phone calls from patient's families	
9:30–10:00	Rechecked Mrs. Green; break, 9:30–9:45; finished treatments; finished 9:00 AM medications	
10:00–10:30	Documented treatments; documented Mrs. Green's shortness of breath episode	
10:30–11:00	Made rounds; took pharmacy calls and called lab	
11:00–11:30	Postponed NA's performance appraisal; evaluated Mrs. Green's chest pain; called doctor	
11:30–12:00	Lunch break	
12:00–12:30	Prepared lunch trays; assisted with distribution and feeding	
12:30–1:00	Delegated noon vitals to NA; doctor to see Mrs. Green; transcribed new orders	
1:00–1:30	Began afternoon treatments	
1:30–2:00	Started 1:00 PM medications; completed NA performance appraisal; interrupted twice for phone calls	
2:00–2:30	Made rounds on patients; transcribed orders—did not finish	
2:30–3:00	Completed afternoon charting	
3:00–3:30	Reported off to evening shift; 10 minutes late for report	

Adapted from Ringsven, M. K., & Bond, D. (1991). *Gerontology and leadership skills for nurses.* Boston: Delmar. Copyright 1997. Reprinted with permission of Delmar Learning, a division of Thomson Learning: www.thomsonrights.com (fax, 800–730–2215).

See the Answer Key in Appendix A for sample answers for this exercise.

SCENARIO: EVALUATING USE OF TIME

Patricia Minor, 62 years of age, was admitted to the nursing unit from surgery yesterday, after having a laparoscopic cholecystectomy. Patricia's history includes chronic atrial fibrillation, urinary incontinence, and diabetes mellitus. During the night, she pulled her urinary catheter and intravenous needle out. The night shift restarted the intravenous line and left the Foley catheter out. The patient complains of being sore in the rectum and is very upset at the night nurse because "she was mean to me." After she stops crying and settles down, she states that she has pain in the calf of her left leg. During assessment, the nurse notes that the area is warm, red, and tender to touch.

The nurse assesses the vital signs, oxygen saturation, level of pain, peripheral vascular status, and Homans' sign.

Determine the priority after performing the assessment.

Use the Daily Time Log provided to plan your nursing activities in order of priority. Doctor's orders include:

Baseline partial thromboplastin time (PTT), International Normalized Ratio (INR), platelet count, hemoglobin, and hematocrit

Repeat PTT per heparin protocol (every 6 hours at first)

Chest radiograph to rule out pulmonary emboli

Intravenous heparin per hospital protocol

Elevate and apply heat to affected extremity

After completing the log, share your plan with another student and offer comments on changes that could have made the day go better.

Daily Time Log

Use this form to plan your day with Patricia.

TIME	ACTIVITIES	EVALUATION OF TIME USE
7:00–7:30		
7:30–8:00		
8:00–8:30		
8:30–9:00		
9:00–9:30		
9:30–10:00		
10:00–10:30		
10:30–11:00		
11:00–11:30		
11:30–12:00		
12:00–12:30		
12:30–1:00		
1:00–1:30		
1:30–2:00		
2:00–2:30		
2:30–3:00		
3:00–3:30		

Adapted from Ringsven, M. K., & Bond, D. (1991). *Gerontology and leadership skills for nurses*. Boston: Delmar. Copyright 1997. Reprinted with permission of Delmar Learning, a division of Thomson Learning: www.thomsonrights.com (fax, 800–730–2215).

See the Answer Key in Appendix A for sample answers for this exercise.

Clinical Daily Time Log

Use this log to organize your clinical day. At the end of the day, evaluate how you could have organized better.

TIME	ACTIVITIES	EVALUATION OF TIME USE
7:00–7:30		
7:30–8:00		
8:00–8:30		
8:30–9:00		
9:00–9:30		
9:30–10:00		
10:00–10:30		
10:30–11:00		
11:00–11:30		
11:30–12:00		
12:00–12:30		
12:30–1:00		
1:00–1:30		
1:30–2:00		
2:00–2:30		
2:30–3:00		
3:00–3:30		

Adapted from Ringsven, M. K., & Bond, D. (1991). *Gerontology and leadership skills for nurses*. Boston: Delmar. Copyright 1997. Reprinted with permission of Delmar Learning, a division of Thomson Learning: www.thomsonrights.com (fax, 800–730–2215).

Answers will vary with student experience.

UNIT TWO

COGNITIVE SKILLS IN THE NURSING PROCESS

CHAPTER 5

NURSING PROCESS Applications

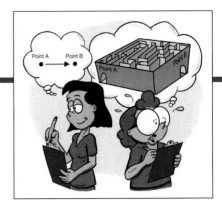

OBJECTIVES

1. Define the role of the nursing process as it pertains to nursing practice.

2. Describe how critical thinking, decision making, and priority setting relate to the nursing process.

3. Discuss how the American Nurses Association (ANA) Standards of Practice influence patient care decisions.

4. Describe the steps in the nursing process and how they influence nursing care.

5. Describe how the North American Nursing Diagnosis Association (NANDA), Nursing Interventions Classification (NIC), and Nursing Outcomes Classification (NOC) terms are used in the nursing process to direct the care of patients.

6. List possible pitfalls in the application of the nursing process.

The nursing process is a problem-solving method that is unique to nursing. It is an organized plan that facilitates the use of sound judgment in care delivery. According to Alfaro-LeFevre (1999, p. 64), "The nursing process is the framework for providing professional, quality nursing care." This chapter explains the basic principles of this framework and how they relate to the American Nurses Association (ANA) Standards of Practice (Box 5-1). These standards illustrate the application of the concepts discussed in previous chapters. For example, the use of critical thinking skills is essential to the assessment phase of the nursing process. Priority setting occurs throughout all the steps of the nursing process, and the formulation of interventions in the plan of care is a key step in the decision-making process.

DEFINITION

"Nursing process is considered to be a specialized form of systematic inquiry or problem solving process used in drawing conclusions about the patient's problems and the corresponding nursing actions to resolve problems." (Saucier, Stevens, & Williams, 2002, p. 246). The major steps of the nursing process are assessment, analysis, outcome identification, planning, implementation, and evaluation. The aim of the process is the performance of actions that maintain and promote health and resolve or prevent patient problems. A schematic drawing of the nursing process can be seen in Figure 5-1.

Box 5-1 AMERICAN NURSES ASSOCIATION STANDARDS OF NURSING PRACTICE

STANDARD 1. ASSESSMENT

The nurse collects comprehensive data pertinent to the patient's health or the situation.

1. Collects data and identifies patterns in a systematic and ongoing process
2. Involves the patient, family, other health care providers, and environment, as appropriate, in holistic data collection
3. Determines the priority of data collection activities by the patient's immediate condition, or anticipated needs of the patient or situation
4. Uses appropriate evidence-based assessment techniques and instruments in collecting pertinent data
5. Uses analytical models and problem-solving tools
6. Documents relevant data in a retrievable format

STANDARD 2. DIAGNOSIS

The nurse analyzes the assessment data to determine the diagnosis or issues.

1. Derives the diagnoses or issues based on assessment data
2. Validates the diagnoses or issues with the patient, family, and other health care providers when possible and appropriate
3. Documents diagnoses or issues in a manner that facilitates the determination of the expected outcomes and plan

STANDARD 3. OUTCOMES IDENTIFICATION

The nurse identifies expected outcomes for a plan individualized to the patient or the situation.

1. Involves the patient, family, and other health care providers in formulating mutually expected outcomes when possible and appropriate
2. Derives expected outcomes from the diagnoses that are culturally appropriate
3. Identifies expected outcomes with consideration of associated risks, benefits, costs, and current scientific and clinical practice knowledge
4. Defines expected outcomes in terms of the patient, environment, or situation
5. Includes a time estimate for attainment of expected outcomes
6. Develops expected outcomes that provide direction for continuity of care
7. Modifies expected outcomes based on changes in the status of the patient or evaluation of the situation
8. Documents expected outcomes as measurable goals

STANDARD 4. PLANNING

The nurse develops a plan that prescribes strategies and alternatives to attain expected outcomes.

1. Develops an individualized plan considering patient characteristics or the situation
2. Develops the plan in conjunction with the patient, family, and others
3. Includes strategies within the plan that address each of the identified diagnoses or issues, which may include strategies for promotion and restoration of health and prevention of illness, injury, and disease
4. Provides for continuity within the plan
5. Incorporates an implementation pathway or timeline within the plan

6. Establishes the plan priorities with the patient, family, and others, as appropriate
7. Uses the plan to provide direction to other members of the health care team
8. Defines the plan to reflect current statutes, rules and regulations, standards, trends, and research affecting care
9. Considers the economic impact of the plan
10. Uses standardized language or recognized terminology to document the plan

STANDARD 5. IMPLEMENTATION

The nurse implements the identified plan.

1. Implements the plan in a safe, timely, and appropriate manner
2. Documents implementation and any modifications, including changes or omissions, from the identified plan
3. Uses evidence-based interventions and treatments unique to patient need
4. Uses community resources and systems to implement the plan
5. Collaborates with nursing colleagues and others to implement the plan

STANDARD 5A: COORDINATION OF CARE

The nurse coordinates care delivery.

STANDARD 5B: HEALTH TEACHING AND HEALTH PROMOTION

The nurse employs strategies to promote health and a safe environment.

STANDARD 5C: CONSULTATION

The advanced practice registered nurse and the nursing role specialist provide consultation to influence the identified plan, enhance the abilities of others, and effect change.

STANDARD 5D: PRESCRIPTIVE AUTHORITY AND TREATMENT

The advanced practice registered nurse uses prescriptive authority, procedures, referrals, and treatments in accordance with state and federal laws and regulations.

STANDARD 6. EVALUATION

The nurse evaluates progress toward attainment of outcomes.

1. Conducts a systematic, ongoing, and criterion-based evaluation
2. Systematically evaluates outcomes in relation to the structures and processes prescribed by the plan
3. Includes the patient and others involved in the care or situation in the evaluative process
4. Uses ongoing assessment data to revise the diagnoses, outcomes, and the plan, as needed
5. Evaluates the effectiveness of the planned strategies in relation to patient responses and the attainment of the expected outcomes.
6. Documents and disseminates, as appropriate, the results of the evaluation, including any need for administrative action.

Adapted from American Nurses Association. (2003). *Nursing: Scope and standards of practice.* Washington, DC: Nursesbooks.org. Reproduced with the permission of the American Nurses Association.

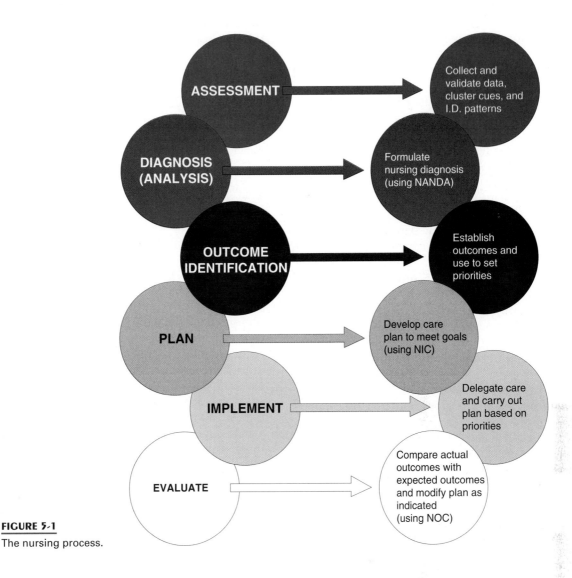

FIGURE 5-1
The nursing process.

ROLE OF THE NURSING PROCESS

The nursing process is integral to nursing practice and nursing language. To be considered a profession, an occupation must possess a unique language and universal processes. For years, nursing functioned under the medical model, leading to a lack of autonomy in the nursing profession. In the past, nurses were considered subservient to physicians. Since then, real strides have been made in the development of nursing as a profession. The movement toward a universal language in nursing supports this growth. The consistent use of standards and standardized language provides a measurable way to quantify the effect of nursing interventions and nursing activities. Future use of this system can facilitate a change in staffing ratios, improve the quality of patient care, improve reimbursement for nursing care, and change health care policies.

The language of a profession should be universal to all its practitioners. The use of a "localized" nursing language is not measurable. Therefore, the ANA recognizes the terms developed by North American Nursing Diagnosis Association (NANDA), Nursing Interventions Classification (NIC), and Nursing Outcomes Classification (NOC) as a universal language for nurses.

NANDA is a professional association that continually prepares a list of accepted nursing diagnoses. The association was formed in 1973. By 1982, a list of 50 accepted nursing diagnoses was selected for use. This list is updated every other year. "NANDA terminology has been translated into nine languages and is used in more than 20 countries throughout the world" (Johnson, Bulechek, McCloskey, Maas, & Moorhead, 2001, p. 4). By using this language, nurses can clearly communicate clinical judgments to other health care professionals.

NIC is a standardized classification of nursing interventions. Each intervention contains a list of possible nursing activities. NIC interventions have been linked with the nursing diagnoses classification system and are frequently used in documentation systems.

NOC is a system for evaluating nursing practice. It presents a method for measuring the patient's progression toward a specific outcome. NOC uses a Likert-type scale to quantify the status of the patient and evaluate the effectiveness of the interventions. When using Likert scales, a person is asked to rate an item according to a given scale. These scales are frequently used as evaluation tools. For example, a participant might be asked to circle one of the following responses to a question: 1. Strongly disagree, 2. Somewhat disagree, 3. Somewhat agree, or 4. Strongly agree. A typical question might be: "I feel my orientation to the clinical setting was adequate." A sample NOC outcome measurement for pain control behavior might be written as follows: "Reports pain controlled." The evaluation scale would be the following options: 1. Never, 2. Rarely, 3. Sometimes, 4. Often, 5. Consistently demonstrated. The NOC evaluation measures enhance the knowledge base of nursing, promote interdisciplinary communication and participation in care, and provide a means for measuring the effectiveness of new techniques.

NIC and NOC promote the standardization of interventions and evaluation. The interventions in NIC are based on research involving current best practices. This is referred to as *evidence-based practice*. Health care delivery decisions should be based on evidence instead of merely tradition and habits. The use of NANDA, NIC, and NOC classifications in the nursing process for assessments, care plans, and daily charting of care leads to standardization and evidence-based practice.

STEPS OF THE NURSING PROCESS

ASSESSMENT

Assessment is the first step of the nursing process. In the ANA Standard of Practice I, it is stated that: "The nurse collects comprehensive data pertinent to the patient's health or the situation." (see Box 5-1.) This collection of significant, relevant data in an organized manner provides a clearer picture of the patient. It provides necessary baseline information and data regarding current patient status. Data can be organized in different ways. A common method is to place the data into subjective and objective categories. Observable data (objec-

tive data) or the signs manifested by the illness that can be observed or measured are placed together. For example, the patient's temperature, diagnostic lab results, or an emesis are objective data. Subjective symptoms are based on the perceptions of the patient. For example, complaints of pain or anxiety are subjective data. The following steps provide a detailed description of the important components of assessment.

1. COLLECT DATA FROM ALL AVAILABLE SOURCES

The initial assessment of the patient's physical status, psychological state, self-care abilities, learning needs, spiritual needs, and discharge-planning needs facilitates the development and accuracy of nursing diagnoses, priorities, expected outcomes, and nursing interventions. Sources of data collection should include the patient, family, other health care providers, and medical records. Poor assessment techniques can result in failure to treat the immediate problems or failure to direct care toward the patient's priority needs. The nurse should use appropriate evidence-based assessment techniques and instruments in collecting data.

Although thorough assessments are important, there are emergency situations in which the nurse must act, based on a partial assessment. In life-threatening cases, quick action is required for patient safety. The nurse may need to proceed to the intervention step following a mini-assessment. As soon as the patient's condition permits, the nurse should finish the assessment.

2. IDENTIFY PERTINENT DATA

A thorough assessment will result in the collection of both important data and data that are not pertinent to the needs of the patient. For instance, during assessment, the nurse may note the presence of a scar in the right lower quadrant of the abdomen. The scar is the result of surgery for an appendectomy in childhood. However, because the previous surgery has no bearing on the current admission, the nurse must focus on data more relevant to current needs.

After all significant data have been gathered, they should be examined for inconsistencies or knowledge gaps.

3. RECOGNIZE DEVIATIONS FROM NORMAL

The signs and symptoms should be sorted into normal data and data that deviate from normal standards. To recognize abnormalities, the nurse must possess adequate background knowledge in disease processes and normal anatomy and physiology.

The nurse should also note diagnostic test results and risk factors, such as a patient's smoking habit.

4. VALIDATE THE DATA WITH THE PATIENT

The nurse should validate the data for accuracy and recognize any assumptions. For instance, if the patient is pacing, the nurse may assume that he or she is upset. This should be clarified with the patient by asking, "I notice you are pacing. Is there something you would like to talk about?" In this way, the nurse does not make inferences from preconceived notions, but rather verifies the meaning of data to this particular patient.

5. SORT AND ORGANIZE DATA IN A LOGICAL SEQUENCE

It is easier to interpret the meaning of data if related concepts are arranged together. This enables the nurse to visualize the total picture and make inferences regarding the meaning of assessment data. To accomplish this organization, the nurse takes data (cues) and places them in clusters.

Data that help the nurse form an initial impression are called *cues*. A cue can also be defined as "a signal that indicates a possible need/direction for care" (Doenges, Moorhouse, & Burley, 2000, p.42). Cues may also be called *defining characteristics*. The following example demonstrates the identification of cues.

A 29-year-old man is 2 days postoperative laminectomy for a herniated disk. He is alert and oriented to person, place, and time. His pupils are equally responsive and react to light. Motor and cognitive functions are within normal limits (WNL). There are no involuntary tremors. His vital signs are as follows: blood pressure, 126/72 mm Hg; temperature, 98.4°F (36.9°C); pulse, 76 beats/min; and respirations, 18 breaths/min. The patient has a steady gait as he ambulates with the use of a back brace. One hour after returning from a walk, the unlicensed assistive personnel (UAP) informs the nurse that the patient is restless, moaning, and crying. As the nurse enters the room, the patient is lying in bed guarding and protecting the incision. He has a facial grimace. Cues include:

Had surgery 2 days ago
Guarding and protective behavior of injured body part
Restless, moaning, and crying
Facial grimacing

The nurse then organizes cues into clusters of related information. In the example above, the cues related to pain or discomfort have been clustered together. A cluster could also be formed regarding neurologic cues:

Alert and oriented to the three spheres
Pupils are equally responsive and react to light
Motor function is WNL
No involuntary tremors.

Clusters organize information in a systematic manner and facilitate the formation of nursing diagnoses. There are several different frameworks for clustering data. The cluster framework developed by Doenges and Moorhouse (2000) is used in this chapter. This framework is outlined in Box 5-2. Other available frameworks for clustering data are Gordon's functional health problems and the NANDA human response patterns (Gordon, 1995; Guzetta, Bunton, Prindey, Sherer, & Seifert, 1989). Students should consult the framework preferred by their school of nursing.

After data are clustered, it is again important to determine relevancy and to discount the value of irrelevant data. The nurse should review the cluster for inconsistencies or missing data. If gaps in knowledge are discovered, further assessment is essential.

6. IDENTIFY PATTERNS IN THE DATA

Pattern identification involves the application of prior knowledge and experience in solving problems that are similar, but not identical. This process allows nurses to categorize problems and needs even though individuality exists among patients. Pattern identification assists in the development of nursing diagnoses.

A good example of pattern identification is demonstrated by examining the use of common doorknobs. Some doorknobs are round, whereas others have levers or handles. When confronted

---

Box 5-2 CLUSTERS BY DIAGNOSTIC DIVISIONS

Activity/Rest
Circulation
Ego Integrity
Elimination
Food/Fluid
Hygiene
Neurosensory
Pain/Discomfort
Respiration
Safety
Sexuality
Social Interaction
Teaching/Learning

Adapted from Doenges, M. E., Moorhouse, M. F., & Burley, J. T. (2000). *Application of nursing process and nursing diagnosis: An interactive text for diagnostic reasoning* (p. 29). Philadelphia: F.A. Davis.

with an unfamiliar doorknob, a problem solver can usually open the door. By recognizing similarities from prior exposure, the individual applies previously learned information to open the door.

Nurses proceed through a similar process in assessing patients. The clustered data lead to an identifiable pattern. Recognizing the cues (symptoms) of a disease process is based on the nurse's knowledge of diseases. Individual patients respond to disease processes by displaying various symptoms in a characteristic way. The nurse is able to recognize the disease or illness, although it can present differently in various people. This goal is accomplished by the use of pattern recognition.

Analysis (Diagnosis)

In the second step of the nursing process, the nurse analyzes data obtained in the assessment step and formulates nursing diagnoses. This step is described in the second ANA Standard of Practice. A nursing diagnosis differs from a medical diagnosis. Nursing diagnoses focus on patient needs and problems. A medical diagnosis is based on the disease process. A distinguishing characteristic of the language of nursing is that nursing diagnoses focus on patient needs and problems. Nursing diagnoses are patient problems that can be addressed by nursing, and therefore, the language used in nursing diagnoses avoids medical terminology.

Suggestions for completing the analysis step are described in the five sections that follow.

1. EXAMINE THE CLUSTERS TO DETERMINE UNMET NEEDS AND THE PATIENT'S STRENGTHS AND HEALTH CONCERNS

The assessment findings should result in the identification of the patient's problems and needs. A sound judgment about the needs of the patient results from the analysis of the data and resulting clusters. Whenever possible, these problems should be validated with the patient and family or significant others during the assessment phase. This information will be used to formulate nursing diagnoses.

2. FOCUS ON PROBLEMS FOR WHICH THE NURSE CAN FACILITATE CHANGE

It may not be possible for the nurse to solve all the patient's problems. For example, the nurse cannot cure the terminally ill patient. However, the nurse can focus on important patient needs, such as pain control. Knowing the principles of effective problem solving is essential to patient care.

3. DEVELOP NURSING DIAGNOSES BASED ON FACTS AND SUPPORTING DATA (CONSULT NANDA)

The nurse should select appropriate nursing diagnoses based on identified cues and clusters. To be effective, nursing diagnoses must be consistent with NANDA nomenclature. Use of NANDA to describe patient problems is essential to promote continuity of care. The focus of nursing activities may vary in different settings (such as pediatrics, obstetrics, long-term care, and home care nursing to name a few), but a nursing diagnosis means the same across all settings.

Correctly composing a nursing diagnosis statement does require practice. The diagnostic statement for an actual problem that already exists includes three parts:

1. The problem (actual or potential)
2. The contributing factors (related to [R/T] factors)
3. The signs and symptoms (as evidenced by [AEB])

The problem portion must be worded with NANDA nomenclature. An example of a correctly worded problem would be: *disturbed thought processes*. A list of available nursing diagnoses can be found in Appendix B at the end of this book.

The contributing factors are often called the *etiology* of the problem. This portion of the statement describes the cause of the problem or things that contributed to the problem. The etiology should not be a medical diagnosis. The contributing factors are preceded by the words "related to." For example, a correctly worded etiology is: Risk for injury related to lack of awareness of hazards secondary to cognitive impairment.

The signs and symptoms that support the choice of this nursing diagnosis are preceded by the words "as evidenced by."

The form for a correctly written nursing diagnosis is:

The problem R/T the contributing factors AEB the signs and symptoms.

Examples include:

Acute pain R/T tissue trauma and dissection of muscles secondary to surgical incision AEB complaints of abdominal pain rated at 8 per patient

Ineffective airway clearance R/T tracheobronchial secretions AEB abnormal breath sounds (crackles and rales) and labored breathing

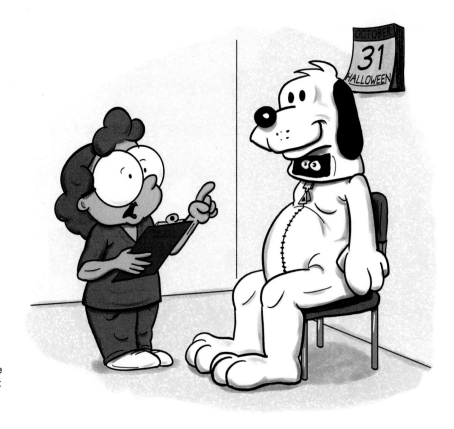

"The diagnosis? Obviously, you're a large canine who has had recent open heart surgery. We should really wait for the vet, however."

Nursing diagnoses are used to describe both actual and potential health problems. Potential problems involve needs that, left unmet, can result in actual health problems. These problems, called *risk diagnoses,* do not include an AEB because the problem has not occurred yet. For example, for the diagnosis of Risk for infection R/T compromised immune system secondary to chemotherapy, the nursing interventions will focus on prevention.

There are five types of nursing diagnoses: actual, risk, possible, wellness, and collaborative. This discussion, however, is limited to actual and risk diagnoses because these are the most common.

4. VALIDATE THE NURSING DIAGNOSES

After nursing diagnoses are selected, the nurse should consult with the patient and family regarding the appropriateness of the selections. The patient may wish to add diagnoses to the list or delete diagnoses that the patient does not consider important. If indicated, other health care workers and third-party payers may also be consulted.

5. ESTABLISH PRIORITIES OF NURSING DIAGNOSES

Nursing diagnoses are listed in order of priority. Frequently, Maslow's Hierarchy of Needs is used to establish priority (see Chapter 4, Figure 4-1). Multiple problems fall into the physiologic category based on Maslow. Figure 5-2 organizes nursing diagnoses for physiologic needs into Doenges' Diagnostic-Related Groups to assist the novice nurse in selecting priorities. This concept is covered more thoroughly in Chapter 4, Priority Setting.

Outcome Identification

In the third step of the nursing process, the nurse identifies expected outcomes, which give direction in planning care. Outcomes also provide the evaluative measurement at the end of the process. Suggestions for selecting outcomes follow.

1. ESTABLISH PATIENT OUTCOMES THAT ARE REALISTIC, ACHIEVABLE, AND MEASURABLE USING NURSING OUTCOMES CLASSIFICATION

Goals and outcomes, based on recognized patient needs, should be determined. These are necessary to give direction and, later, to guide the evaluation of nursing care effectiveness. Although the terms are used interchangeably, goals and outcomes are not identical. *Goals* are broad descriptions of the

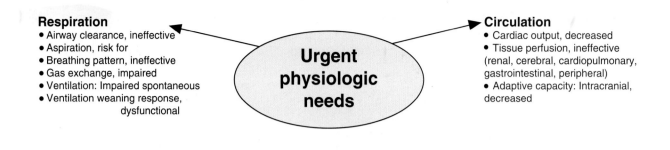

Respiration
- Airway clearance, ineffective
- Aspiration, risk for
- Breathing pattern, ineffective
- Gas exchange, impaired
- Ventilation: Impaired spontaneous
- Ventilation weaning response, dysfunctional

Urgent physiologic needs

Circulation
- Cardiac output, decreased
- Tissue perfusion, ineffective (renal, cerebral, cardiopulmonary, gastrointestinal, peripheral)
- Adaptive capacity: Intracranial, decreased

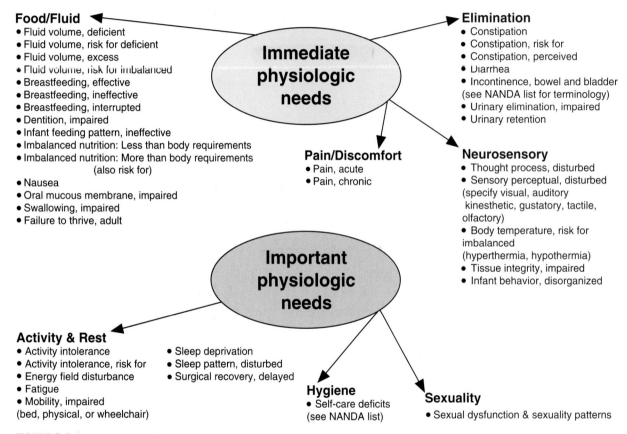

Food/Fluid
- Fluid volume, deficient
- Fluid volume, risk for deficient
- Fluid volume, excess
- Fluid volume, risk for imbalanced
- Breastfeeding, effective
- Breastfeeding, ineffective
- Breastfeeding, interrupted
- Dentition, impaired
- Infant feeding pattern, ineffective
- Imbalanced nutrition: Less than body requirements
- Imbalanced nutrition: More than body requirements (also risk for)
- Nausea
- Oral mucous membrane, impaired
- Swallowing, impaired
- Failure to thrive, adult

Immediate physiologic needs

Elimination
- Constipation
- Constipation, risk for
- Constipation, perceived
- Diarrhea
- Incontinence, bowel and bladder (see NANDA list for terminology)
- Urinary elimination, impaired
- Urinary retention

Pain/Discomfort
- Pain, acute
- Pain, chronic

Neurosensory
- Thought process, disturbed
- Sensory perceptual, disturbed (specify visual, auditory kinesthetic, gustatory, tactile, olfactory)
- Body temperature, risk for imbalanced (hyperthermia, hypothermia)
- Tissue integrity, impaired
- Infant behavior, disorganized

Important physiologic needs

Activity & Rest
- Activity intolerance
- Activity intolerance, risk for
- Energy field disturbance
- Fatigue
- Mobility, impaired (bed, physical, or wheelchair)
- Sleep deprivation
- Sleep pattern, disturbed
- Surgical recovery, delayed

Hygiene
- Self-care deficits (see NANDA list)

Sexuality
- Sexual dysfunction & sexuality patterns

FIGURE 5-2

Priority setting: Physiologic needs using diagnostic divisions. Adapted from Doenges, M. E., Moorhouse, M. F., & Burley, J. T. (2000). *Application of nursing process and nursing diagnosis: An interactive text for diagnostic reasoning.* Philadelphia: FA Davis.

desired final result. Goals tend to be stated in more general terms. For instance, a patient goal might be to "maintain compliance with the medication regime."

Outcomes are the steps in achieving a goal. Frequently, a goal will have more than one outcome. In the earlier goal example, an outcome might be "By next Tuesday, the patient will describe all the steps in refilling a prescription" or "The patient will list the appropriate times for self-administration of medications with 100% accuracy by 1/10."

Patient outcomes must be realistic. For example, if the patient has Alzheimer's disease, an outcome describing the restoration of cognitive functioning to pre-illness levels would be inappropriate.

Outcomes are also specific and measurable. To judge successful attainment of an outcome, the nurse must be able to measure the results. In writing a measurable outcome, an action verb should be used. Terms such as *explain, list, increase, demonstrate,* and *identify* are action verbs. Specific verbs could also include *sit, stand, exercise,* and *cough.*

Terms such as *understand, know,* and *feel* are not action verbs. They would be difficult to measure. The criteria identifying success must be stated specifically. For example, "The patient will ambulate without assistance 50 feet by discharge date." Another example might be, "After receiving dietary instructions, the patient will lose 5 pounds this month." For further listing of action verbs, see Chapter 8, Box 8-3.

A correctly written outcome statement usually has four parts: behavior, measure, condition, and time frame. The book, *Charting Made Incredibly Easy* (2002, p. 27), states that each outcome should contain:

The specific behavior that shows the patient has reached his goal
Criteria for measuring that behavior
Conditions under which the behavior should occur
When the behavior should occur.

Another method of composing an outcome statement is to use the correct NOC indicator. NOC results from evidence-based practice. It is used to standardize outcomes and can be incorporated into documentation procedures.

Table 5-1 contains a sample NOC concerning asthma control. The nurse might use this NOC definition in the outcome statement. It may be written like this: "The patient will demonstrate personal actions to reverse inflammatory condition resulting in bronchial constriction of the airways, as evidenced by appropriate use of inhalers, spacers, and nebulizers at a level of 5 by January 10." There may also be variations in the way the outcome is worded. For example, in some institutions, it might be shortened to: "The patient will demonstrate asthma control by the appropriate use of inhalers, spacers, and nebulizers at a level of 5 by January 10." This method uses the NOC category instead of the definition. It might also be stated: "The patient will demonstrate asthma control as demonstrated by the standards included in Asthma Control (NOC 0704)." In whichever method is chosen, the outcome statement can be used to evaluate progress. If using the asthma control example, a copy of NOC (0704) could be included in the chart. As a method of evaluation, the nurse would be required to indicate at what level the patient was functioning for certain indicators. Obviously, not all indicators listed in this NOC category would be appropriate for every patient. For example, if support or advocacy groups were not available, indicator 070416, which refers to those groups, would not be an appropriate outcome measure. Therefore, it should not be used. At specified intervals, the nurse should reevaluate progress toward successful outcome attainment. The patient may be required to reach certain levels on important indicators before discharge. For instance, a 5 may be required on the indicator 070413—demonstrates appropriate use of inhalers, spacers, and nebulizers.

2. COLLABORATE WITH THE PATIENT TO REVIEW GOALS FOR MEETING PATIENT NEEDS

The nurse must remember to consult with others when establishing goals. The patient should have input if possible. Patients may possess values and routines that differ from those of the nurse. Therefore, a plan made without consulting the patient may be built on assumptions. Other people who can contribute information are family members and other health care workers. The ANA Standards of Practice propose that outcomes should be individualized to the patient. Individualized outcomes should be culturally appropriate.

PLAN

The ANA Standards of Practice dealing with planning state: "The nurse develops a plan of care that prescribes strategies and alternative interventions to attain expected outcomes." Accordingly, the plan of care should include strategies for nursing interventions. Delaune and Ladner describe a nursing intervention as "the activity that the nurse will execute for and with the patient to enable accomplishment of the goals." (2002, p. 87). These interventions should be based on the identified nursing diagnoses and priorities. They are planned to reduce or remove the contributing factor (R/T) portion of the nursing diagnosis.

1. USE NURSING INTERVENTIONS CLASSIFICATION TO IDENTIFY NURSING INTERVENTIONS IN RESPONSE TO RELATED NURSING DIAGNOSES

Nursing interventions are "any treatment, based upon clinical judgment and knowledge, that a nurse performs to enhance patient outcomes." (McCloskey & Bulechek, 2000, p. xvii) Nursing interventions are determined using the NIC system. This system matches nursing interventions with nursing diagnoses to facilitate improved patient care. The NIC was developed for several reasons (McClosky & Bulechek, 2000, pp. 16–19):

■ Standardization of nomenclature of nursing treatments
■ Expansion of nursing knowledge about the links between diagnoses, treatments, and outcomes

Domain—Physiologic health (II)
Class—Immune response (H)
Scale—Never demonstrated to consistently demonstrated (m)

Definition: Personal actions to reverse inflammatory condition resulting in bronchial constriction of the airways

ASTHMA CONTROL	NEVER DEMONSTRATED 1	RARELY DEMONSTRATED 2	SOMETIMES DEMONSTRATED 3	OFTEN DEMONSTRATED 4	CONSISTENTLY DEMONSTRATED 5
INDICATORS					
070401 Initiates action to avoid personal triggers	1	2	3	4	5
070402 Initiates action to manage personal triggers	1	2	3	4	5
070403 Makes appropriate environmental modifications	1	2	3	4	5
070404 Seeks early treatment of infections	1	2	3	4	5
070405 Participates in age-appropriate activities	1	2	3	4	5
070406 Sleeps through the night with no nocturnal cough or wheeze	1	2	3	4	5
070407 Wakes up rested	1	2	3	4	5
070408 Experiences no medication side effects	1	2	3	4	5
070409 Reports symptom-free state with minimal medication regimen	1	2	3	4	5
070410 Monitors peak flow routinely	1	2	3	4	5
070411 Monitors peak flow when symptoms occur	1	2	3	4	5
070412 Makes appropriate medication choices	1	2	3	4	5
070413 Demonstrates appropriate use of inhalers, spacers, and nebulizers	1	2	3	4	5
070414 Self-manages exacerbations	1	2	3	4	5
070415 Contacts health care professional when symptoms not controlled	1	2	3	4	5
070416 Accesses support and advocacy groups	1	2	3	4	5
070417 Other _____	1	2	3	4	5

Adapted from Johnson, M., Maas, M., & Moorhead, S. (2000). *Nursing outcomes classification (NOC)*. St. Louis: Mosby.

- Development of nursing and health care information systems
- Teaching decision making to nursing students
- Determination of the costs of services provided by nurses
- Planning for resources needed in nursing practice settings
- Language to communicate the unique function of nursing
- Articulation with the classification systems of other health care providers

Each NIC intervention has a label name, a definition, and a list of nursing activities. The nurse selects interventions appropriate to the nursing diagnoses. This process is demonstrated in the following scenario:

A nurse is assigned a 92-year-old female patient admitted from a long-term care facility due to pneumonia. The transfer sheet reveals chronic bowel and bladder incontinence and the need for two people to assist with transfers. During assessment, the nurse notes that the patient is incontinent of urine. When turning the patient, the nurse notes that the skin on the sacral area is pale and intact, but there is a reddened area on the right ischium that persists throughout the turning and linen change.

In this case, the nurse might select the following diagnosis: Risk for impaired skin integrity R/T general debilitation, reduced mobility, altered circulation, and excretions/secretions (bowel and bladder incontinence). The nurse can then consult a book containing diagnoses, outcomes, and interventions for guidance regarding appropriate interventions. Table 5-2 contains a sample of the appropriate section on skin integrity located in the book *Nursing Diagnosis, Outcomes, and Interventions* (Johnson et al., 2001). It is necessary to include interventions related to skin care in the plan of care. A review of the NIC list reveals an intervention listed as "skin surveillance," which is geared toward maintaining skin integrity (Table 5-3). Activity

statements for nursing interventions should use an action verb. The effectiveness of nursing care can then be evaluated.

Another appropriate NIC intervention related to skin care deals with activities pertaining to the application of topical treatments on the skin. This example can be found in Table 5-4.

Each intervention has a list of activities. The nurse selects activities appropriate for each particular patient. This is reflective of the patient's changing database and his or her surrounding circumstances as care is provided and results in an individualized care plan. Successful strategies learned from previous situations may also be incorporated. By using scientific principles, alternative approaches to situations that do not respond to routine interventions can also be developed. Principles of critical thinking and decision making should always be used to facilitate the formation of an appropriate list of interventions.

2. WRITE APPROPRIATE NURSING PLAN OF CARE USING STANDARDIZED LANGUAGE

Every patient must have an individualized plan of care. The forms of the plans may differ, but the plan must be based on the nursing process. Required documentation should also be derived from the nursing process. When charting, the nurse needs to include an evaluation of the patient's response

---

TABLE 5-2 **List of Possible Interventions Appropriate for the Nursing Diagnosis of Skin Integrity: Risk for Impaired**

Nursing Diagnosis: Skin integrity, Risk for impaired
Definition: A state in which an individual's skin is at risk for being adversely altered.
Outcome: Immobility consequences: Physiologic

MAJOR INTERVENTIONS	SUGGESTED INTERVENTIONS	OPTIONAL INTERVENTIONS
Bed rest care	Circulatory precautions	Skin care: Topical treatments
Pressure management	Embolus care: Peripheral	Surveillance
	Embolus precautions	Vital signs monitoring
	Exercise promotion: Strength training	
	Exercise promotion: Stretching	
	Exercise therapy: Joint mobility	
	Exercise therapy: Muscle control	
	Positioning	
	Positioning: Intraoperative	
	Positioning: Wheelchair	
	Pressure ulcer prevention	
	Simple massage	
	Skin surveillance	
	Traction/immobilization care	

Adapted from Johnson, M., Bulechek, G., McCloskey, J., Maas, M., & Moorhead, S. (2001). *Nursing diagnosis, outcomes, and interventions: NANDA, NOC, and NIC linkages* (p. 437). St. Louis: Mosby.

TABLE 5-3   Sample Intervention, Nursing Interventions Classification (NIC) Skin Surveillance (3590)

Definition: Collection and analysis of patient data to maintain skin and mucous membrane integrity

ACTIVITIES:

Inspect condition of surgical incision, as appropriate

Observe extremities for color, warmth, swelling, pulses, texture, edema, and ulcerations

Inspect skin and mucous membranes for redness, extreme warmth, or drainage

Monitor skin for areas of redness and breakdown

Monitor for sources of pressure and friction

Monitor for infection, especially of edematous areas

Monitor skin and mucous membranes for areas of discoloration and bruising

Monitor skin for rashes and abrasions

Monitor skin for excessive dryness and moistness

Inspect clothing for tightness

Monitor skin color

Monitor skin temperature

Note skin or mucous membrane changes

Institute measures to prevent further deterioration, as needed

Instruct family member/caregiver about signs of skin breakdown, as appropriate

---

to treatments and the patient's progress toward achieving the desired outcomes.

The plan of care is not static. It is modified to reflect changing patient needs, newly acquired information, and the correction of critical thought processes. The nurse who monitors the patient's condition well uses inference to determine a change in patient condition (Ignatavicius, 2001). This results in a change in the plan of care.

3. COLLABORATE WITH OTHER HEALTH CARE TEAM MEMBERS WHEN PLANNING DELIVERY OF PATIENT CARE

Nurses use dependent, independent, and collaborative actions in meeting the needs of the patient. Dependent actions are based on the physician's orders. When the patient does not have orders to treat the problem and the situation cannot be managed within the scope of nursing practice, the appropriate response is to call the physician. Independent interventions are those that are within the scope of nursing practice. For example, an intravenous line has infiltrated and needs to be restarted. Interdependent interventions are shared with other members of the health care team. Sharing knowledge and using the expertise of other disciplines is beneficial to administering quality nursing care. For example, the nurse should collaborate with the social service department for the transfer of the patient to a long-term care facility.

Implementation

Interventions consistent with the plan of care should be initiated after mutual agreement with the patient. In the implementation step, the nurse coordinates the actions necessary to accomplish the goals established during outcome identification. Strategies are selected that promote health and a safe environment.

1. INITIATE AND COMPLETE ACTIONS NECESSARY TO ACCOMPLISH DEFINED GOALS SAFELY AND EFFECTIVELY

Nursing actions may vary, based on individual variations in presenting problems, diagnostic tests, and medical diagnoses. It is important to select strategies that reflect the transfer of theory knowledge to the practice setting. The application of knowledge to the real-world setting results in improved nursing care. Nurses should select interventions that reflect knowledge of cause-and-effect relationships. For instance, critical thinking skills must be used to examine the cause of symptoms. If a patient is confused, the interventions selected will vary, depending on the cause of the problem. If confusion were caused by an acute problem such as an elevated blood urea nitrogen (BUN), the interventions would be based on alleviating the medical problem. On the other hand, if the confusion were related to Alzheimer's disease,

TABLE 5-4	Sample Intervention, Nursing Interventions Classification (NIC): Skin Care: Topical Treatments (3584)

Definition: Application of topical substances or manipulation of devices to promote skin integrity and minimize skin breakdown

ACTIVITIES:

Avoid using rough-textured bed linens

Clean with antibacterial soap, as appropriate

Dress patient in nonrestrictive clothing

Dust the skin with medicated powder, as appropriate

Remove adhesive tape and debris

Provide support to edematous areas (e.g., pillow under arms and scrotal support), as appropriate

Apply lubricant to moisten lips and oral mucosa, as needed

Administer back rub/neck rub, as appropriate

Change condom catheter, as appropriate

Apply diapers loosely, as appropriate

Place on incontinent pads, as appropriate

Massage around the affected area

Apply appropriately fitting ostomy appliance, as needed

Cover the hands with mittens, as appropriate

Provide toilet hygiene, as needed

Refrain from giving local heat applications

Refrain from using an alkaline soap on the skin

Soak in a colloidal bath, as appropriate

Keep bed linen clean, dry, and wrinkle free

Turn the immobilized patient at least every 2 hours, according to a specific schedule

Use devices on the bed (e.g., sheepskin) that protect the patient

Apply heel protectors, as appropriate

Apply drying powders to deep skinfolds

Initiate consultation services of the enterostomal therapy nurse, as needed

Apply clear occlusive dressing (e.g., Tegaderm or Duoderm), as needed

Apply topical antibiotic to the affected area, as appropriate

Apply topical antiinflammatory agent to the affected area, as appropriate

Apply emollients to the affected area

Apply topical antifungal agent to the affected area, as appropriate

Apply topical débriding agent to the affected area, as appropriate

Paint or spray skin warts with liquid nitrogen, as appropriate

Inspect skin daily for those at risk for breakdown

Document degree of skin breakdown

Add moisture to environment with a humidifier, as needed

interventions should focus on safety. It should not be assumed that the same interventions will work for all disoriented patients.

When providing care, the nurse uses cognitive, psychomotor, and interpersonal skills to achieve established goals in a safe and effective manner. Cognitive skills involve knowledge and the ability to think critically. Obviously, this is important to the administration of safe nursing care. Skills in the psychomotor domain (technical skills) are also nec-

essary. Skillful performance of nursing procedures is vital to quality care. Finally, nurses should possess good interpersonal skills. The ability to communicate effectively with the patient and colleagues is essential.

Critical thinking involves the ability to process information with clarity, accuracy, and precision, giving appropriate significance to each piece of data to produce reasoned judgments. The nurse must determine the significance of individual

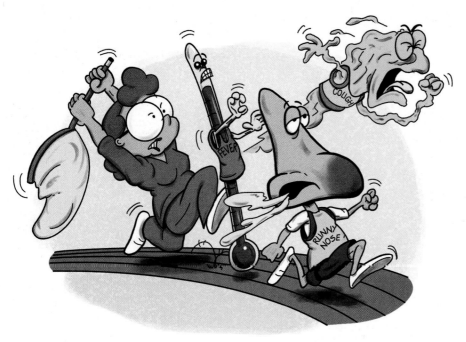

Chasing the symptoms instead of the problem leaves you running in circles!

pieces of information. The cognitive skills used to process this information include interpretation, analysis, evaluation, inference, explanation, and self-regulation. These skills are used in processing information to solve problems, make decisions, and set priorities within the framework of the nursing process. Cognitive skills involve knowledge and the ability to think critically for managing the patient's care.

2. MANAGE PATIENT'S CARE IN ORDER OF PRIORITY

The patient's care should be organized with appropriate consideration of priorities. Actions can be divided into high, medium, and low priority. The nurse must ensure that high-priority activities, such as safety measures, are performed before focusing on lower-priority or comfort measures. (See Chapter 4 for more detailed information on this topic.)

3. DELEGATE CARE AS APPROPRIATE, BASED ON THE CAPABILITY OF THE CAREGIVER, THE ACUITY OF THE PATIENT, THE PATIENT'S NEEDS, AND THE PLAN OF CARE

Implementation involves performing or delegating activities. Delegation is based on several factors, including the capability of the caregiver, the acuity and needs of the patient, and the plan of care.

This concept is further addressed in Chapter 6, Delegation.

4. INTERVENE AS THE PATIENT'S ADVOCATE WHEN NECESSARY

The nurse is obligated to function as the patient's advocate. At times, a conflict may exist between the patient and the desires of the family. The primary duty of the nurse is to the patient. For example, an alert, oriented patient has supplied the institution with an advance directive stating he does not wish to be resuscitated. However, the family requests that all extraordinary measures be performed. In this dispute, the nurse's role is to be an advocate for the patient and uphold the advance directive.

5. DOCUMENT NURSING INTERVENTIONS AND THE PATIENT'S RESPONSES TO THE THERAPEUTIC MODALITIES IN USE

All nursing interventions should be documented, including the patient's response to the treatment modalities. Forms for documentation vary among institutions. However, use of NIC, NOC, and NANDA provides standardized language in measuring progress toward goals and in completing documentation.

Evaluation

The ANA Standards of Practice state, "The nurse evaluates the patient progress toward attainment of outcomes."

1. COMPARE ACTUAL OUTCOMES WITH EXPECTED OUTCOMES OF PATIENT CARE, BASED ON CURRENT CIRCUMSTANCES

A comparison of expected outcomes with actual outcomes should be performed. Because outcomes are building blocks of goals, the nurse is also measuring the extent to which goals have been achieved. The measurement of progress toward outcomes can occur by examining the results on the appropriate NOC indicator.

When examining the success of outcomes, the nurse is provided with information regarding the effectiveness of the interventions. If they are ineffective, a revision of the plan of care may be necessary.

2. COMMUNICATE FINDINGS TO THE APPROPRIATE HEALTH CARE TEAM MEMBERS

Evaluation involves communicating with colleagues. If a certain intervention was successful, sharing this information during shift report can contribute to the continuity of care. Ongoing progress toward goals should be discussed. As goals are reached, other team members should be notified. Those goals should be deleted from the plan of care and perhaps a new goal formulated.

3. RECORD JUDGMENT AND MEASUREMENT OF GOAL ATTAINMENT

Evaluation includes the measurement of progress toward goal attainment. Documentation of evaluation is an aspect that will be scrutinized carefully by accrediting and funding agencies. Programs that can demonstrate successful goal achievement are more likely to continue and to be funded.

4. REVIEW AND MODIFY NURSING PLAN OF CARE AS INDICATED; SET PRIORITIES BASED ON CHANGING NEEDS

The care plan must be reviewed and changed continually to include changes in the health status of the patient. Constantly evaluating and reevaluating is essential to quality care. Throughout the process, nurses must examine their own critical thinking to ensure logical conclusions.

CARE PLAN

A plan of care is a written documentation of the nursing process. It validates that appropriate care has been given.

Institutions use various methods for plan of care documentation. A traditional care plan can be written for each individual patient. Another option is to use a standardized care plan. In this method, preprinted plans are available for each nursing diagnosis. The nurse selects the appropriate nursing diagnosis and individualizes or tailors the interventions to the particular patient. Other institutions use preprinted care pathways and primarily document only variations from the established pathways. This is commonly referred to as *charting by exception.*

The care plan includes columns for nursing diagnosis, outcomes, activities, rationale, and evaluation. All the above-mentioned components have been discussed earlier in this chapter, except for rationale. Student nurses are often required to supply the scientific rationale justifying the selection of an intervention. "The rationale—the 'why' of the intervention—describes a research-based reason for performing the intervention" (Craven & Hirnle, 2003, p. 191). Many reliable sources of data, such as medical-surgical textbooks, nursing care plan books, pharmacology books, and other nursing references, provide evidence-based rationales for interventions. Students should consult their instructor for further information if unable to locate appropriate resources.

The scenario described in Box 5-3 demonstrates the formation of a plan of care. Explanations of the various sections of the care plan are provided with the scenario. Table 5-5 provides a sample plan of care for the patient in this scenario. Practice exercises designed to strengthen these skills can also be found at the end of this chapter.

PITFALLS

As is the case with any process, the nursing process does not always flow smoothly. Errors can occur during the execution. Therefore, nurses need to be aware of the following pitfalls identified by Costello-Nickitas (1997; as cited in Delaune & Ladner [2002, p.82]):

- Jumping too quickly toward a conclusion before exploring all the aspects of a problem

Box 5-3   Sample Care Plan

PHYSICAL DATA

John Davis, 46 years of age, was admitted with a medical diagnosis of left tibia/fibula fracture following a minor auto accident. He had a closed reduction of the fracture with a long leg cast application last night. He states that the pain in the left leg occurs with movement and ambulation. John rates the pain at 7 to 8 during movement and ambulation and at 1 to 2 at rest. During transfer to the chair and ambulation to the bathroom, the patient moans, and the nurse notes facial grimacing. Physical therapy is scheduled in 1 hour for gait training with crutches, and discharge is scheduled for this evening. He verbalizes concern about having some difficulty getting to work because he works in a building that has several steps to gain entry into the building. Also, he has expressed concern about how he will get his pants on over the bulky cast. He works as an accountant and will be able to make other accommodations for the cast.

DIAGNOSTIC DATA

Left leg anteroposterior and lateral radiographs show comminuted distal tibial/fibula fracture with large butterfly fragment. Tibial fragment is displaced posteriorly approximately 8 mm, with posterior angulation at fracture site.

	PATIENT VALUES	NORMAL RANGE
WBC	12.7	5,000–10,000
RBC	4.71	4.7–6.1
Hemoglobin	15.2	14–18
Hematocrit	43.8	42%–52%
Platelets	284,000	150,000–400,000

After reviewing the available data, the nurse would identify pertinent cues and place them into clusters. Three clusters are present in this example.

PAIN/DISCOMFORT

Rates pain 7–8 during ambulation
Moaning and facial grimace noted during transfer and ambulation

HYGIENE

Verbalizing needs for assistance to get pants over cast
Observed having difficulty getting pants and shoes on

ACTIVITY/REST

Has a long leg cast on the left leg
Verbalizes the fear of difficulty ambulating on stairs
Uses crutches for ambulation

At this stage, the nurse must consider immediate problems first. If the physical therapist will arrive in 1 hour, the nurse may need to medicate now for anticipated pain during therapy. The medication will have time to take effect before physical therapy arrives for gait training and crutch-walking activities. After completion of this task, the nurse can continue with the assessment. As this scenario points out, there will be times when the nurse notices gaps in the assessment. The white blood cell count (WBC) is elevated. Therefore, the nurse should obtain a set of vital signs. The graphic sheet should be reviewed to determine the course of the temperature. After assessing the general physical status of the patient, the nurse may be able to infer the source of the elevated WBC. Physician's orders should be reviewed for antibiotic orders. Calling the physician may be indicated if orders are not in place to meet the needs of this abnormal finding.

ANALYSIS

During this step, the nurse has identified three priority nursing diagnoses and listed them in order of priority. These diagnoses are:

- Pain RT muscle spasm, edema, trauma AEB patient rating pain at 7–8 during ambulation and moaning and facial grimace noted during transfer and ambulation
- Ineffective health maintenance RT deficient knowledge regarding care of fracture AEB patient verbalizing fear of ambulating on steps with long leg cast and using crutches and patient needing assistive devices for dressing
- Risk for peripheral neurovascular dysfunction RT mechanical compression, treatment of fracture. (A "risk for" diagnosis has no AEB factors because it has not been demonstrated as a problem.)

For the purpose of illustration, only the priority nursing diagnosis will be included on Mr. Davis' sample plan of care.

OUTCOME IDENTIFICATION

Identify appropriate goal for the plan of care and list indicators (based on NOC) to be used to measure progress toward the goal. A suggestion would be pain control (NOC 1605). If the following evaluative statement were used, the nurse would have parameters for later evaluation:

The patient will verbalize pain upon movement decreased to a level of 1–2 by discharge.

PLAN

This information is then placed in the format selected by the institution. A sample care plan for this patient would be attached.

IMPLEMENTATION

The nurse may implement the following actions: Initiate the assessment of pain and give the medication in anticipation of therapy. Assess neurovascular status. Collaborate with therapy to plan gait training while medication is at peak levels for pain management. Monitor the patient's response to medication and activity and evaluate readiness for self-care in the event of discharge later today.

Delegate personal hygiene and grooming and taking vital signs to the UAP.

EVALUATION

Monitor the patient for responses to interventions. Evaluate level of outcome attainment by rating performance level based on NOC. Selected indicators from Pain Control (NOC 1605) include:

- Recognizes causal factors.
- Uses nonanalgesic relief measures.
- Uses analgesics appropriately.
- Uses warning signs to seek care.
- Reports pain controlled.

All aspects of the nursing process are included in the plan of care. Therefore, formulation of a plan can synthesize knowledge regarding a patient. See Table 5-5 for a sample plan of care for Mr. Davis.

TABLE 5·5   LIPPINCOTT'S INTERACTIVE CARE PLAN CREATOR

NAME: STUDENT	ID: 123	COURSE: COGNITIVE SKILLS IN NURSING		INSTRUCTOR: SAUNDRA	DATE: 07/01/2005
MEDICAL DIAGNOSES	**NURSING DIAGNOSES**	**PATIENT OUTCOMES/ GOALS**	**NURSING ACTIVITIES**	**RATIONALE**	**EVALUATIONS**
SUTURES	PAIN (ACUTE)				
	DEFINING CHARACTERISTICS: Guarding	Pain Control (NOC 1605) Consistently demonstrate personal actions to control pain. The patient will verbalize pain decreased to a level of 1–2 upon movement by discharge. Demonstrate participation in physical therapy for gait training and crutch walking.	Medications or drugs, teach about	Regardless of the patient's cultural background, pain rated at >4 on a 0–10 pain-rating scale interferes significantly with daily function. (McCaffery, 1999; McCaffery, Pasero, 1999) Administering medication before a pain-producing activity will minimize the pain experienced. Analgesics are more effective if given before pain becomes severe. Pain diminishes activity. (McCaffery, Pasero, 1999)	Recognizes causal factors
	Pain, facial mask		Health problem (etiology, pathology, & signs & symptoms), teach about	Compliance with the medical regimen for diagnoses involving pain improves the likelihood of successful management (Humphrey, 1994)	Uses nonanalgesic relief measures
	Pain, measurement		Guided imagery or meditation, teach about	Cognitive-behavioral strategies can restore the patients' sense of self-control, personal efficacy, and active participation in own care. (Acute Pain Management Guideline Panel, 1992)	Uses analgesics appropriately
	Blood pressure, abnormal		Comfort, physical, assess	The intensity of pain and discomfort should be assessed and documented after any known pain-producing procedure, with each new report of pain, and at regular intervals. (JCAHO, 2000)	Uses warning signs to seek care
	Pulse rate change				Reports pain controlled Performance Level 5

- Failing to obtain critical facts about either the problem or proposed change
- Selecting problems or changes that are too general, too complex, or poorly defined
- Failing to articulate a rational solution to the problem or proposed change
- Failing to implement and evaluate the proposal appropriately

To avoid these pitfalls, it is very important to define the problem clearly, analyze the data, understand the cause of the problem, and create new ideas. The effective use of cognitive skills (critical thinking) is essential. A review of the six cognitive skills necessary in the practice of bedside nursing demonstrates how important these abilities are to the nursing process. Ignatavicius (2001) identified these skills as interpretation, analysis, evaluation, inference, explanation, and self-regulation.

Interpretation involves the clarification of meaning. The nurse uses this skill when determining the significance of laboratory values, vital signs, and physical assessment data. It also includes understanding the meaning of patient behavior or statements. In the sample plan of care (see Box 5-3), the patient was noted to exhibit moaning and facial grimacing. These are classic indicators of pain. The nurse assesses pain using the standard pain scale of 1 to 10 (with 10 being the worst pain ever experienced) and records the patient's perception of the pain.

In *analysis,* the patient's problems are determined, based on assessment data. At times, the actual problem cannot be validated initially, but several possibilities can be identified. In this case, the nurse would consider the pain characteristics and the importance of therapy participation in the discharge plan. A neurovascular assessment should also be performed. The nurse may determine that the best plan of care includes medicating the patient before physical therapy to progress further toward the desired outcome.

When using the cognitive skill of *evaluation,* the nurse identifies expected patient outcomes and assesses the degree of successful completion. If outcomes were not met, the nurse investigates possible reasons.

Inference involves drawing conclusions. For example, the nurse determines when the patient's health status improves or declines through careful monitoring. This patient's pain is based on the tissue trauma related to the fracture and the fact that movement of the traumatized tissue increases the pain and discomfort. The patient may refuse to participate in physical therapy unless appropriate pain management is implemented. Pain is ap-

propriate as a nursing diagnosis because it is a significant problem in the treatment plan.

Explanation entails the ability to justify actions. The nurse implements interventions based on research or other sources of evidence. Procedures that increase the pain may cause a patient's unwillingness to cooperate with care. Pain management is essential to gain patient participation in restorative therapy. Neurovascular assessment is also important to rule out more serious problems before assuming it is normal pain that the patient is experiencing.

A very important critical thinking skill is the process of examining one's practice and correcting or improving it, if necessary; this is known as *self-regulation.* In the sample scenario (see Box 5-3), assessing neurovascular status to determine adequate vascular supply will enable earlier intervention in the hope of avoiding further damage. The nurse should also determine the onset of action for the specific medication ordered. The medication should be administered before the scheduled therapy session, after collaboration with the physical therapy team. The following questions would also be appropriate for the nurse to ask:

Do I have all the facts?
Is my thinking biased?
Have I evaluated accurately?

The relationship of cognitive skills to the entire nursing process is evident. Therefore, improving one's cognitive skills can be beneficial to nursing practice. Activities are presented at the end of the chapter to practice these skills.

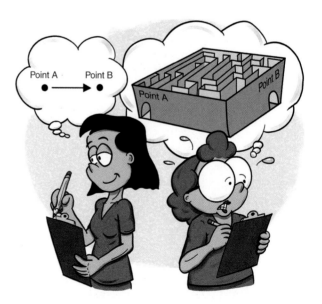

Simplify problems with the nursing process.

SUMMARY

The nursing process is an important element in organizing thought processes for problem solving and decision making. Although the six steps in the nursing process are presented as separate steps, they are interrelated in a dynamic process to ensure ongoing quality nursing service. This is an essential part of the changing health care environment.

Skill checklists are included at the end of this chapter, which can be used to evaluate abilities in this area. Instructors can also combine the lists with scenarios as a learning tool to provide student guidance.

KEY POINTS

- The nursing process is an organized problem-solving method that facilitates the use of sound judgment in care delivery. The steps of the nursing process are assessment, analysis, outcome identification, planning, implementation, and evaluation.
- The American Nurses Association (ANA) recognizes the terms developed by the North American Nursing Diagnosis Association (NANDA), Nursing Interventions Classification (NIC), and Nursing Outcomes Classifications (NOC) as being included in the universal language for nurses.
- The interventions in NIC are based on research into current best practices, which is called *evidence-based practice*.
- The nurse collects pertinent health data during the assessment step. The data are sorted and organized into clusters of related information.
- Nursing diagnoses are formulated in the analysis step. A properly composed nursing diagnosis normally has three parts: the problem (in NANDA terms), the contributing factors (related to), and the signs and symptoms (as evidenced by).
- Patient outcomes should be realistic, achievable, and measurable using NOC. A correctly written outcome statement usually has four parts: behavior, measure, condition, and time frame.
- In the planning stage, nursing interventions are matched with nursing diagnoses to facilitate improved patient care. A plan of care is developed, which can be modified to reflect changing patient needs, newly acquired information, or the corrections of critical thought processes.
- During the implementation step, the nurse initiates and completes actions necessary to accomplish the defined goals in a safe, effective manner.
- All nursing interventions, including the patient's response to the treatment modalities, should be documented.
- Evaluation involves a comparison of expected outcomes with actual outcomes.
- A plan of care is a written documentation of the nursing process.

REFERENCES

Acute Pain Management Guideline Panel. (1992). *Acute pain management operative or medical procedures and trauma: Clinical practice guideline.* Agency for Health Care Policy and Research Pub No 92-0032. Rockville, MD: Public Health Service, U.S. Department of Health and Human Services.

Alfaro-LeFevre, R. (1999). *Critical thinking in nursing: A practical approach.* Philadelphia: W.B. Saunders.

Alfaro-LeFevre, R. (2002). *Applying nursing process: Promoting collaborative care.* Philadelphia: Lippincott Williams & Wilkins.

American Nurses Association. (2003). *Nursing scope and standards of practice.* Washington, DC: American Nurses Publishing.

Aquilino, M. L., & Keenan, G. (2000). Having our say: Nursing's standardized nomenclatures. *American Journal of Nursing, 100*(7), 33–38.

Bersky, A., Krawczak, J., & Kumar, T. (1999). *Lippincott's interactive care plan creator.* Co-developed by the National Council of State Boards of Nursing. (Version: Multimedia PC Level 11) [Computer software] Philadelphia: Lippincott Williams & Wilkins.

Catalano, J. T. (1996). *Contemporary professional nursing.* Philadelphia: F.A. Davis.

Charting made incredibly easy. (2002). Philadelphia: Lippincott Williams & Wilkins.

Costello-Nickitas, D. (1997). *Quick reference to nursing leadership.* Albany, NY: Delmar.

Craven, R. F., & Hirnle, C. L. (2003). *Fundamentals of nursing: Human health and function* (4th ed.). Philadelphia: Lippincott Williams & Wilkins.

Daly, J. M., Maas, M., McCloskey, J. C., & Bulechek, G. M. (1996). A care planning tool proves what we do. *RN, 59*(6), 26–29.

Delaune, S. C., & Ladner, P. K. (2002). *Fundamentals of nursing: Standards and practice.* Albany, NY: Delmar.

Dexter, P., Applegate, M., Backer, J., Claytor, K., Keffer, J., Norton, B., & Ross, B. (1997). A proposed framework for teaching and evaluating critical thinking in nursing. *Journal of Professional Nursing, 13*(3), 160–167.

Doenges, M. E., & Moorhouse, M. F. (2000). *Nurse's pocket guide: Diagnoses, interventions, and rationales.* Philadelphia: F. A. Davis.

Doenges, M. E., Moorhouse, M. F., & Burley, J. T. (2000). *Application of nursing process and nursing diagnosis: An interactive text for diagnostic reasoning.* Philadelphia: F.A. Davis.

Dracup, K. (1996). Clinical practice guidelines. *Nursing, 26*(2), 41–47.

Gordon, M. (1995). *Nursing diagnosis: Process and application.* St. Louis: Mosby.

Guzetta, C. E., Bunton, S. D., Prindey, L. A., Sherer, A. P., & Seifert, P. C. (1989). *Clinical assessment tools for use with nursing diagnoses.* St. Louis: Mosby.

Humphrey, C. (1994). *Home care nursing handbook.* Gaithersburg, MD: Aspen.

Ignatavicius, D. D. (2001). Critical thinking skills for at-the-bedside success. *Nursing Management, 32*(1), 37–39.

Johnson, M., Bulechek, G., McCloskey, J., Maas, M., & Moorhead, S. (2001). *Nursing diagnosis, outcomes, and interventions: NANDA, NOC, and NIC linkages.* St. Louis: Mosby.

Johnson, M., Maas, M., & Moorhead, S. (2000). *Nursing outcomes classification (NOC).* St. Louis: Mosby.

Joint Commission on Accreditation of Healthcare Organizations (JCAHO). (2000). *2000 Hospital accreditation standards.* Oakbrook, IL: Author.

Lunney, M. (2001). *NANDA: Critical thinking and nursing diagnosis.* Philadelphia: North American Nursing Diagnosis Association.

McCaffery, M. (1999). Culturally sensitive pain assessment. *American Journal of Nursing, 99*(8), 18.

McCaffery, M., & Pasero, C. (1999). *Pain: Clinical manual.* St. Louis: Mosby.

McCloskey, J. C., & Bulechek, G. M. (2000). *Nursing interventions classification (NIC).* St. Louis: Mosby.

North American Nursing Diagnosis Association. (2001). *NANDA nursing diagnosis: Definitions and classifications (2001–2002).* Philadelphia: Author.

Rubenfeld, M. G., & Scheffer, B. K. (1999). *Critical thinking in nursing: An interactive approach.* Philadelphia: Lippincott Williams & Wilkins.

Saucier, B. L., Stevens, K. R., & Williams, G. B. (2002). Critical thinking outcomes of computer-assisted instruction versus written nursing process. *Nursing and Health Care Perspectives, 21*(5), 240–246.

Wycoff, J. (1991*). Mindmapping: Your personal guide to exploring creativity and problem-solving.* New York: Berkley Books.

Student Worksheets

SKILL SHEET: NURSING PROCESS

Purpose

1. To provide a framework for planning and delivering patient care.
2. To enable the student to draw accurate conclusions based on relevant data.
3. To enable the student to formulate an individualized plan of care based on NIC, NOC, and NANDA.
4. To facilitate priority setting and decision making regarding care for assigned patients.

Objectives

The student will demonstrate the ability to do the following:

1. Collect information, from all available sources.
2. Organize data in a logical sequence.
3. Examine the patterns to identify possible problems and causes for the patient's symptoms.
4. Make an inference based on data gathered.
5. Use sound priority-setting and decision-making principles.
6. Utilize NIC, NOC, and NANDA to increase accountability for interventions selected and measuring outcomes of care.
7. Develop a comprehensive plan of care.

Steps: Nursing Process

ASSESSMENT

1. Collect data from all available resources (i.e., review nursing history, perform physical assessment, interview patient's family, and study health record).
2. Identify pertinent data.
3. Recognize deviations from the normal.
4. Validate the data with the patient.
5. Sort and organize data in logical sequence.
6. Identify patterns in the data.

ANALYSIS

1. Examine the clusters to determine unmet needs as well as patient's strengths and health concerns.
2. Focus on problems that can be changed.
3. Develop nursing diagnoses based on facts and supporting data (consult NANDA).
4. Validate the nursing diagnoses.
5. Establish priorities of the nursing diagnoses.

OUTCOME IDENTIFICATION

1. Establish patient outcomes that are realistic, achievable, and measurable using NOC.
2. Collaborate with the patient to review goals for meeting patient needs.

PLAN

1. Use NIC to identify nursing interventions in response to related nursing diagnoses.
2. Develop an individualized written nursing care plan with strategies to achieve these goals.
3. Collaborate with other health care team members when planning delivery of patient's care.

IMPLEMENTATION

1. Initiate and complete actions necessary to accomplish the defined goals in a safe and effective manner.
2. Manage patient's care to satisfy high-priority or life-threatening needs first, then medium-priority needs, and finally low-priority needs.
3. Delegate care as appropriate, based on the capability of the caregiver, the acuity of the patient, the patient needs, and the plan of care.
4. Intervene when necessary as the patient's advocate.
5. Document nursing interventions and the patient's responses to the therapeutic modalities in use.

EVALUATION

1. Compare actual outcomes with expected outcomes of patient care based on current circumstances.
2. Communicate findings to the appropriate health care team members.
3. Record judgment and measurement of goal attainment.
4. Review and modify plan of care as indicated.

The steps of nursing process are completed as a sequence of set steps. Activities within these steps can be performed in a different order.

COMPETENCY VALIDATION: NURSING PROCESS

COMPETENCY STATEMENT

Identify common needs and problems, formulate individualized care plan, and deliver nursing care based on the plan.

The student demonstrated the ability to do the following:

1. Assess and observe both physiologic and psychological needs of the patient.
2. Describe the problem and provide supporting data for its identification.
3. Focus on problems that are controllable.
4. Use NOC to identify goals that are plausible and measurable.
5. Use scientific principles and rationale to develop alternative courses of action.
6. Perform safe and effective nursing care.
7. Document the effectiveness of the plan of care for the individual patient based on current circumstances.
8. Develop nursing diagnoses based on facts and supporting data according to NANDA.
9. Use NIC to identify nursing interventions in response to related nursing diagnoses.
10. Establish a plan of care outlining appropriate independent nursing actions based on assessment data and analysis for goal attainment.
11. Evaluate extent to which goals had been achieved.
12. Revise and modify plan of care.

COMPETENT

- Understands reason for task and is able to perform task independently
- Understands reason for task but needs supervision
- Understands reason for task and is able to perform task with assistance

NOT COMPETENT

- Understands reason for task but performs task at provisional level
- Is unable to state reason for task and performs task at a dependent level

SKILL CHECKLIST: NURSING PROCESS

NURSING PROCESS	SATISFACTORY	UNSATISFACTORY	NI/COMMENTS
ASSESSMENT			
1. Gather information through nursing history, physical assessment, interviews, and chart review.			
2. Identify pertinent data.			
3. Recognize deviations from normal.			
4. Validate the data with the patient.			
5. Sort and organize data in a logical sequence.			
6. Identify patterns in the data.			
ANALYSIS			
1. Examine the clusters to determine unmet needs, strengths, and health concerns.			
2. Focus on problems that can be changed.			
3. Develop nursing diagnosis.			
4. Validate nursing diagnosis.			
5. Establish priorities of nursing diagnosis.			
OUTCOME IDENTIFICATION			
1. Establish patient outcomes that are realistic, achievable, and measurable using NOC.			
2. Collaborate with the patient to review goals for meeting patient needs.			
PLAN			
1. Use NIC to identify nursing interventions in response to related nursing diagnosis.			
2. Write appropriate nursing plan of care.			
3. Collaborate with other health care team members to plan delivery of care.			
IMPLEMENTATION			
1. Initiate and complete actions based on plan of care and defined goals.			
2. Manage care in order of priority.			
3. Delegate care as appropriate.			
4. Intervene as necessary as patient's advocate.			
5. Record nursing interventions and patient responses to the therapeutic modalities.			

NURSING PROCESS	SATISFACTORY	UNSATISFACTORY	NI/COMMENTS
EVALUATION			
1. Compare actual outcomes with expected outcomes of patient care based on current circumstances.			
2. Communicate findings to the appropriate health care team members.			
3. Record judgment and measurement of goal attainment.			
4. Review and modify nursing plan of care as indicated. Set priorities based on the changing needs.			

 # SCENARIOS TO ACCOMPANY STUDENT WORKSHEETS

Identifying and clustering cues

SCENARIO 1

A 72-year-old woman was admitted following a motor vehicle accident. In the emergency department (ED), an x-ray revealed that the head of the left femur was fractured. She is scheduled for an open reduction and internal fixation (ORIF) later today. At present, she rates the pain at 8 on a 1 to 10 scale. The son mentioned during the assessment that his mother is forgetful sometimes.

Vital signs include the following: blood pressure, 168/92 mm Hg; temperature, 98°F (36.7°C); pulse, 102 beats/min and irregular; respirations, 26 breaths/min. Breath sounds are clear bilaterally, respirations even and unlabored, and peripheral pulses present and palpable at 2+ except left foot. The left pedal pulse is weak and barely palpable, and capillary refill response is 5 seconds. The patient is alert and oriented, is able to move all extremities except the left leg, and verbalizes appropriate responses to all questioning. She relates allergies to sulfa and ampicillin.

During the assessment, the patient is very anxious and states that she has never been in the hospital before. She did confide that she had spent a lot of time at the hospital when her husband died from cancer last year. Significant medical history includes high blood pressure controlled with medication.

1. Underline all of the cues and problems in the above scenario.

2. Sort and cluster the relevant data using Diagnostic-Related Groups.

Circulation: _____

_____

_____

_____

_____

Activity/Rest: _____

_____

_____

_____

_____

Neurosensory: _____

_____

_____

_____

_____

Pain/Discomfort: _____

_____

_____

_____

_____

Safety: _____

_____

_____

_____

_____

Ego Integrity: _____

_____

_____

_____

_____

Teaching/Learning: _____

_____

_____

_____

_____

Scenario 2

A 68-year-old man presented in the ED with an acute epistaxis (nosebleed) 2 hours earlier. At the time the bleeding started, he also experienced blurred vision, which he stated had never happened before. Upon questioning, the patient related that he has been experiencing early-morning headaches for the past 3 to 4 months. The initial blood pressure of 198/116 mm Hg was treated with medication in the ED, and the epistaxis subsequently stopped without specific intervention. The patient was admitted for further diagnostic tests and follow-up care.

On arrival to the medical-surgical unit, the following vital signs were obtained: blood pressure, 142/88 mm Hg; temperature, 98.2°F (36.8°C); pulse, 98 beats/min; respirations, 28 breaths/min. The patient verbalizes weakness and fatigue gradually increasing during the past 4 months. He ambulates with a steady gait, and muscle strength and hand grasp are equal and strong bilaterally. He also relates feeling "palpitations" and shortness of breath on exertion. He attributes his symptoms to working a lot of overtime and being stressed because of his wife's illness. He states he did not seek medical attention because he thought he was just tired. Current body weight is 328 pounds; height is 5 feet, 10 inches. On the lab draw, his blood sugar was 228 mg/dL (he states he had not eaten this morning before arriving in the ED). He has a history of smoking since the age of 23 years, and he always adds salt to his food at the table.

1. Underline all of the cues and problems in the above scenario.

2. Sort and cluster the relevant data using the Diagnostic-Related Groups.

Ego Integrity: _____

_____

_____

_____

_____

Food/Fluid: _____

_____

_____

_____

_____

Neurosensory: _____

_____

_____

_____

_____

Pain/Discomfort: _____

_____

_____

_____

_____

Respirations: _____

_____

_____

_____

_____

Circulation: _____

_____

_____

_____

_____

_____

Teaching/Learning: _____

_____

_____

_____

_____

_____

See the Answer Key in Appendix A for sample answers for this exercise.

Practice Exercises: Advanced Nursing Process Applications

IDENTIFYING AND CLUSTERING CUES

Scenario 1

A 53-year-old woman was admitted on a 23-hour observation for a laparoscopic cholecystectomy. On the admission database, she verbalized frequent episodes of nausea, belching, and heartburn when eating fatty foods. Immediately before admission, the severity of the epigastric distress and right upper abdominal pain had increased. The patient has a saline lock in the left hand; Steri-Strips to the four puncture wound sites on the abdomen, and pain management with oral medication. She is scheduled for discharge today.

1. Underline all of the cues and problems in the above scenario.

   _____

   _____

   _____

2. Select the appropriate Diagnostic-Related Groups. Sort and cluster the relevant data into the groupings.

   _____

   _____

   _____

3. Identify the priority nursing diagnosis.

   _____

   _____

   _____

4. What is the expected outcome?

   _____

   _____

   _____

Scenario 2

A 28-year-old woman was admitted with a diagnosis of recurrent inflammatory bowel disease. She has been on prednisone for 10 years and experienced a gradual weight loss of 30 pounds in the past year. Symptoms include 5 to 10 loose stools per day, nausea, and frequent, intermittent pain. During the physical assessment, the patient described patterns of fatigue with normal daily chores and sleep patterns being disturbed at night as a result of the frequent episodes of diarrhea. Anxiously, she reported recently quitting her job because of inability to cope with all of the problems the disease causes at work. Her current body weight is 106 pounds, and her height is 5 feet, 7 inches. She has poor muscle tone, pale mucous membranes, and poor skin turgor. There are visible hemorrhoids and a fissure noted in the anal area, and she verbalizes noting small amounts of red blood during bowel movements.

1. Underline all of the cues and problems in the above scenario.

2. Identify the appropriate diagnostic groups. Sort and cluster the relevant data using the groupings.

_____

_____

_____

_____

_____

_____

_____

_____

_____

_____

_____

_____

_____

_____

_____

_____

_____

_____

3. Based on these clusters, identify the priority nursing diagnoses and place in order of priority.

_____

_____

_____

_____

_____

_____

_____

_____

_____

4. What are the expected outcomes for the two top-priority nursing diagnoses?

_____

_____

_____

_____

_____

Scenario 3

Marie Kelly, who is 53 years old, was admitted from the emergency room with chronic renal failure, has a long history of diabetes mellitus and hypertension, and is on hemodialysis. Her symptoms include extreme fatigue, general malaise, and occasional confusion from the chronic uremia. She has no known allergies. Physical assessment reveals generalized tissue and pitting edema of feet and legs, pallor, and bronze-gray, yellow skin. She verbalizes that urine output is normally anuric and that constipation is always a problem. Her skin has numerous crusted areas on both arms, and she is scratching during the assessment. She complains of frequent nausea and vomiting and an unpleasant metallic taste in her mouth.

1. Underline all of the cues and problems in the above scenario.

2. After identification of the cues (defining characteristics), sort them into appropriate data clusters.

_____
_____
_____
_____
_____
_____
_____
_____
_____
_____
_____
_____
_____
_____
_____
_____
_____
_____
_____

3. Identify two priority nursing diagnoses (write in three-part format) and list in order of urgency.

_____
_____
_____
_____
_____

4. What are the expected outcomes for the priority nursing diagnoses?

_____

_____

_____

_____

Scenario 4

Ronald Johnson, a 73-year-old man, was seen in the emergency room for the following symptoms: right-sided hemiparesis, expressive aphasia, and dysphagia. He is drowsy and demonstrates slurred speech and altered mental status. The wife states, "I found him in the hallway outside the bathroom." She also requests a laxative because he has been constipated all morning. A computed tomography (CT) scan and angiogram completed in the ED revealed a blockage in the middle cerebral artery.

1. Underline all of the cues and problems in the above scenario.

2. After identification of the cues (defining characteristics), sort them into appropriate data clusters.

_____

_____

_____

_____

_____

_____

_____

_____

_____

_____

_____

_____

3. Identify three priority nursing diagnoses (write in three-part format) and list in order of urgency.

_____

_____

_____

_____

_____

_____

_____

4. Use your critical thinking skills to develop another nursing diagnosis that is implied in the above scenario. This one will only have two parts because it is a "risk for" diagnosis and no cues are present.

_____

_____

_____

5. What are the expected outcomes for the priority nursing diagnoses?

_____

_____

_____

_____

See the Answer Key in Appendix A for sample answers for this exercise.

ADVANCED APPLICATIONS: USING THE NURSING PROCESS

SCENARIO

Jimmy Little, 61 years old, presented in the emergency room with a temperature of 100.2°F and complaints of abdominal pain. He rated the pain at 10 on a 1 to 10 scale and was admitted for urinary tract infection and urosepsis. Past medical history included cancer of the prostate.

Mr. Little reports incontinence related to a long-term indwelling catheter left in place during chemotherapy and removed last week. The nurse obtained only 30 mL of dark-brown urine, with no visible blood noted upon catheterization in the emergency room. The 18-gauge Foley catheter was attached to a drainage bag after insertion. The patient verbalized that he has not been drinking fluids because it hurts when he voids. He reports no unintentional weight loss or gain of 10 pounds or greater. There is no visible or palpable edema noted. A saline lock was placed in the left forearm for antibiotic therapy while he was in the ED. The lock is patent and free of signs of infection.

ASSESSMENT

1. Identify the cues (defining characteristics) for the nursing diagnosis and place into data clusters.

_____

_____

_____

_____

_____

_____

_____

_____

_____

_____

_____

_____

ANALYSIS (DIAGNOSIS)

2. Identify the two priority nursing diagnoses (based on NANDA and written in three-part format).

_____

_____

_____

_____

3. Which data definitely need further discussion with the patient?

_____

_____

_____

_____

OUTCOME IDENTIFICATION

4. Identify the outcome desired and the indicators (based on NOC) that the outcomes have been achieved.

_____

_____

_____

_____

PLAN

5. Develop a nursing plan of care based on this patient's current health care needs.

_____

_____

_____

_____

IMPLEMENTATION

_____

_____

_____

_____

EVALUATION

_____

_____

_____

_____

See the Answer Key in Appendix A for sample answers for this exercise.

Lippincott's Interactive Care Plan Creator

Name: _____

Client Initials: _____

ID: _____

Admission Date: _____

Course: _____

Age: _____

Sex: _____

Instructor: _____

Date: _____

MEDICAL DIAGNOSES	NURSING DIAGNOSES	PATIENT OUTCOMES/GOALS	NURSING ACTIVITIES	RATIONALE	EVALUATIONS

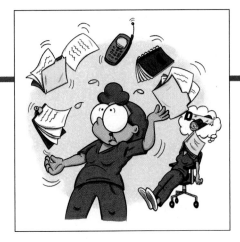

CHAPTER 6

DELEGATION

OBJECTIVES

1. Define delegation.

2. Analyze the legal and regulatory relationships of delegation and supervision.

3. Describe factors the nurse must consider before delegation.

4. Identify the five rights of delegation.

5. Explain the procedure to select the right person for the right task.

6. Identify the process necessary to achieve desired outcomes in the plan of care.

7. Assign patients based on desired outcomes in the plan of care.

8. Describe ways to facilitate performance of tasks by the delegate.

9. Describe the procedure for comparing accomplished tasks with the plan of care outcomes.

Delegation is an essential decision-making skill, necessary for the effective use of available personnel. The need to transfer tasks to another individual is a reality in the world of work. One person can only do so much. The appropriate use of human resources is critical in the health care industry to produce cost-effective care with an acceptable quality of patient outcomes. Today's patients tend to have complex health care needs requiring a higher level of care. To meet the demand, nurses are increasingly being asked to coordinate care with unlicensed assistive personnel (UAP) because fewer institutions are using primary care nursing. This trend is expected to continue because of nationwide concern over health care costs.

DEFINITION

Delegation is "transferring to a competent individual the authority to perform a selected nursing task in a specific situation. The nurse retains accountability for the delegation" (National Council of State Boards of Nursing [NCSBN], 1995, p. 2). Central to the definition of delegation is the concept that the nurse retains accountability. To be accountable is to be legally responsible.

The nurse delegating the task (the *delegator*) remains accountable for the delegation and may be held liable for any related consequences. The delegator is held responsible for his or her own acts, the decision to delegate, an assessment of the situation, planning desired outcomes, providing proper communication and adequate supervision, and initiating any necessary corrective actions. The nurse must provide adequate supervision of individual patients to ensure progression toward the desired outcomes in their plan of care. Supervision has been defined by the NCSBN as the "provision of guidance or direction, evaluation and follow-up by the licensed nurse for the accomplishment of a nursing task delegated to unlicensed assistive personnel." (NCSBN, 1995, p. 1). The person accepting the task (the delegate) is answerable for his or her own acts, the decision to accept the delegation, and proper communication.

PRINCIPLES OF DELEGATION

Frequently, the registered nurse (RN) must delegate tasks when the skill levels of personnel are mixed. These levels may include UAP, licensed practical nurse/licensed vocational nurse (LPN/LVN), and RN staff members. Before delegation, it is essential to identify the roles of available staff. The RN is responsible for providing care to the public within the legal and professional standards of nursing practice. There are three distinct sources that provide guidelines for safe delegation.

The state (provincial) Nurse Practice Act provides the legal definition of nursing practice and the Scope of Practice for that state (province). Each state (province) varies in the definition, but the primary purpose of this law is to protect the health and safety of the public, while achieving quality patient outcomes. The duties of the state (provincial) Board of Nursing include the approval of nursing schools, the regulation of nursing practice, and the authority to grant and revoke licenses. Each state's (province's) Board of Nursing interprets and enforces the rules set forth in the Nurse Practice Act. Understanding legal authority, responsibilities, and accountability in the delegation process is essential to nursing practice. Nurses should be familiar with the delegation aspects of the Nurse Practice Act. A violation occurs when a nurse delegates responsibility to someone who does not have the appropriate qualifications. The Board of Nursing uses the National Council Licensure Examination (NCLEX) as an advance assessment of a graduate's knowledge and ability to apply the principles of delegation.

Standards of practice can be found in the Board of Nursing regulations, the American Nurses Association (ANA) literature, and the literature of other specialty organizations. Professional standards of

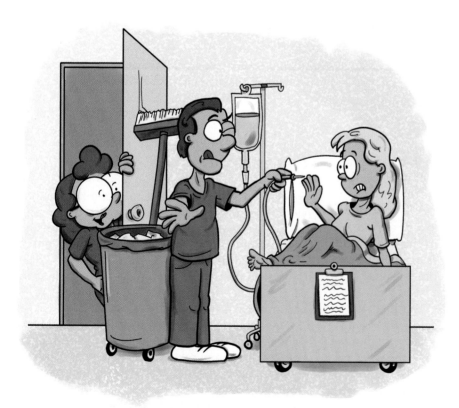

"We're a little short-handed right now, so Nurse Charles will insert your IV. Call if you need anything!"

practice have been set forth in *Nursing's Social Policy Statement* (ANA, 2003), *Nursing: Scope and Standards of Practice* (ANA, 2003), and the *Code for Nurses With Interpretive Statements* (ANA, 2001). These sources define standards of nursing care. They serve as a guide for practice decisions and are used to determine incompetent, unethical, or illegal practice.

Institutional policies and procedures and job descriptions are other sources of guidelines used in making delegation decisions. Each institution is charged with establishing standards of care to be applied within the facility. Accrediting bodies such as the Joint Commission on Accreditation of Healthcare Organizations (JCAHO) and state and local government regulators provide guidelines for these standards. The state legislature empowers the Board of Nursing to define and monitor nursing practice. If the agency policy conflicts with the Nurse Practice Act, the Act always prevails.

The delegator must also consider the job description of the delegate. Individuals cannot be expected to perform tasks above the expectations delineated in their job description. The individual competency of the caregiver should be evaluated before delegation. Caregiver competency includes level of experience and familiarity with performing the procedure involved. Performance evaluations are a part of the institution's responsibility as an ongoing assessment of staff ability. Standards for competency of individual caregivers are essential components for the institution to maintain.

As the issues of cost control and downsizing continue to be a major focus in health care, the rules for skill mix and competencies will continue to change. Every nurse must be responsible for the continued self-development and maintenance of his or her own competency.

Five Rights of Delegation

Before practicing delegation, the nurse must have a working knowledge of the five rights of delegation. The five rights are outlined by the NCSBN to assist the professional nurse in establishing the parameters for delegation. They are also intended to facilitate the delivery of safe and effective care while maximizing utilization of all available resources.

The five rights of delegation are:

1. Right task
2. Right circumstance
3. Right person
4. Right direction and communication
5. Right supervision and evaluation

RIGHT TASK

The delegator starts by determining the tasks that need to be completed. Decisions are then made regarding who should perform the task. The first criterion is that the task can be legally delegated as defined by the state (provincial) Nurse Practice Act and the ANA Standards of Care.

RNs should not delegate their own personal accountability for the patient outcome. Neither should they delegate management skills such as employee discipline, recognition, or praise. The nurse must not delegate nursing actions that require professional judgment, including teaching, assessment, decision making, priority setting, critical thinking, and the nursing process. The checklist developed by Huber (2000), depicted in Box 6-1, is a helpful tool that can be used to identify questions the nurse should ask before the act of delegation.

RIGHT CIRCUMSTANCE

The right circumstance pertains to factors related to patient condition. To delegate a task, the outcome of care needs to be reasonable and predictable, and the task must be one that does not require an ongoing assessment or critical decision making. Consideration is given to the plan of care, the individual patient needs, the desired outcomes, and the resources required to complete the care.

RIGHT PERSON

The RN is accountable and responsible for determining the best way to meet the patient's needs through the effective use of resources. Therefore, the RN may delegate to staff members with various levels of education and abilities. The job classification of each staff member should be considered before delegation. The comparison of the role of the LPN/LVN and the RN in the nursing process developed by Harrington, Smith, and Spratt (1996) is a useful aid for differentiating the role of the LPN/LVN (Table 6-1).

Box 6-1 Delegation Checklist
■ How is the task to be done?
■ When is the task to be done?
■ Where is the task to be done?
■ By whom is the task to be done?
■ What is the responsibility and authority for decision making (approves, is responsible, is consulted, is informed)?
Adapted from Huber, D. (2000). *Leadership and nursing care management.* Philadelphia: W. B. Saunders

TABLE 6-1

TABLE 6-1 COMPARISON OF THE ROLE PLAYED BY LICENSED PRACTICAL NURSES/LICENSED VOCATIONAL NURSES (LPN/LVNs) AND REGISTERED NURSES (RNs) IN THE NURSING PROCESS AND NURSING DIAGNOSIS

NURSING PROCESS PHASE	ROLE OF LPN/LVN	ROLE OF RN BEYOND LPN/LVN SCOPE OF PRACTICE
Assessment	Gather data Perform patient assessment Identify patient strengths	Gather more extensive bio-psychosocial data Group and analyze data Research additional data needed Identify client resources
Nursing diagnosis	Not applicable	Draw conclusions Use judgment Make diagnoses
Planning	Contribute to development of care plans	Set short- and long-term patient goals Establish priorities Collaborate and refer
Implementation	Provide basic therapeutic and preventative nursing measures Provide client teaching Record client information	Manage patient care (perform and delegate) Provide patient and family teaching Provide referrals Record and exchange patient information with health team
Evaluation	Evaluate effects of care given	Evaluate effectiveness of overall plan; analyze new data Modify, redesign plan Collaborate with other health team members

Adapted from Harrington, N., & Terry, C. L. (2003). *LPN to RN transitions* (p. 107). Philadelphia: Lippincott Williams & Wilkins.

The UAP requires special considerations. Unlicensed workers are regulated by each state; however, there are some common guidelines. The UAP is the least skilled of all the workers. Care delegated to the UAP should be for stable patients. Also, the patient's reaction to illness and hospitalization should not be threatening to his or her mental health. Examples of tasks that can be delegated to the UAP include bathing patients, making beds, taking routine vital signs, feeding patients, and transferring patients. Box 6-2 identifies guidelines for appropriate assignments for the UAP. The UAP is accountable for accepting the delegation and reporting to the RN information regarding areas in which the professional nurse has requested notifi-

cation. The UAP is also responsible and accountable for accomplishing the tasks assigned. The RN is responsible for supervision and follow-up of the care delivered by the UAP and for the definition of the parameters for reporting back to the RN. Defining these parameters includes providing specific guidelines for the worker to follow in performing the task and in reporting to the nurse. The following is an example of well-defined parameters: "At 12:00, take the vital signs on Mr. Green in Room 103." In addition to being clear and precise, the RN should identify any limitations such as, "Do not use the left arm for a blood pressure because the patient has a dialysis graft on that arm." Finally, the information should be very specific about what to do with the results. This may include reporting information with directions such as, "Report the readings to me, as soon as you have completed the vitals," or "Report the readings to me and record them on the clipboard at the nurse's station before the patient's lunch tray arrives." Being clear and precise with established limits and guidelines for reporting results minimizes the chance for a negative result.

Certain tasks can be delegated to the LPN/LVN. The primary role of the LPN/LVN is to provide nurs-

Box 6-2 UNLICENSED ASSISTIVE PERSONNEL SKILLS

Competencies: Basic nursing skills that include standard reoccurring procedures
Appropriate assignment: Predictable outcomes
Abilities: Performs care for routine procedures that demonstrate standardized outcomes; for example, feeding, bathing, routine vital signs, transferring patients

ing care for patients in structured health care settings, who are experiencing common, well-defined, health problems. The LPN/LVN must practice under the guidance of an RN or a licensed physician. The LPN/LVN has more competencies with technical skills than the UAP. An appropriate patient assignment for this level of staff would be one that involves care for a stable patient with a predictable outcome. Assignments may include delivering physical care to patients with more complex conditions, using selected treatments including sterile technique, and administering some medications. Medication delivery should be in accordance with the state (provincial) Nurse Practice Act and institutional policies. An example of a patient that could be delegated to an LPN/LVN is an individual admitted for a fractured femur who is in balanced suspension traction. Box 6-3 identifies appropriate assignments for the LPN/LVN.

Being an RN involves giving care by delegating to others. However, there are competencies that must remain RN duties. The RN possesses skill in assessment, evaluation, and the knowledge base for nursing judgment. The RN cannot give this responsibility away. An RN assignment would include the unstable patient with the least predictable outcome. Examples of more complex procedures that RNs perform include central line care, parenteral nutrition, blood infusion, patient-controlled analgesia, and the development of the plan of care.

The RN makes assignments based on the staff member's Scope of Practice and competency. Nursing activities that include the components of nursing process and require higher-level knowledge and judgment should not be delegated. The RN assignment includes performing the most complex procedures, applying the nursing process, and coordinating the plan of care. The RN also performs patient and family teaching, ensures appropriate documentation, and acts as a patient advocate. Box 6-4 outlines skills unique to the RN.

RNs are also responsible for directing and supervising care delivered by others. They must di-

---

Box 6-4 REGISTERED NURSE Skills

Competencies: Assessment, evaluation, clinical reasoning and nursing judgment

Appropriate assignment: Unstable patients with least predictable outcomes

Abilities: Acts as a patient advocate, directs and supervises care delivered by others, provides patient/family teaching, and collaborates with other health team members on the patient's behalf. The RN applies the nursing process and coordinates the plan of care; for example, the RN administers intravenous medications, interprets laboratory data, monitors patient for change in status, develops plans of care, and processes physician's orders

---

rect, manage, control, and make decisions about the treatment and interventions needed for patients assigned to their care. The delegator should assess the delegate's competency and the amount of supervision required.

While directing the work of others, the RN is acting in a supervisory capacity. The RN supervisory role includes encouragement, observation, support, and evaluation of care. When an RN is working with another RN and one is not designated as charge nurse, neither nurse is accountable for supervision of the other.

RIGHT DIRECTION AND COMMUNICATION

Communication is very important in the delegation process. In addition to identifying the task, the nurse must communicate expectations. The delegator needs to evaluate whether or not instructions were understood. Directions should be thorough and unambiguous. The four Cs of communication are clear, concise, correct, and complete. Questions that Hansten and Washburn (1994) identified to evaluate the four Cs are presented in Figure 6-1.

RIGHT SUPERVISION AND EVALUATION

When delegating, the nurse should use appropriate monitoring and provide feedback. While monitoring care delivery, the nurse is responsible for providing guidance and direction. Interventions necessary for achieving the desired outcomes are derived from the plan of care. Quality of care is evaluated by the patient's progress toward the desired outcomes.

Nursing Interventions Classification (NIC) 7650 provides standardized nursing activities to use in the delegation of tasks. These have been developed to facilitate patient safety and to achieve desirable patient outcomes. Box 6-5 identifies standard

---

Box 6-3 LICENSED PRACTICAL NURSE/LICENSED VOCATIONAL NURSE Skills

Competencies: Technical skills

Appropriate assignment: Stable patient with predictable outcomes

Abilities: Performs physical care for the more complex conditions; for example, sterile technique, selected treatments, and medication administration (depending on state Nurse Practice Act)

Four Cs of Initial Direction

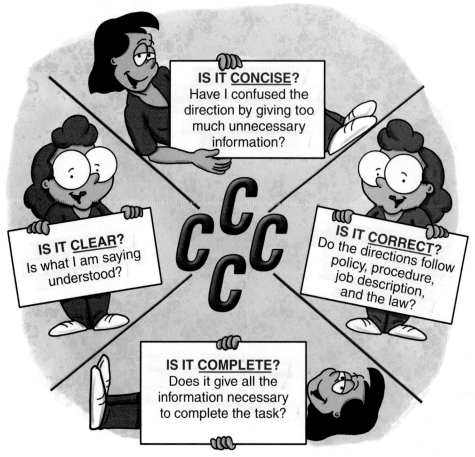

FIGURE 6-1

Four C's of initial direction. Adapted from Zerwekh, J., Claborn, J. C., & Miller, C. J. (1997). Concepts of nursing practice. *Basic care: memory notebook of nursing* (Vol. II). Dallas: Nursing Education Consultants.

Box 6-5 DELEGATION

Definition: Transfer of responsibility for the performance of patient care while retaining accountability for the outcome.

ACTIVITIES:

- Determine the patient care that needs to be completed.
- Identify the potential for harm.
- Evaluate the complexity of the care to be delegated.
- Determine the problem-solving and innovative skills required.
- Consider the predictability of the outcome.
- Evaluate the competency and training of the health care worker.
- Explain the task to the health care worker.

- Determine the level of supervision needed for the specific delegated intervention or activity (e.g., physically present or immediately available).
- Institute controls, so that the nurse can review the interventions or activities of the health care worker and intervene as necessary.
- Follow up with health care workers on a regular basis to evaluate their progress in completing the specific tasks.
- Evaluate the outcome of the delegated intervention or activity and the performance of the health care worker.
- Monitor the patient's and family's satisfaction with care.

Adapted from McCloskey, J. C., & Bulechek, G. M. (2000). *Nursing interventions classification (NIC)* (p. 244). St. Louis: Mosby.

---

nursing activities used in delegation. (McCloskey & Bulechek, 2000).

A well-developed plan of care is essential to directing the nurse's decisions regarding appropriate delegation. Although the Nursing Outcomes Classification (NOC) was developed to evaluate the patient's response, an appropriate application is to use the indicators in Decision Making (NOC 0906) when selecting optimum choices for patient care assignments. Table 6-2, developed by Johnson, Maas, and Moorhead (2000), identifies standard indicators used to evaluate the quality of a decision.

OBSTACLES TO DELEGATION

Three areas contribute to delegation failure. First, the delegator might be reluctant to take the risk and to give up control of every aspect of care. Second, the subordinate could fail to accept responsibility for the delegated duties. Finally, delegation failures could be related to workplace issues.

When work is delegated, there is risk taking and a loss of control. Getting caught in the "I can do it better myself" trap is an avoidance technique. In delegation, a lack of skill frequently results from the inability to direct, from low self-confidence, or from low-risk taking ability. Inadequate experience and education in delegating can also cause difficulties. Other behaviors that inhibit the delegation process are a lack of confidence in subordinates, a need to feel indispensable, and a fear of losing authority. It is demoralizing to subordinates when the manager undercuts their authority. Lack of time for delegation planning also inhibits appropriate application of this skill. Development of competent managerial skill is essential to being able to follow through with delegation.

When subordinates avoid the delegated responsibilities, several issues must be examined. The reluctance to accept responsibility may be due to fear of criticism for mistakes or lack of self-confidence. Another issue may be a lack of time. The manager may have given inadequate infor-

TABLE 6-2	DECISION MAKING (0906)

DOMAIN—PHYSIOLOGIC HEALTH (II)
CLASS—NEUROCOGNITIVE (J)
SCALE—NEVER DEMONSTRATED TO CONSISTENTLY DEMONSTRATED (M)

Definition: Ability to choose between two or more alternatives

DECISION MAKING	NEVER DEMONSTRATED 1	RARELY DEMONSTRATED 2	SOMETIMES DEMONSTRATED 3	OFTEN DEMONSTRATED 4	CONSISTENTLY DEMONSTRATED 5
INDICATORS					
090601 Identifies relevant information	1	2	3	4	5
090602 Identifies alternatives	1	2	3	4	5
090603 Identifies potential consequences of each alternative	1	2	3	4	5
090604 Identifies resources necessary to support each alternative	1	2	3	4	5
090605 Recognizes contradiction with others' desires	1	2	3	4	5
090606 Acknowledges social context of the situation	1	2	3	4	5
090607 Acknowledges relevant legal implications	1	2	3	4	5
090608 Weighs alternatives	1	2	3	4	5
090609 Chooses among alternatives	1	2	3	4	5
090610 Other _____ (Specify)	1	2	3	4	5

Adapted from Johnson, M., Maas, M., & Moorhead, S. (Eds.). (2000). *Nursing outcomes classification (NOC)*. St. Louis: Mosby.

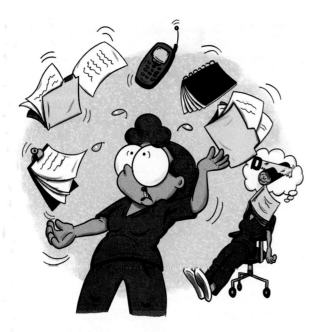

Delegate tasks when you're overloaded.

mation and resources to perform the assignment. The subordinate may sense a lack of trust from the manager. Positive incentives may be inadequate as motivators.

Other common barriers that interfere with the effective application of delegation skills include poorly written job descriptions and a lack of an adequate skill mix of assigned workers. Skills and competencies of the workers are further discussed in Chapter 11, Applying Nursing Judgment in Clinical Settings.

DELEGATION PROCEDURE

To delegate properly, the nurse needs a plan. Without a plan, it is difficult to reach the proper destination. Just as a road map is important for a journey, a plan is important for delegation. The plan for delegation utilizes the nursing process; that is, assessment, analysis, outcome identification, planning, implementation, and evaluation. The nurse needs to know what patient care is required in order to delegate these tasks. This is accomplished in the assessment phase. During the analysis phase, the nurse considers the patient's condition and the qualities of the delegate. The nurse should establish the desired outcomes in the outcome identification phase and assign patients to available personnel in the planning phase. Implementation involves the communication about the

assignment, supervision, and assistance. By the end of the shift, the nurse needs to evaluate outcomes.

ASSESSMENT

During this phase, the nurse creates a list of patient needs. The source of this list includes information gained from shift reports, the patient's record and plan of care, and, in some cases, an initial assessment. During assessment, the nurse should consider the circumstances surrounding the delegation. Factors such as the risk for harm, the stability of the patient, and the complexity of care required to complete the activities need to be considered. Other considerations include the degree of problem solving necessary for resolving each patient's needs and the amount of time the RN has available to the patients. The tool developed by Guido (2001) identifies some useful guidelines for making delegation decisions (Box 6-6).

The RN is responsible for assessing each patient to determine the plan of care. Next, the nurse must assess the available staff. A decision must be made about how best to use the available human resources to provide safe, competent, and effective care for every patient in the group.

Analysis

The nurse must analyze several factors before delegating care. Factors to consider include the level of care and the complexity of each assigned patient's needs. The physical status of the patient should lead to a determination of the level of care required. Pertinent questions also need to be answered, such as the following:

- Are the assessment needs highly complex, or would a simple assessment be adequate without compromising care?
- Is the stability of the patient expected to change?
- What are the risks for complications or change in status for this health state?
- What level of technology is required to complete the care?
- Do the care needs involve routine medication administration, sterile dressings, and catheter insertion, or are discharge planning, high-tech equipment use, or in-depth assessment skills required?
- If assignment is made to the UAP or LPN/LVN, is there adequate supervision available to ensure safe care?

Box 6-6 Guidelines: Delegation

ACTIONS THAT MAY BE DELEGATED INCLUDE THOSE THAT HAVE:

1. A low potential for harm.
2. Minimum complexity of nursing activity.
3. Minimum required problem solving and innovation.
4. High predictability of outcome.
5. Ample opportunity for patient interaction with the staff nurse.
6. Adequate RN ability to supervise the delegated activity and its outcome.

THE NURSE WHO DELEGATES THE ACTION IS RESPONSIBLE FOR:

1. Using a thoughtful decision-making process in deciding to delegate.
2. Providing clear and specific directions.
3. Individualizing the plan of care to meet the patient's unique needs.
4. Communicating the method of performance, expected outcomes, and parameters.
5. Supervising performance of the task.
6. Evaluating the patient outcome.

THE PERSON RECEIVING THE DELEGATION IS RESPONSIBLE FOR:

1. Demonstrating competence to perform the specific task.
2. Asking questions if directions are not understood.
3. Following directions from the RN.
4. Following established protocols and guidelines.
5. Reporting observations and activities to the delegating staff member.

THE EMPLOYER, NURSE-MANAGER, OR SUPERVISOR IS RESPONSIBLE FOR:

1. Providing adequate staffing and other resources needed for safe and effective patient care.
2. Following up on every report of concern for safe staffing or concern for safe practice and taking steps to correct situations that prevent safe or effective care.
3. Providing education and orientation to all employees, including education on delegation.

Adapted from Guido, G. W. (2001). *Legal and ethical issues in nursing* (p. 354). Upper Saddle River, NJ: Prentice Hall.

■ Does the staff have training for specialized procedures such as electrocardiogram interpretation, disease-specific isolation precautions, or central lines that may be needed to provide care for this specific group of patients?

Health care workers should only be assigned duties that they can legally perform. The job description outlines the duties that can be assigned to each category of health care worker. The experience and ability of available health care workers must also be considered, along with the availabil-

ity of resources, including adequate supervision. A tool such as the Delegation Decision-Making Grid developed by the NCSBN should be consulted (Figure 6-2). This tool facilitates the assessment of the level of patient stability, level of UAP competence, level of licensed nurse competence, potential for harm, frequency with which the UAP has performed the task, level of decision making, and ability for self-care (NCSBN, 1997b).

OUTCOME IDENTIFICATION

At this time, the nurse should establish priorities for each patient. A discussion of this process is can be found in Chapter 4, Priority Setting.

Using the list of patient needs prepared in the assessment phase, the nurse develops outcomes for each of the patient's nursing diagnoses. Identification of the tasks or processes necessary to achieve the outcome helps the RN determine which health care worker should receive the assignment.

PLAN

In the planning phase, the nurse specifies the nature of each task and the knowledge and skills required to perform it safely. Patient care requirements must be compared with available human resources. Making assignments based on the expertise and experience of the available staff will produce maximum productivity and cost-effective results. After tasks necessary to achieve the desired outcome have been formulated, the nurse should assign patients to available personnel.

ASSIGNMENT PROCESS EXERCISE

Consider the scenarios listed below. These patients have been selected to allow the student to practice the application of the delegation checklist. Individual nursing diagnoses along with the desired outcomes are provided for each scenario.

SCENARIO: ROOM 101

A 79-year-old woman with a history of type 1 diabetes mellitus was admitted for a right modified radical mastectomy. The biopsy was positive for ductal cell carcinoma. One day after surgery, she is given a patient-controlled analgesia(PCA) pump for pain control, infusing intravenous (IV) fluids, intravenous antibiotics (IVABs), two wound drainage devices, and a dressing over the incision. Her

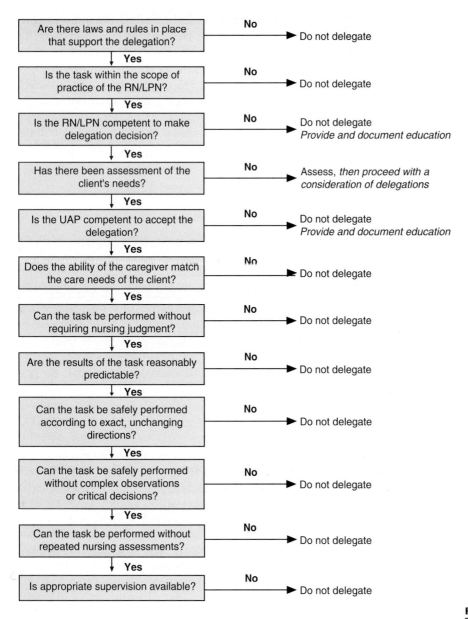

Are there laws and rules in place that support the delegation? — **No** → Do not delegate

↓ **Yes**

Is the task within the scope of practice of the RN/LPN? — **No** → Do not delegate

↓ **Yes**

Is the RN/LPN competent to make delegation decision? — **No** → Do not delegate
Provide and document education

↓ **Yes**

Has there been assessment of the client's needs? — **No** → Assess, *then proceed with a consideration of delegations*

↓ **Yes**

Is the UAP competent to accept the delegation? — **No** → Do not delegate
Provide and document education

↓ **Yes**

Does the ability of the caregiver match the care needs of the client? — **No** → Do not delegate

↓ **Yes**

Can the task be performed without requiring nursing judgment? — **No** → Do not delegate

↓ **Yes**

Are the results of the task reasonably predictable? — **No** → Do not delegate

↓ **Yes**

Can the task be safely performed according to exact, unchanging directions? — **No** → Do not delegate

↓ **Yes**

Can the task be safely performed without complex observations or critical decisions? — **No** → Do not delegate

↓ **Yes**

Can the task be performed without repeated nursing assessments? — **No** → Do not delegate

↓ **Yes**

Is appropriate supervision available? — **No** → Do not delegate

FIGURE 6-2

Delegation decision-making tree. Adapted from National Council of State Boards of Nursing, Inc. (1997).

Note: Authority to delegate varies, so licensed nurses must check the jurisdiction's statutes and regulations. RNs may need to delegate to the LPN the authority to delegate to the UAP.

orders include a Glucoscan with sliding scale insulin and incentive spirometry every 2 hours.

Nursing Diagnoses

Acute pain related to (R/T) tissue trauma, interruption of nerves, and dissection of muscles secondary to surgery as evidenced by (AEB) stiffness, numbness in chest, shoulder and arm pain rated at 5 to 6 on a 1 to 10 scale by patient

Deficient knowledge regarding ongoing care of disease process, care of the incision and drains, follow-up care related to surgical intervention R/T lack of exposure AEB patient's questions and requests for information

Risk for disuse syndrome R/T upper extremity immobilization secondary to tissue trauma, interruption of lymph flow causing lymphedema, radiation-related injuries, or wound infection after surgery

Desired Outcomes

Within 24 hours of discharge, patient will begin to participate in exercises and verbalize pain

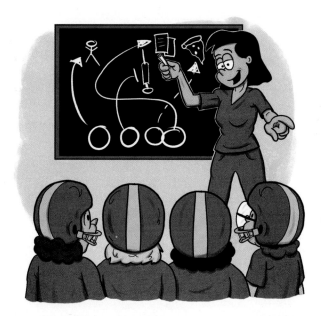

"Connie, go long and interview. Joyce, you know the filing system. Carlos has time for the blood work, and Myra can order lunch. Hut!!"

reduction to less than 3 on a 1 to 10 scale, with oral pain medications.

Within the 24-hour period before hospital discharge, patient will verbalize understanding of disease process, home care of drains, medication, care of surgical incision, potential for complications, and follow-up care necessary to protect the hand and arm.

Before discharge, patient will verbalize understanding of rehabilitation and exercises necessary to put hand, arm, and shoulder through expected range of motion.

SCENARIO: ROOM 102

A 64-year-old male, with a history of type 1 diabetes mellitus and above the knee amputation was admitted 3 days ago with cellulitis of the left stump. Treatments include wet to dry dressings of the left lower extremity, saline lock, IVABs, and fluid restrictions. His orders include Glucoscan with sliding scale insulin and he can be up with assistance.

Nursing Diagnoses

Ineffective peripheral tissue perfusion R/T poor venous circulation secondary to the diabetes mellitus AEB pallor, cyanosis, and presence of infection in stump

Deficient knowledge R/T ongoing care of disease process, care of the incision and infection, medication, and home management AEB

verbalization about lack of understanding of home management

Desired Outcomes

Before discharge, patient will have adequate perfusion AEB absence of pallor and cyanosis; evidence of healing of incision.

Within 24 hours of discharge, patient will demonstrate proper dressing change and verbalize understanding of home care management and follow-up care.

SCENARIO: ROOM 103

A 78-year-old woman with type 1 diabetes mellitus and a history of Alzheimer's disease was admitted with adrenal insufficiency. Treatments include IV fluids, IVABs, fluid restrictions, calorie count, Foley catheter to drainage, and Glucoscan with sliding scale. She has chronic confusion and stage 2 decubitus to the coccyx; with a walker and assistance of one person, she is able to ambulate.

Nursing Diagnoses

Deficient fluid volume R/T active loss through diuresis secondary to adrenal disease AEB low blood pressure, dry mucous membranes, poor skin turgor, and abnormal electrolytes

Infection R/T impaired immune system secondary to decreased adrenal function and poor venous circulation secondary to diabetes mellitus AEB purulent drainage from decubitus on coccyx

Ineffective protection R/T potential for addisonian crisis

Desired Outcomes

Within 24 hours of hospital admission, patient will have stabilized fluid volume AEB balanced intake and output, urinary output of more than 30 mL/hour, vital signs within normal limits (WNL), stable blood pressure with position change, normal skin turgor, capillary refill time longer than 3 seconds, stable weight, and moist mucous membranes.

At discharge, signs of infection will subside AEB normothermia; clear, straw-colored urine; absence of abnormal breath sounds; and no further purulent drainage from coccyx

During hospitalization, the patient will be free of symptoms of addisonian crisis AEB normal temperature, normal heart rate (60 to 100 beats/min), normal breath sounds, and usual mental status, and patient will verbalize no complaints of headache, nausea, or vomiting.

SCENARIO: ROOM 104

A 61-year-old woman with a history of colon cancer and metastasis was admitted for a kidney stone. Two days after cystoscope, her treatments include IV fluids, IVABs, Foley to straight drainage and irrigate catheter as needed (PRN). She is up *ad lib*, and her temperature this morning was 102.6°F (39.2°C)

Nursing Diagnoses

Impaired urinary elimination R/T obstruction of the ureter secondary to tissue trauma AEB presence of Foley catheter, visible sediment in urine, and complaints of intermittent spasms and flank pain

Health-seeking behaviors regarding dietary regimen and its relationship to calculus (stone) formation

Desired Outcomes

Each shift, patient will have adequate urinary output AEB normal volume of urinary output and will report pain at less than 3 on a 1 to 10 scale, within 30 to 60 minutes after medication.

Before discharge, patient will verbalize knowledge of foods and liquids to limit in order to prevent calculus (stone) formation.

SCENARIO: ROOM 105

A 53-year-old woman was admitted for a laparoscopic cholecystectomy performed yesterday. Treatments include a saline lock and oral pain medication. She has Steri-Strips over the incision and probably will be discharged today.

Nursing Diagnoses

Deficient knowledge R/T home management of postoperative status secondary to cholecystectomy AEB verbalized questions about follow-up care and dietary prescription

Desired Outcomes

Before discharge, patient will verbalize knowledge about self-care, indicators to report to primary health care provider, components of a low-fat diet with gradual introduction of fats over 4 to 6 months, and follow-up care.

SCENARIO: ROOM 106

A 67-year-old woman was admitted for treatment of a rectal hemorrhage. She had a sigmoidoscopy with a polypectomy yesterday. She has a saline lock and probably will be discharged today.

Nursing Diagnoses

Deficient knowledge R/T self-care and discharge needs AEB questions and request for information.

Health-seeking behaviors regarding recommendations for follow-up diagnostic care for malignant polyps.

Desired Outcomes

Within 24 hours of discharge, patient will verbalize signs and symptoms that warrant notification of the health care provider, review limitations of activity, and indicate understanding of follow-up regimen.

Before hospital discharge, patient will verbalize accurate information about recommendations for follow-up preventive diagnostic care.

Before making assignments, the nurse must undertake a detailed analysis of the tasks and activities involved in these patient scenarios. When making assignments, it is essential to analyze the skills and activities necessary to achieve each outcome. The outcomes of the interventions are frequently used to determine who should do specific aspects of the care assignment. This method provides an effective means by which to evaluate whether the delegation is appropriate. Table 6-3 provides sample answers to using outcomes as a basis for delegation decisions.

The final step in the assignment process involves a written assignment sheet. The key question is: Who can perform each task? A well-developed plan of care guides the nurse in making appropriate delegation decisions. Box 6-7 contains a completed assignment sheet that breaks down the tasks assigned to each level of staff in these scenarios.

Using the outcomes as a guide assists the RN to measure the effectiveness of interventions at the end of the shift. Describing the expected outcomes enables the new nurse to recognize the desired results of nursing actions. When outcomes are not met, the plan should be reevaluated, modified, and changed to meet the patient's individual needs or condition.

IMPLEMENTATION

During this phase, communication and supervisory skills are key elements. Using the grid as a plan, the nurse delegates tasks. Now the nurse needs to facilitate the performance of these tasks. Clear and concise directions must be given to the delegate. Appropriate nursing interventions should

TABLE 6-3	Using Outcomes as a Basis for Delegation Decisions

PATIENT	OUTCOME	TASK/PROCESS	WHO WILL PERFORM IT?
Room 101	Patient will verbalize knowledge about disease process, home care of drains, medication, care of surgical incision, and potential complications.	Perform patient teaching and discharge planning.	RN: teaching plan
		Evaluate emotional status and coping mechanisms.	RN: evaluation and nursing judgment
		Collaborate with Reach for Recovery (breast cancer support group).	RN: collaborate with support group
	Within 24 hours of discharge, patient will verbalize pain reduction to less than 3 on a 1 to 10 scale, with oral pain medication.	Manage pain control with PCA pump.	RN: pain management for PCA
		Monitor fluid volume status.	LPN: data gathering and reporting
			RN: evaluate the fluid volume status
			LPN: collect data and report
			UAP: obtain intake and output and report
Room 102	Patient has adequate perfusion of left lower extremity.	Assess vital signs, monitor tissue perfusion, and quality of output.	RN: assessment and interpretation of data
			LPN: data gathering and reporting
			UAP: comfort measures and report of progress
		Monitor fluid volume status and fluid restrictions.	RN: evaluate the fluid volume status
			LPN: collect data and report
			UAP: obtain intake and output and report
		Manage diabetic control with Glucoscan and sliding scale insulin.	LPN: perform Glucoscan and give sliding scale insulin
		Perform wet to dry dressing change.	LPN: perform dressing change and report progress
	Patient will demonstrate proper dressing change and verbalize understanding of home care management and follow-up care.	Teach dressing change and home care of extremity.	RN: initial wound assessment
			RN: teaching plan
Room 103	Patient will maintain hemodynamic stability with normovolemia.	Monitor fluid volume status.	RN: evaluate the fluid volume status
			LPN: collect data and report
			UAP: obtain intake and output and report
		Manage diabetic control with Glucoscans and sliding scale insulin.	LPN: perform glucoscan and give sliding scale insulin
	Signs of infection will subside, with WBC returning to normal and patient becoming afebrile before discharge.	Perform initial baseline vital signs and assessment of wound; monitor labs.	RN: assessment and interpretation of data
			LPN: perform dressing change and report progress
		Collaborate with the dietitian.	RN: collaboration
		Monitor for change in vitals, alteration in mental status, headaches, nausea, and vomiting.	RN: assessment and interpretation of data
	Patient will be free of symptoms of addisonian crisis. Patient will have no hospital-acquired injuries.	Provide for safety needs.	All staff to monitor for safety

(continued)

PATIENT	OUTCOME	TASK/PROCESS	WHO WILL PERFORM IT?
Room 104	Patient has adequate urinary output and is pain free.	Monitor and manage pain with oral medication. Monitor fluid volume status.	RN: pain management for PCA LPN: data gathering and reporting RN: evaluate the fluid volume status LPN: collect data and report UAP: obtain intake and output and report
	Patient will verbalize knowledge about food and fluid to limit to prevent calculus formation.	Perform patient teaching and discharge planning.	
Room 105	Patient will verbalize knowledge about self-care, indicators to report to primary health provider, and follow-up care.	Prepare discharge plan and patient teaching.	RN: teaching plan
Room 106	Patient will demonstrate care of incision, indicators to report to primary health provider, and follow-up care. Patient will verbalize information and recommendations for follow-up diagnostic care related to diagnosis.	Prepare discharge plan and patient teaching.	RN: teaching plan RN: teaching plan LPN: provide pamphlets and review content

Adapted from Zerwekh, J., & Claborn, J. C. (2000). *Nursing today: Transitions and trends.* Philadelphia: W. B. Saunders.

Box 6-7   **Shift Assignment Sheet**

RN:

All initial assessments
All IVs and IV medications (101–106)
Discharge planning (101, 104–106)
Collaborate with dietitian (103, 108)
Monitor labs (101, 103)
Irrigate Foley PRN (104)
Collaborate with Reach for Recovery (101)
Wound assessment (103)
Patient teaching (all patients)
Pain management (101)
Plan work assignment for oncoming shift

LPN:

All medications (except IVs)
Glucoscan (101–103)
Dressing change (102)
Monitor and empty drains (101)
Manage pain (102–106)
Assist UAP with hygienic care

UAP:

Obtain vital signs and intake and output (all patients)
Hygienic care (all patients)
Assist with admissions, discharges, and transfers
Pass meal trays

*All staff to share answering call lights. All staff monitor for safety Room 103

be described. The delegate needs to understand the ability of the patient to participate in care and the role of ancillary departments. After the delegation, the nurse continues to monitor the progress of the patients toward outcomes specified in their plan of care.

The nurse provides assistance and support to the delegates being supervised. The delegate, in turn, needs to understand what to do to obtain assistance and what things to report to the nurse. The nurse listens carefully to the suggestions and concerns of the delegates. Expectations of job performance require communication and subsequent monitoring.

Evaluation

Evaluation is an essential step in the delegation process. At the end of the shift, outcomes are compared with the plan of care. If outcomes were not attained, the process is examined. Were the outcomes appropriately written? Were the tasks properly delegated? Did the delegation result in safe, effective care? Answers to these questions can lead to improvements in the delegation process.

Evaluation of care is sought from many sources. This usually includes input related to satisfaction with care from the patient and significant others. Input from other health care workers is also important. Direct observation is yet another source for the evaluation of care. The nurse communicates the results of the evaluation to workers on the next shift.

The nurse provides the delegates with positive or negative feedback on their job performance. If feedback is negative, it should be presented in a constructive manner.

SUMMARY

Delegation is an important nursing skill. It requires a systematic plan to ensure optimal patient care. The plan should be based on the nursing process.

Delegation is a skill that can be learned. Many of today's nurses were trained with an emphasis on primary nursing. Some were not taught the principles of delegation. Systematic delegation is a skill that can benefit professional practice. Over the years, employers have expressed concern about a deficiency of delegation skills with new graduates (Beasley, 1998; Cicatiello, 1974).

It is very important that patient care not be compromised as cost cutting and that productivity continue to be the driving force in health care. Other issues that are major concerns are early discharge without adequate preparation for self-care and short-staffing, which compromises patient outcomes. Another issue of concern is the lack of adequate time to assess and deliver care in certain situations, which interferes with the ability of the nursing staff to deliver care according to standards established by the profession and licensing bodies. Every nurse should have a working knowledge of the ANA Code of Ethics, the ANA Standards of Practice, and the ANA Standards of Performance.

For the student nurse, delegation practice gives a clearer picture of nursing roles and the scope of nursing practice. A delegation checklist has been provided at the end of this chapter to identify the essential steps in the delegation process. Students can use this checklist as a guide or use it in a lab setting accompanied by a scenario.

KEY POINTS

- Delegation is planning or controlling activities through others.

- Delegation does not transfer accountability.
- The state (provincial) Nurse Practice Act must be consulted to determine the legality of delegation.
- The delegated task must be included in the staff member's job description.
- The plan for delegation uses the nursing process.
- A list of patient needs is created in the assessment phase.
- In analysis, the characteristics of the health care worker and the patient condition are considered.
- The nurse develops a plan of care based on the desired outcome for each patient need.
- Tasks are delegated based on the patient stability and the predicted outcomes.
- During implementation, the nurse communicates expectations to team members.
- Support and supervision are provided for delegates.
- At the end of the shift, the delegation process is evaluated.

REFERENCES

American Nurses Association. (1996). *Registered professional nurses and assistive personnel.* Washington, DC: American Nurses Publishing.

American Nurses Association. (2001). *Code of ethics for nurses with interpretive statements.* Washington, DC: American Nurses Publishing.

American Nurses Association. (2003a). *Nursing: Scope and standards of practice.* Washington, DC: American Nurses Publishing.

American Nurses Association. (2003b). *Nursing's social policy statement.* Washington, DC: American Nurses Publishing.

Beasley, S. K. (1998). Employer ratings of competencies of licensed practical nurses. *Digital dissertations,* AAT 9916984 (DAI-A 60/01, p. 107, July 1999).

Cicatiello, J. S. A. (1974). Expectations of the associate degree nurses. *Journal of Nursing Education, 13*(2), 22–25.

Ellis, J., & Hartley, C. (2000). *Managing and coordinating nursing care.* Philadelphia: Lippincott Williams & Wilkins.

Guido, G. W. (2001). Legal and ethical issues in nursing. Upper Saddle River, NJ: Prentice Hall.

Hansten, R., & Washburn, M. (1998). *Clinical delegation skills.* Gaithersburg, MD: Aspen.

Hansten, R., & Washburn, M. (1994). *Clinical delegation skills: A handbook for nurses.* Gaithersburg, MD: Aspen.

Harrington, N., Smith, N. E., & Terry, C. (1996). *LPN to RN transitions.* Philadelphia: Lippincott-Raven.

Huber, D. (2000). *Leadership and nursing management.* Philadelphia: W. B. Saunders.

Johnson, M., Maas, M., & Moorhead, S. (Eds.). (2000). *Nursing outcomes classification (NOC)*. St. Louis: Mosby.

McCloskey, J. C., & Bulechek, G. M. (Eds.). (2000). *Nursing interventions classification (NIC)*. St. Louis: Mosby.

National Council of State Boards of Nursing (NCSBN). (1995). *Delegation: Concepts and decision-making process*. Chicago: Author.

National Council of State Boards of Nursing (NCSBN). (1997a). *Delegation decision-making tree*. Chicago: Author.

National Council of State Boards of Nursing (NCSBN). (1997b). *Delegation decision-making grid*. Chicago: Author.

Perry, A. G., & Potter, P. A. (2002). *Clinical nursing skills and techniques*. St. Louis: Mosby.

Swearingen, P. L. (2003). *Manual of medical-surgical nursing care: Nursing interventions and collaborative management*. St. Louis: Mosby.

Tappen, R., Weiss, S., & Whitehead, D. (2001). *Essentials of nursing leadership and management*. Philadelphia: F. A. Davis.

Zerwekh, J., Claborn, J. C., & Miller, C. J. (1997). *Basic care: Memory notebook of nursing* (Vol. II). Dallas: Nursing Education Consultants.

Zerwekh, J., & Claborn, J. (2000). *Nursing today: Transitions and trends*. Philadelphia: W. B. Saunders.

Student Worksheets

SKILL SHEET: DELEGATION

Purpose

To develop the student's skill in planning and directing the activity of others in the delivery of safe, effective, quality care to patients.

Objectives

The student will demonstrate the ability to:

1. List criteria the nurse must consider before delegation.
2. Identify the five rights of delegation.
3. Explain the procedure to select the right person for the right task.
4. Develop plan of care outcomes.
5. Assign patients based on plan of care outcomes.
6. List ways to facilitate performance of tasks by delegation.
7. Describe how to compare the tasks accomplished with the plan of care outcomes for evaluation.

Steps: Delegation*

ASSESSMENT

1. Make a list of patient care that needs to be completed.
2. Perform initial assessment of physical status if necessary to determine the needs of patients.

ANALYSIS

1. Examine the level of care and complexity of needs for each patient to be assigned.
2. Identify the experience and ability of the health care workers available to provide care.

OUTCOME IDENTIFICATION

1. Establish priorities of care.
2. Establish patient goals and outcomes desired.

PLAN

1. Determine level of skill required to provide safe and effective care for each patient.
2. Develop an assignment sheet for delegating tasks within the guidelines of the NCSBN decision-making tree.
3. Assign patients to the available personnel.
4. Assign the tasks within the scope of practice and job description of the delegate.
5. Assign the person most competent using the certification or licensure, job description, skills checklist, and demonstrated skill as a measuring tool.

IMPLEMENTATION

1. Give clear, concise, correct, and complete direction about the assignment to each caregiver.
2. Work collaboratively with the delegate by seeking input, recognizing efforts, and learning the delegate's solutions to the problem.
3. Supervise the delivery of care during the completion of the delegated task.
4. Provide assistance and support to the delegates in the performance of tasks.

EVALUATION

1. Evaluate the tasks accomplished with the plan of care outcomes.
2. Provide feedback on job performance to the delegates.

---

*Prior knowledge to complete this task includes a working knowledge of the Nurse Practice Act, familiarity and knowledge of the job description for each worker's classification, and knowledge and skill of available personnel.

 COMPETENCY VALIDATION: DELEGATION

COMPETENCY STATEMENT

1. Assesses all activities to be accomplished.
2. Delegates activities according to Nurse Practice Act, ANA Standards of Practice, ANA Standards of Performance, and protocol of the health care facility.
3. Delivers nursing care based on the established plan of care.

The student demonstrated the ability to do the following:

1. Identify all activities and care to be completed.
2. Perform initial assessment of physical status as necessary to determine the needs of the patients.
3. Identify the level of care and complexity of needs for each patient.
4. Identify the experience and ability of the health care team available to provide care using appropriate resources.
5. Develop the plan of care outcomes for each patient based on priorities and outcome criteria established.
6. Use the five rights to assign activities according to state (provincial) Nurse Practice Act, NCSBN decision-making tree, job description of each worker's classification, and knowledge and skill of available personnel.
7. Develop a realistic assignment for each worker that reflects a quantity of work that could be performed by an individual during a shift.
8. Give clear, concise, accurate, and complete direction to personnel to complete activities.
9. Supervise the delivery of safe and effective care for the delegated tasks, giving support and assistance for completion in a timely manner.
10. Review effectiveness of plan in the accomplishment of the identified plan of care outcomes.
11. Provide feedback on job performance to the delegates.
12. Document completion of assigned activities and the therapeutic and nontherapeutic effects.
13. Demonstrate accountability for own decision and actions and for nursing care delegated to peers and assistive personnel.

COMPETENT

- Understands reason for task and is able to perform task independently
- Understands reason for task but needs supervision
- Understands reason for task and is able to perform task with assistance

NOT COMPETENT

- Understands reason for task but performs task at provisional level
- Is unable to state reason for task and performs task at a dependent level

---

SKILL CHECKLIST: DELEGATION

DELEGATION	SATISFACTORY	UNSATISFACTORY	NI/COMMENTS
ASSESSMENT			
1. Make a list of patient care that needs to be completed.			
2. Perform initial assessment of physical status if necessary to determine the needs of patients.			
ANALYSIS			
1. Examine the level of care and complexity of needs for each patient to be assigned.			
2. Identify the experience and ability of the health care workers available to provide care.			
OUTCOME IDENTIFICATION			
1. Establish the desired outcomes for each nursing diagnosis in the plan of care.			
2. Prioritize the desired outcomes for each patient.			
PLAN			
1. Determine level of skill required to provide safe and effective care for each patient.			
2. Develop an assignment sheet of patients for available personnel.			
IMPLEMENTATION			
1. Give clear, concise, correct, and complete direction about the assignment to each caregiver.			
2. Supervise the delivery of care during the completion of the delegated task.			
3. Provide assistance and support to the delegates in the performance of tasks.			
EVALUATION			
1. Evaluate the tasks accomplished with the desired outcomes for the plan of care.			
2. Provide feedback on job performances to the delegates.			

SCENARIOS TO ACCOMPANY STUDENT WORKSHEETS

Consider the following patient scenarios. The individual nursing diagnoses with expected outcomes have been identified. Carefully review each patient. The Activity Sheets are presented in the appropriate order for completion.

SCENARIO: ROOM 101

An 83-year-old woman with a history of Alzheimer's disease was admitted for a gastrointestinal bleed. Her orders include nothing by mouth (NPO) for an esophagogastroduodenoscopy (EGD), Foley catheter and a saline lock, and hemoglobin and hematocrit tests every 12 hours. The next lab draw is scheduled for 10:00 AM.

NURSING DIAGNOSES

Ineffective protection R/T potential reoccurrence of bleeding and obstruction secondary to scar tissue formation

Deficient knowledge regarding EGD R/T lack of exposure AEB questions by patient's family and request for more information

Risk for injury R/T lack of awareness of hazards secondary to cognitive impairment

DESIRED OUTCOMES

Within 24 hours of discharge, the patient will be free of symptoms of bleeding AEB negative occult test, stable hemoglobin and hematocrit, passing stool and flatus, and soft, nondistended abdomen.

Before the EGD, the patient's family will verbalize their understanding of potential complications and follow-up care before signing the informed consent.

The patient will be free of physical injury during hospitalization.

SCENARIO: ROOM 102

A 39-year-old woman was admitted for a right modified radical mastectomy. Two days after surgery, the patient-controlled analgesia (PCA) and IV fluid line is to be removed. She has a saline lock, a wound drainage device in the incision line, and a dressing over the incision. Her activity is as tolerated.

NURSING DIAGNOSES

Acute pain R/T tissue trauma, interruption of nerves, and dissection of muscles secondary to surgery AEB stiffness, numbness in chest, shoulder and arm pain rated at 4 to 5 on a 1 to 10 scale by patient

Deficient knowledge R/T ongoing care of disease process, care of the incision and drains, follow-up care related to surgical intervention, and lack of exposure AEB patient's questions and requests for information

Risk for disuse syndrome R/T upper extremity immobilization secondary to tissue trauma, interruption of lymph flow causing lymphedema, radiation-related injury, or wound infection after surgery

DESIRED OUTCOMES

Within 24 hours of discharge, the patient will begin to participate in exercises and verbalize pain reduction to less than 3 on a 1 to 10 scale, with oral pain medications.

Within the 24-hour period before hospital discharge, the patient will verbalize understanding of disease process, home care of drains, medication, care of surgical incision, potential for complications, and follow-up care necessary to protect the hand and arm.

Before discharge, the patient will verbalize understanding of rehabilitation and exercises to put hand, arm, and shoulder through expected range of motion.

SCENARIO: ROOM 103

A 43-year-old woman with a history of end-stage renal disease (ESRD) who receives dialysis treatments was admitted with a clotted left arm arteriovenous (AV) graft. She also has a history of type 1 diabetes mellitus. Her orders include a saline lock, Glucoscans with sliding scale insulin, and NPO for a surgical declotting procedure.

NURSING DIAGNOSES

Ineffective peripheral tissue perfusion R/T interrupted blood flow AEB clotting in the vascular access
Deficient knowledge R/T impending surgical procedure AEB patient's questions

DESIRED OUTCOMES

After surgical intervention, the patient will have adequate tissue perfusion AEB positive bruit and thrill in the left arm AV graft and warmth and sensation in left hand.
Before signing the informed consent, the patient will verbalize understanding of procedure and complications.

SCENARIO: ROOM 104

A 64-year-old woman with a history of lung cancer was admitted for dehydration secondary to intractable nausea, vomiting, and diarrhea. Her orders include IV fluids, stool specimen, and NPO for an ultrasound of the gallbladder.

NURSING DIAGNOSES

Deficient fluid volume R/T active loss through nausea, vomiting, and diarrhea secondary to chemotherapy AEB low blood pressure, dry mucous membranes, poor skin turgor, and abnormal electrolytes
Deficient knowledge R/T lack of exposure to diagnostic test AEB questions
Risk for infection R/T compromised immunologic status secondary to chemotherapy

DESIRED OUTCOMES

Within 24 hours of hospital admission, the patient's fluid volume will have stabilized AEB balanced intake and output, urinary output of more than 30 mL/hour, vitals within normal limits WNL, stable blood pressure with position change, normal skin turgor, capillary refill time longer than 3 seconds, stable weight, and moist mucous membranes.
Patient will verbalize understanding of procedure and preparation before scheduled test.
At discharge, no signs of infection will be present AEB vital signs WNL; clear, straw-colored urine; and absence of abnormal breath sounds.

SCENARIO: ROOM 105

A 79-year-old man with a history of bladder and prostate cancer was admitted for altered level of conscious (LOC). His orders include IV fluids, IVABs, and consult with the nursing home for discharge. He is incontinent of bowels and bladder, alert to person only, and needs to be fed meals.

NURSING DIAGNOSES

Relocation stress syndrome R/T move to the nursing home and unpredictability of the experience AEB fear "they won't take care of me like I get here" and worry about impending transfer verbalized by patient

DESIRED OUTCOME

By discharge, patient will demonstrate effective coping strategies AEB verbalized comfort with the move.

Scenario: Room 106

A 42-year-old woman was admitted with Crohn's disease exacerbation, sepsis, and pyelonephritis. Her orders include IV fluids, IVABs, blood transfusion of 3 units, and hemoglobin and hematocrit tests after transfusion. She has a temperature of 100.3°F (37.9°C) and diarrhea, and Hemoccult test of stool is positive. Her current hemoglobin is 7.2 and hematocrit is 21.5.

NURSING DIAGNOSES

Deficient fluid volume R/T impaired absorption of fluid and active loss secondary to diarrhea AEB low blood pressure, increased pulse, abnormal electrolytes, low urinary output, and frequent liquid stools

Infection R/T lowered resistance associated with malnutrition and steroid treatments AEB elevated temperature, chills, and presence of pathogens in urine

DESIRED OUTCOMES

Within 24 hours of admission, patient will stabilize fluid volume AEB balanced intake and output, urinary output of more than 30 mL/hour, normal vital signs, stable blood pressure with position change, good skin turgor, capillary refill time of less than 3 seconds, moist mucous membranes, and diarrhea controlled.

Patient will be free from indicators of infection by discharge AEB normal vital signs; soft, nondistended abdomen; white blood cell count WNL; normal breath sounds; and normal urine specimen on recheck.

PATIENT	OUTCOMES	TASK/PROCESS	WHO WILL PERFORM IT?
Room 101	Within 24 hours of discharge, the patient will be free of symptoms of bleeding AEB labs and physical data. Before the EGD, the patient will verbalize understanding of the procedure, complications, and follow-up care before signing the informed consent. The patient will have no hospital-acquired injuries.		
Room 102	Within 24 hours of discharge, the patient will verbalize pain reduction to less than 3 on a 1 to 10 scale with oral pain medications. Within 24 hours of discharge, the patient will verbalize knowledge about disease process, home care of drains, medication, care of the surgical incision, and potential complications.		
Room 103	After surgical intervention, perfusion of left arm and hand will be adequate AEB a positive bruit and thrill. The patient will verbalize understanding of the need for an AV graft revision and the risks, benefits, and complications involved before signing the consent form.		
Room 104	Within 24 hours of discharge, the patient will have vital signs WNL and other signs of stable fluid volume. No signs of infection will be present on discharge.		
Room 105	By discharge, the patient will demonstrate effective coping strategies AEB diminished anxiety with the transfer.		
Room 106	Within 24 hours of discharge, the patient will have vital signs WNL and other signs of stable fluid volume. Signs of infection will subside, with white cell count returning to normal and patient becoming afebrile before discharge.		

Adapted from Zerwekh, J., & Claborn, J. C. (2000). *Nursing today: Transitions and trends*. Philadelphia: W. B. Saunders.

The final step in the process involves a written assignment sheet. Who can perform each task?

RN:
LPN/LVN:
UAP:

See the Answer Key in Appendix A for sample answers to this exercise.

PRACTICE EXERCISES: DELEGATION

 SCENARIOS: DELEGATING TASKS

SCENARIO 1

You are the RN for a team of 14 patients. Your members include one LPN/LVN and one UAP. The patients include a newly admitted patient who needs to be prepared for the operating room, a new postoperative cholecystectomy patient, and two patients 1 day after appendectomy who need to be ambulated.

1. Identify the tasks for the new admission that could be delegated to the UAP.

_____

_____

_____

The following tasks need to be completed during your shift in addition to other tasks of assessing patients, passing medications, completing documentation, processing physician's orders, and performing discharge planning.

A. Teach a patient to give own insulin
B. Assist the physician with a paracentesis
C. Write the plan of care for a newly admitted patient
D. Perform wound assessment and photo-documentation
E. Perform blood glucose tests for three patients
F. Phone report of labs to the physician
G. Insert Foley catheter
H. Collect intake and output data
I. Evaluate patient response to pain medication

2. Identify those tasks that you as the RN could not delegate and explain why.

_____

_____

_____

3. Identify those tasks that you could delegate to an experienced LPN/LVN who has demonstrated competent skills.

_____

_____

_____

_____

_____

_____

4. The RN delegates the vital signs, baths, and intake and output for eight patients to the UAP. What is the RN's accountability for the delegated work?

_____

_____

_____

5. Describe the directions and communication you would use in defining the patient parameters to be reported by the UAP.

_____

_____

_____

_____

_____

See the Answer Key in Appendix A for sample answers to this exercise.

Scenario 2

You are the RN on a 32-bed adult medical-surgical unit for the evening shift. You have been working on the unit for 4 months since you completed a 6-week orientation program after graduating from nursing school. Your assignment this evening includes 14 patients on your team. You have yourself, one LPN/LVN with 6 years of experience, and one UAP with 10 years of experience on the unit. The unit secretary has called with a flat tire and will be 1 to 2 hours late reporting for duty.

In report, you learn that there are two postoperative patients complaining of nausea and one postoperative patient complaining of incisional pain who has not voided since returning to the unit 6 hours ago. A patient, 2 days after surgery, who just tore off her colostomy bag and is screaming that the nurses are trying to kill her. Another patient is complaining about a painful IV site. A new patient has just arrived from the emergency room with a diagnosis of asthma, and a geriatric patient from the nursing home requires feedings every 4 hours through a gastrointestinal tube and wound care for multiple decubitus ulcers on the coccyx and right hip.

1. Identify the tasks for the new admission that could be delegated to the UAP.

_____

_____

_____

The following tasks need to be completed during your shift in addition to other tasks of assessing patients, passing medications, documentation, processing physician's orders, and discharge planning.

A. Incentive spirometry every 4 hours for postoperative patients
B. Pain management for postoperative patients
C. Remove IV from painful IV site
D. Restart IV
E. Apply oxygen setup for new admission
F. Obtain oxygen saturation level on new admission
G. Perform admission assessment on new admission
H. Develop plan of care for new admission
I. Perform blood glucose tests for two patients
J. Administer tube feeding every 4 hours for geriatric patient
K. Perform wound reassessment and dressing changes for decubitus sores

2. Identify those tasks that you as the RN could not delegate and explain why.

_____

_____

_____

_____

3. Identify those tasks that you could delegate to the LPN/LVN.

_____

_____

_____

_____

4. Identify those tasks that you would delegate to the UAP.

_____

_____

_____

_____

See the Answer Key in Appendix A for sample answers to this exercise.

EVALUATING SKILLS AND COMPETENCIES OF THE CAREGIVER

First, describe the desired outcome for each patient; then determine interventions necessary to achieve the outcome. Next, identify the skills needed to accomplish the tasks required to complete the activities in the assignment. Determine appropriate assignments based on physical status, stability, and acuity level of the patient. Place the abbreviation for the appropriate caregiver assignment in the space using the following: UAP, LPN/LVN, RN.

1. An 11-year-old female diabetic patient running a blood sugar of 800 is severely dehydrated.

_____

2. A 67-year-old female patient with a gastrointestinal tube for feeding with a diagnosis of congestive heart failure and debilitating arthritis

_____

3. An 89-year-old female patient with bladder incontinence and a diagnosis of dementia who needs hygienic care

_____

4. A 52-year-old female patient experiencing abdominal discomfort and abdominal distention, who has had 50 mL urine output in past 24 hours

_____

5. A 14-year-old patient admitted 2 days ago with a tibial fracture and an external fixator that requires pin site care

_____

6. An 85-year-old patient, 2 days after gastrointestinal tube placement, with a methicillin-resistant *Staphylococcus aureus* (MRSA)–positive culture, who needs a dressing change to a pressure ulcer to the coccyx

_____

7. A 36-year-old female patient, 2 days after appendectomy, who needs to be ambulated

_____

8. A 78-year-old patient, admitted with a fractured hip, 4 days after surgery, who requires a sterile dressing change

_____

9. A new colostomy patient who requires fitting of the appliance and the first irrigation procedure

_____

10. A 38-year-old patient, 2 days after an above-the-knee amputation, who is receiving peritoneal dialysis

_____

11. A 29-year-old female patient admitted for a cardiac catheterization today, in need of an informed consent, lab work to be drawn, and patient teaching

_____

12. A patient with a right-sided cerebral vascular accident who requires assistance with feeding

_____

13. A 46-year-old new-onset diabetes patient being discharged today

_____

14. A 37-year-old female patient in need of a blood glucose test before meals (ac) and at bedtime (hs)

_____

15. A 29-year-old patient, 2 days after a right total-knee operation, in need of having intake and output recorded

_____

16. A 33-year-old female patient, 3 days after an open-reduction, internal-fixation right leg operation, who needs the catheter discontinued today

_____

17. A 27-year-old male patient positive for hepatitis C, with urine positive for illegal drugs, who is threatening to leave against medical advice if he "doesn't get pain medication now"

_____

18. An 89-year-old female patient admitted with dementia and urinary incontinence needing hygienic care

_____

19. A 24-year-old patient, 2 days after appendectomy, who needs vital signs taken

_____

20. A 21-year-old patient, 2 days after appendectomy, who ran a fever last night and needs to be ambulated today

_____

See the Answer Key in Appendix A for sample answers to this exercise.

CHAPTER 7

COMMUNICATION

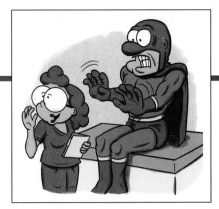

OBJECTIVES

1. List the three levels of communication.
2. Define collaboration and how it relates to nursing care.
3. Describe the important aspects of communicating during delegation.
4. Explain the steps involved in giving change-of-shift report.
5. Delineate methods for conflict resolution.
6. Describe the procedure for contacting a physician.
7. List important items that are included in the documentation of patient care.

An essential element of the critical thinking skill is the organization and communication of thoughts. To communicate effectively, the nurse must be able to clarify and express his or her ideas and listen to the input of others. Communication is a skill that underlies many of the processes described in this book, including delegation, problem solving, and the nursing process.

LEVELS OF COMMUNICATION

There are three levels of communication: social, therapeutic, and collegial. Social communication involves interactions for the purpose of accomplishing tasks or building social relationships, such as friendships. During therapeutic communication, the nurse listens to patient problems and focuses on patient needs. Descriptions of these communication skills can be found in most introductory psychiatric nursing textbooks. The focus of this

chapter is on collegial communication, especially the skills that result in enhanced relationships with colleagues, improved patient care, and better documentation. Collegial communication can take place in both verbal and written forms. Nonverbal communication, including such things as body language, eye contact, and personal space, is an aspect of all three levels of communication. The astute nurse observes nonverbal communication closely.

Verbal Communication

The possibility of miscommunication exists with the verbal transmission of information. The person receiving the message hears it within the context of his or her own knowledge and past experiences. To correct this situation, the sender must give clear messages and, at the same time, verify that these messages are being accurately interpreted by the receiver.

Effective communication may be particularly difficult when the participants are from different cultures. In such situations, the nurse must accept different communication norms, seek to understand others, and verify that communication was successful.

The health care workforce is composed of individuals representing numerous cultures that vary in their beliefs and values. Andrews and Boyle (2003) include communication among the areas influenced by values. The areas listed include: "time orientation, family obligations, communication patterns (including etiquette, space/distance, touch), interpersonal relationships (including long-standing historic rivalries), gender/sexual orientation, education, socioeconomic status, moral/religious beliefs, hygiene, clothing, meaning of work, and personal traits" (p. 373). The effects of cultural values on communication range from distance between conversational participants to meanings placed on individual words. An example of cultural differences is the use of eye contact. Some cultures value steady eye contact and view it as a sign of interest or honesty. Others believe that steady eye contact is disrespectful. An increased knowledge of other cultures enhances collegial communication.

COLLABORATION

Many verbal exchanges in health care settings involve collaboration. A useful definition of collaboration is "two or more people working together to a common end" (Adams & Jones, 2000, p. 220). Nurses collaborate with nursing personnel and other health care workers to improve patient care. Failure to communicate effectively can result in serious consequences. For example, a nurse's failure to communicate deterioration in a patient's condition could have severe repercussions for the patient. The nurse must keep all involved personnel apprised of changes by using effective communication.

Nursing Personnel

With the ultimate goal of quality care, nursing personnel must function as a team. Communication is the basis for effective team building. Nurses routinely communicate patient needs, outcomes, and goals. This is best accomplished in an atmosphere of openness and honesty. The team must embrace the diversity and creativity of its members, recognizing that each individual has strengths and weaknesses. A well-functioning team uses this individuality to its advantage. For instance, the team member who writes well may be assigned the job of composing meeting plans or notes. A creative member might prefer to generate options to solve a problem. Team members should feel comfortable with their role; respect underlies this collegial relationship. In Table 7-1, Alfaro-LeFevre (1999) lists behaviors that can enhance or impede interpersonal relationships.

DELEGATING

One advantage to working as a team is that tasks can be accomplished more quickly by a group than by an individual. An important key to effective teamwork is the assignment of individual duties. The principles of delegation must be considered when making assignments. Delegation is covered more thoroughly in Chapter 6, Delegation. However, because communication is a vital aspect of delegation, some key concepts will also be discussed in this chapter.

When delegating a task, the nurse is responsible for ensuring that the right direction or communication is given. It is one of the five rights of delegation (National Council of State Boards of Nursing [NCSBN], 1995). The five rights of delegation (right task, right circumstance, right person, right communication, and right supervision and evaluation) are discussed in Chapter 6.

To accomplish effective communication, instructions should be given clearly. These instructions commonly include a timeline for completion, the expected outcome, and any necessary performance guidelines. For example, consider the following effective communication: "Before noon, I want you to ambulate Mr. Jones to the door of his room. Be sure to use the gait belt and his walker." The delegate also needs to be given any parameters that require reporting. For example: "He should be able to do that without any shortness of breath. If he becomes short of breath, assist him back to bed. Then notify me immediately." Or, the communicator might say: "Please notify me immediately if Mr. Smith's blood pressure drops below 106/70." At times, the delegate may nod or indicate understanding, when in fact, instructions were not completely understood. The nurse should observe for this occurrence. If there is any doubt that the communication was understood, it may be appropriate to ask the delegate to repeat or write down the instructions. The nurse may also ask questions to verify that the communication was understood. However, these questions should not be ones that can be answered with one word.

TABLE 7-1   Behaviors Enhancing and Impeding Interpersonal Relationships

BEHAVIORS THAT ENHANCE INTERPERSONAL RELATIONSHIPS	BEHAVIORS THAT INHIBIT INTERPERSONAL RELATIONSHIPS
Conveying an attitude of openness	Conveying an attitude of doubt, mistrust, or negative judgment
Being honest	Giving false information
Taking initiative and responsibility	Conveying an "it's not my job" attitude
Being reliable	Not meeting commitments, only partially meeting commitments, or not being punctual
Demonstrating humility	Demonstrating self-importance
Showing respect for what others are, have been, or may become	"Talking down," or assuming familiarity
Accepting accountability	Making excuses or placing blame where it doesn't belong
Being confident and prepared	Being unsure, and trying to "wing it"
Showing genuine interest	Acting like you're only doing something because it's a job
Conveying appreciation for others' time	Assuming others have more time than you do
Accepting expression of positive and negative feelings	Demonstrating annoyance when negative feelings are expressed
Taking enough time	Rushing
Being frank and forthright	Sending mixed messages, saying things just because you think it's what the other person wants to hear, or talking behind others' backs
Admitting when you've been wrong	Denying or ignoring when you've made an error
Apologizing if you've caused distress or inconvenience	Acting like nothing happened or making excuses

Adapted from Alfaro-LeFevre, R. (1999). *Critical thinking in nursing: A practical approach* (p. 221). Philadelphia: W. B. Saunders.

Questions with one-word answers are called *closed questions*. It is generally more difficult to ascertain understanding with closed questions.

Report Skills

An important aspect of communication among nursing personnel is "giving report." At the end of each shift, nurses report essential information about the assigned patients to nurses working the next shift. The purpose of this report is the continuity of care. For instance, if one nurse discovers that an activity is particularly beneficial to the patient, this knowledge should be shared with the next shift. The format for giving report can vary from institution to institution. The three most common methods of giving report are oral, audiotape, and walking rounds. Each method has its own advantages and disadvantages.

Oral report is a verbal exchange often occurring in a conference room. It permits immediate feedback on questions because both nurses are present. However, this form of report may take more time if nurses choose to socialize at the same time.

An audiotape report is sometimes more convenient because the end of shift is a very busy time. Nurses can tape their report close to the end of their shift, whenever time is available. Audiotaping also allows the novice nurse to edit or redo his or her report, resulting in a more organized delivery.

Walking rounds, conducted at the patient's bedside, is another popular form of report. A major advantage of this method is that it allows for patient and family input. The oncoming nurse can also perform a mini-assessment at the bedside at the same time. The two nurses can check such things as intravenous line site, type of fluids, oxygen concentration, and safety measures. One disadvantage of walking rounds may be a lack of privacy for the patient. The nurses may also need to speak in low tones so as not to disturb sleep.

The organization of patient information is a key element in any reporting method selected by an institution. Important facts may be written on special forms to facilitate report delivery. Recent changes in patient status or priority situations concerning patient conditions should be discussed during report.

Shift report can be organized by using the nursing process format. Box 7-1 contains a sample shift report following this format.

Under assessment, the nurse identifies demographic data such as patient name, age, room number, medical diagnosis, chief complaint, and physician. This information can be obtained from a written patient Kardex or a patient care profile (PCP). A PCP is used with computerized records. The nurse should also consult worksheets and treatment plans. The patient condition should then be assessed and information collected regarding

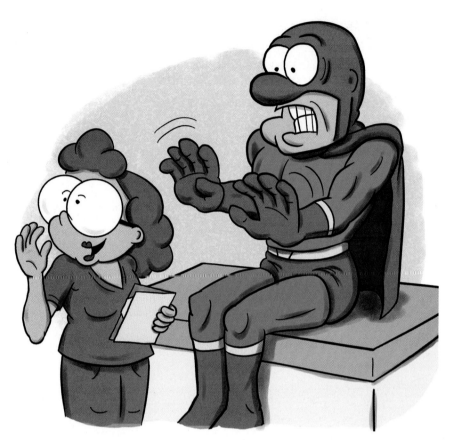

"Hey, everyone! Check it out! Captain Steroid's real identity is John Nerdly!"

completed and scheduled diagnostic tests, current nursing diagnoses, and significant health history. The information obtained should be analyzed for relevancy and significance to determine its appropriateness for report.

During planning, the nurse organizes and prioritizes the information obtained. The actual giving of report occurs in the implementation phase. Report should not consist of just reading the complete Kardex because the oncoming nurse has access to the Kardex. Instead, the following descriptions should be included in report: patient progress during the shift, therapies or treatments administered during the shift, patient teaching, the effectiveness of the discharge plan, consultations with other disciplines, the status of identified outcomes, and any changes in patient status.

Evaluation is an examination of report for factors such as organization, length of presentation, and thoroughness. The activities involved in shift report as identified in NIC 8140 can be found in Box 7-2. A performance checklist that can be used for shift report practice has been included as an exercise at the end of this chapter.

Interdisciplinary Communication

Interdisciplinary communication is the communication that occurs among practitioners from different disciplines. "To be effective and efficient, nurses must be willing and able to work collaboratively with other members of the health-care team to provide consistently high quality care to the consumer" (Bastable, 1997, p. 14). Nurses will have the opportunity to interact with other practitioners during multidisciplinary care conferences and during patient care delivery.

Just as establishing a good working relationship with other nursing personnel is important, a good rapport with individuals from other disciplines is also crucial. In both cases, communication begins with respect for the staff member and his or her role in the health care team. Some nurses lose sight of the contributions made by other disciplines.

Because good communication is the basis for quality care, nurses must share patient knowledge with other disciplines. For example, if the patient is cognitively impaired and requires special ob-

Box 7-1 Sample Shift Report Using the Nursing Process Format

Rosa Hernandez, 52 years of age, was admitted into Room 101 with a diagnosis of left leg deep vein thrombosis (DVT). Her chief complaint is pain and tenderness to her left calf.

ASSESSMENT:

Assess patient's physical and mental conditions.

Obtain worksheets from delegates, which may contain information such as vital signs and intake and output.

Consult the Kardex or treatment plan for previously recorded problems and nursing diagnoses.

Check the chart for test results.

Review information supplied in report received at beginning of shift.

ANALYSIS:

During the assessment, the nurse notes the following things:

Both hands are contracted. The patient discussed her history of rheumatoid arthritis.

The IV site has no signs of infiltration. The IV containing heparin is infusing at the required rate.

The left calf is reddened. It measures 2 cm larger in diameter than the right calf. Bilateral popliteal and pedal pulses are palpable.

The patient answered questions pleasantly.

She likes to cross her legs while in bed.

Her abdomen is soft.

She has a bunion at the base of the right great toe.

She has a scar from repair of a cleft lip as an infant.

The nurse decides the following data are not significant for this patient and will not be mentioned in report: presence of the bunion and the scar, condition of the abdomen, and pleasant attitude.

OUTCOME IDENTIFICATION:

The nurse wishes to deliver a concise, organized report, which accurately reflects the patient's condition.

PLAN:

The nurse organizes the information. It may be beneficial to use a report form or a computer printout of patient information or simply to make organized notes. Priority information is identified so that it is not overlooked.

IMPLEMENTATION:

The sample report on Ms. Hernandez follows:

In Room 101, bed two, the patient is Rosa Hernandez, 52 years of age. She was admitted with a diagnosis of left DVT. Her chief complaints are pain and tenderness to the left calf. Dr. Jones admitted her about an hour ago. Dr. Perez is to see her on a consult, and he said he would be in tonight. Lab drew a baseline activated partial thromboplastin time (aPTT) and complete blood count at 1330 hours. I started her IV in the right cephalic vein at 1400 hours. She had a bolus of 5,000 units of heparin at 1415 hours. The IV of D-5-W with heparin is infusing at 1,000 units per hour. There is no sign of infiltration at the site. I ordered a repeat aPTT for 2015 hours. Her respirations are 20 breaths/min and nonlabored. As for her leg, the left calf is warm to touch. Her left calf measures 2 cm larger than the right calf. Bilateral pedal and popliteal pulses are palpable, with capillary refill time of less than 3 seconds. She had a venous Doppler performed, but the results have not been received yet. She tolerated being up to the bedside commode without difficulty. She has bilateral elastic hose applied. She has rheumatoid arthritis, and both her hands are contracted, but she does not require assistance with activities of daily living (ADLs). We managed to get a late lunch tray sent up, and she ate 100%. I identified a nursing diagnosis of Ineffective protection 363 R/T risk for prolonged bleeding secondary to anticoagulant therapy. I went over a list of precautions with anticoagulant therapy with her. She verbalized understanding. I also explained the rationale behind not crossing her legs. She has a habit of crossing her legs.

EVALUATION:

The nurse reviews notes to make sure all vital information has been communicated. If the report is taped, it can be reviewed. If not, feedback can be obtained from oncoming staff.

servation, the x-ray technician needs to know. Likewise, physical therapy should be notified if a patient who is scheduled to ambulate has experienced severe vomiting during the day. This exchange of information enhances patient care.

Conflict Resolution

Conflict is always a possibility when dealing with interdisciplinary interactions. Personality differences can be a factor, and turf wars between disciplines may occur. Some people consider conflict to be an uncomfortable situation. However, it is important to remember that conflict is not always a negative thing; it can result in growth. New knowledge and better interpersonal skills can be obtained through the process. Because conflicts are the result of problems, conflict resolution can be thought of as following a problem-solving or nursing process format.

The first step in conflict resolution should be an assessment of the facts. It is very important at this stage to listen actively to all participants. Basing decisions on preconceived notions ignores the underlying critical thinking process. In most cases, discussions regarding conflicts should be conducted in private. Public displays of conflict may serve to further deteriorate the situation.

DEFINITION:

Exchanging essential patient care information with other nursing staff at the change of shift.

ACTIVITIES:

Review pertinent demographic data, including name, age, and room number.

Identify chief complaint and reason for admission as appropriate.

Summarize significant past health history, as necessary.

Identify key medical and nursing diagnoses, as appropriate.

Identify resolved medical and nursing diagnoses, as appropriate.

Present information succinctly, focusing on recent and significant data needed by nursing staff assuming responsibility for care.

Describe treatment regimen, including diet, fluid therapy, medications, and exercise.

Identify laboratory and diagnostic tests to be completed during the next 24 hours.

Review recent pertinent laboratory and diagnostic test results, as appropriate.

Describe health status data, including vital signs and signs and symptoms present during the shift.

Describe nursing interventions being implemented.

Describe patient and family response to nursing interventions.

Summarize progress toward goals.

Summarize discharge plans, as appropriate.

Adapted from McCloskey, J. C., & Bulechek, G. M. (2000). *Nursing interventions classification (NIC)* (p. 585). St. Louis: Mosby.

When identifying and analyzing the problem, participants should be careful to use "I" messages. Blaming others does not help resolve disagreements. Therefore, an individual might say, "I become anxious when this procedure is not performed by 3:00." In blaming, the same individual might say, "You make me so angry. You never get your work done on time."

Outcome identification is a very important step in conflict resolution. The participants should ask themselves, "Where do I want to end up with this situation?" Several options exist. For example, the individual might think compromise is a viable option. This might be the desired direction, but it is important to remember that with compromise, both sides can lose. Usually, participants begin with a desire to win. Winning is normally considered a good thing. However, winning at the expense of others may be detrimental in the long run. Relationships with other participants could definitely suffer. Steven Covey (1989) advises people to look for "synergistic solutions" or "win–win solutions." When participants work together on

problems, solutions can be generated that neither would have considered if working alone. During the planning stage, participants should identify all possible solutions and look toward mutually beneficial decisions.

Several concepts should be remembered during the implementation of conflict resolution. All parties involved must seek to communicate clearly. Active listening is essential. This involves careful listening, processing what is heard, and conveying this understood meaning to the sender. While one participant is talking, the others should truly listen instead of thinking about what to say next or assuming what will be said. Each party should seek clarity and listen for underlying themes. Steven Covey advises to "seek first to understand."

In evaluating conflict resolution, participants should look at ways to avoid unnecessary conflicts through establishing rapport, focusing on the needs of others, and using effective communication skills. Methods to facilitate the resolution process in the future may also be considered. Box 7-3 presents an example of conflict resolution using the nursing process steps.

Physician Notification

Physicians are important participants in interdisciplinary communication. Open, direct communication between doctors and nurses should be encouraged. Box 7-4 contains a copy of NIC 7710: Physician Support, which describes nursing activities that facilitate building rapport. A physician is more likely to respond positively if he or she trusts the nurse's judgment. Therefore, developing critical thinking and decision-making skills can facilitate a good working relationship.

CALLING A PHYSICIAN

Novice nurses are often required to telephone a physician with a patient report or to obtain orders. This procedure becomes easier with practice. In learning situations, instructors may practice this skill on real phones and employ a colleague to role-play the position of doctor. Before placing a call, the nurse should be aware of the institutional policy and check the procedure manual for guidance in determining who may contact the physician.

The first step in phoning a physician is to assess the necessity of the call. When assessing, the nurse might ask several questions, such as, "Is medication ordered for this problem? Has the medication had time to work?"

Before phoning, the nurse must obtain all available results of the patient's diagnostic tests.

Box 7-3 Conflict Resolution Using the Steps of the Nursing Process

Three West is a busy medical-surgical unit. Recently, several nurses have complained about patients returning from the radiology department with infiltrated IVs. This has led to tension among staff from both departments. The following is an example of an attempt to resolve this conflict.

ASSESSMENT:

A meeting is called to assess the facts. Invited participants include representatives from the following departments: nursing, radiology, and the transport team. All participants are allowed to present their interpretation and any mitigating factors. The mediator listens to all participants respectfully. Questions are asked to complete the assessment.

ANALYSIS:

The mediator investigates the complaint thoroughly, including such issues as how often has this occurred, is there a pattern, and do infiltrations occur more frequently with transport to radiology than to other departments.

OUTCOME IDENTIFICATION:

The desired outcome is to decrease the number of IV infiltrations that occur when a patient is transported to radiology.

PLAN:

Possible solutions are generated. These might include:

- The nurse could accompany patients.
- The transport team and x-ray technicians could receive instructions on proper IV care.
- X-ray technicians could obtain the patients instead of using transport services.
- Methods to secure the tubing more effectively could be used.
- An extra transporter could be assigned to guide the IV pump.
- Equipment could be selected that tolerates transfers well.

One solution is selected. In this case, it is to educate the x-ray technicians and transport team on IV care during transfers.

IMPLEMENTATION:

This education is carried out as a mandatory inservice conducted by the education department.

EVALUATION:

A study may be conducted to determine whether the inservice had an affect on the number of infiltrations. The participants could also identify methods to avoid similar conflicts in the future such as communicating needs more effectively with other departments.

It is also important to be aware of which tests were performed. A patient assessment should be performed with the results available. Calling a doctor without knowledge of the patient's vital signs and current status will not accomplish the desired results. The doctor, who is not present, is depending on information supplied by the nurse to make decisions. The nurse needs to collect, organize, and analyze all patient data before making the call.

The nurse should also inform other colleagues before placing the call because other nurses may

---

Box 7-4 NIC 7710 Physician Support

DEFINITION:

Collaborating with physicians to provide quality patient care.

ACTIVITIES:

Establish a professional working relationship with the medical staff.
Participate in orientation of medical staff.
Help physicians to learn routines of the patient care unit.
Participate in educational programs for the medical staff.
Encourage open, direct communication between physicians and nurses.
Coach residents and physicians through unfamiliar routines.
Alert physicians to changes in scheduled procedures.
Discuss patient care concerns or practice-related issues directly with physicians involved.
Assist patient to voice concerns to physician.
Report changes in patient status, as appropriate.
Report variation in physician practice within the quality assurance or risk management system, as appropriate.

Participate on multidisciplinary committees to address clinical issues.
Provide information to appropriate physician groups to encourage practice changes or innovations, as needed.
Follow up physician requests for new equipment or supplies.
Process practice changes through the appropriate administrative channels once physician groups have been educated about the need for change.
Provide feedback to physicians about changes in practice, equipment, and staffing.
Include physicians in in-services for new equipment or practice changes.
Encourage physicians to participate in collaborative education programs.
Use multidisciplinary projects and committees as forums to educate physicians about related nursing issues.
Support collaborative research and quality assurance activities.

Adapted from McCloskey, J. C., & Bulechek, G. M. (2000). *Nursing interventions classification (NIC)* (p. 434). St. Louis: Mosby.

also need to talk with the same physician. This avoids making numerous phone calls to the same physician. Informing others of the call also decreases the possibility of interruptions during the call.

When reaching the physician, the nurse should identify himself or herself, the unit, the patient, the purpose of the call, and the actual or potential patient problems. The information should be provided in a clear, concise manner. The nurse should listen carefully and record any orders accurately. Because the possibility exists for misunderstanding with verbal orders, the nurse should repeat any orders back to the physician using his exact words. Clarification should be sought when necessary, even if this requires the physician to repeat the order. The names of medications should be spelled for accuracy. The order should then be checked to ensure that all necessary components have been given, such as dosage, route, and frequency of medications. The nurse must be prepared to answer questions and make any appropriate recommendations. Inappropriate orders should be questioned and should not be accepted. The nurse should identify perceived problems with the order. If the physician insists on the order, the nurse may consult with a supervisor for guidance. The nurse is responsible for any results if he or she

carries out an inappropriate order. After completion of the call, the nurse must write the orders on an order sheet and document the following: T.O. (telephone order), the physician's name, and the nurse's signature and title. Regulations may require that the physician sign this order within 24 hours. The nurse should also document the problem that led to the call and the time that the physician was contacted.

If the nurse is unable to reach the physician, he or she should document contact attempts and the phone numbers called. Agency policy should be followed if the nurse is unable to contact the physician within a reasonable time. A skills checklist and scenario for student practice of this skill can be found at the end of this chapter. Box 7-5 outlines an example of a nurse's call to a physician.

Receiving Phone Calls

Nurses are representatives of their employing agency. The first person a potential patient speaks with could be a nurse. Therefore, phones should be answered quickly and in a courteous manner. The nurse should greet the caller with the appropriate unit name and his or her name and title. All responses should be friendly, helpful, and profes-

---

Box 7-5 Example of a Nurse and Physician Phone Conversation

Lisa Wood, RN, is making her first round of the evening shift. As she approaches the room of Anna Fear, she hears loud, angry voices. Mrs. Fear's daughter stomps out of the room.

Lisa enters the room to begin her assessment. Mrs. Fear is complaining of increasing shortness of breath. Lisa elevates the head of the bed, checks the oxygen level being delivered, and takes a reading with the pulse oximeter. She auscultates lung sounds. This reveals the slight expiratory crackles described by the nurse in report. Lisa assesses Mrs. Fear's level of consciousness while taking vital signs. She speaks with Mrs. Fear in a quiet, calm manner. She asks if there is anything Mrs. Fear would like to talk about. Mrs. Fear briefly discusses her daughter and the disagreement. She states that her daughter is concerned about paying the hospital bills. Lisa listens attentively.

Lisa is concerned about the decreased oxygen saturation of 89% and increased blood pressure. She weighs her options and examines ordered treatments and medication. This problem indicates a deterioration in condition requiring interventions not previously ordered. Therefore, Miss Wood elects to call the physician. Miss Wood calls the physician's office and requests to speak with her.

The following conversation takes place:
Lisa Wood: Dr. Good, this is Lisa Wood, RN, from St. Joseph's second floor. I'm calling about Anna Fear

in Room 2004-1. She is complaining about increasing shortness of breath. The slight expiratory crackles in the lower base of her lungs have not increased since this morning. Her vital signs are blood pressure, 164/94 mm Hg; temperature, 99°; pulse, 110 beats/min; respirations, 28 breaths/min. Pulse oximetry reading is 89%. Were her arterial blood gas results available when you came in the morning?
Doctor: No. Can you give me those?
Lisa Wood: Let me see. The pH was 7.3, the pO_2 is 80, pCO_2 is 45, bicarb 25.
Doctor: Are the results back today from her chest x-ray?
Lisa Wood: Yes, it shows slight pleural effusion in both lungs and cardiomegaly. Evidence supports the diagnosis of congestive heart failure.
Doctor: The lab work looks about the same as yesterday.
Lisa Wood: Well, when her daughter was in this morning, they had a loud argument. Mrs. Fear stated her daughter is concerned about hospital bills.
Doctor: Let's increase her oxygen to 4 liters. Give her Lasix, 40 mg IV now. Arrange a social service consult. Give Ativan, 1 mg p.o. prn for anxiety. Tell her I will be in to see her at about 4:30 PM.
Lisa Wood: (Repeats orders). Thank you.
Lisa records orders on order sheet as a telephone order.
Note: Some institutions may have policies that restrict nurses from taking verbal orders.

---

sional. Telephones do not allow nonverbal cues, making the tone of voice even more important.

WRITTEN COMMUNICATION

DOCUMENTATION

One way to validate critical thinking is to write it down. The thought processes of the nurse must be clear to communicate in written format. The advantage of nonverbal cues does not exist in this medium. The writer must organize and determine the significance of his or her thoughts before writing them down.

The patient's chart is the legal documentation of the quality of care. It is also consulted first in the event of a malpractice suit. Insurance companies base payment or denial of payment on the patient chart; therefore, nurses must document carefully. Charting patient care should follow the requirements of state statutes and accrediting agencies. Institutional policy and procedure books must also be consulted for charting guidance.

There are numerous items that require charting. Patient assessments are very important, as are changes in patient condition. Descriptions of patient behavior should be written in the chart objectively. Statements made by the patient may be quoted directly. Nursing interventions, activities, and diagnoses should also be charted. The nurse must document expected outcomes of care and any deviations from the expected outcome, along with the achievement of outcomes. It is important to note whether nursing activities accomplished desired outcomes. As described earlier, any notification of the physician warrants charting. Other actions that must be charted include procedures and consultations, involvement of significant others, and the use of safety devices or major equipment. Finally, the patient's condition upon discharge should be documented.

Although there are several methods of charting, some standard rules do exist. First, the chart must remain confidential. It should only be viewed by individuals who have the right to the information. Charting should be accurate and objective while avoiding assumptions. For example, charting that a patient is pacing and wringing his hands is much more accurate than stating that he is nervous. Charting needs to be performed promptly after the event, with the time accurately recorded. Also, it is important to avoid duplication in charting because it creates unnecessary work. Generally, the nurse does not have to document the same thing in several different places in the chart. The nurse must carefully check spelling and grammar on charting entries; these areas reflect on professionalism.

SUMMARY

Communication is the basis for forming relationships. Therapeutic relationships are an integral aspect of nursing. Therefore, the importance of clear communication cannot be underestimated.

There are specific nursing activities that require effective communication skills. A nurse must communicate directions and expectations clearly in the delegation process. An organized shift report is more likely to result in continuity of care and increased patient satisfaction. Effective communication skills also enhance collaboration between disciplines. The ability to communicate clearly with the physician can result in increased quality of care.

In addition to verbal communication, nurses should be skilled at written communication. The chart is a legal document used by nursing and other disciplines to monitor patient care. Entries should be made in accordance with the policies of the institution.

KEY POINTS

- The three levels of communication are social, therapeutic, and collegial.
- Nurses collaborate with nursing personnel and other health care workers to improve patient care.
- Failure to communicate can result in serious consequences.
- Nursing personnel need to function together as a team.
- When delegating a task, the nurse is responsible for ensuring that the right direction or communication is given.
- When giving report, the nurse communicates clearly with personnel on the next shift to ensure continuity of care.
- It is important that nurses share knowledge regarding the patient with other disciplines.
- Conflict resolution is a problem-solving process. Outcome identification is an important step in conflict resolution.
- Novice nurses are often required to telephone a physician. This is a skill that can improve with practice.

- Nurses should respond to phone calls in a friendly, helpful, and professional manner.
- The chart provides documentation of the quality of care delivered. Expected outcomes and achievement of those outcomes should be charted.

REFERENCES

Adams, C. H., & Jones, P. D. (2000). *Interpersonal communication skills for health professionals*. New York: Glencoe/McGraw-Hill.

Alfaro-LeFevre, R. (1999). *Critical thinking in nursing*. Philadelphia: W. B. Saunders.

Andrews, M. M., & Boyle, J. S. (2003). *Transcultural concepts in nursing care*. Philadelphia: Lippincott Williams & Wilkins.

Bastable, S. B. (1997). *Nurse as educator: Principles of teaching and learning*. Boston: Jones and Bartlett.

Covey, S. R. (1989). *The seven habits of highly effective people*. New York: Simon and Schuster.

McCloskey, J. C., & Bulechek, G. M. (2000). *Nursing interventions classification (NIC)*. St. Louis: Mosby.

National Council of State Boards of Nursing (NCSBN). (1995). *Delegation: Concepts and decision-making process*. Chicago: Author.

Student Worksheets

 ## SKILL SHEET #1: COMMUNICATION

Change-of-Shift Report

Purpose

To develop the student's skill in communicating important material to oncoming personnel, thereby enabling continuity of care.

Objectives

The student will demonstrate the ability to:

1. List the information that should be gathered in the assessment phase.
2. Determine relevancy of obtained information.
3. Describe criteria for successful report.
4. Prioritize the information.
5. Give report in a systematic, logical fashion.

Steps: Communication

ASSESSMENT

1. Identify demographic data from Kardex or PCP.
2. Gather information from worksheets, treatment plans, UAP report, and current patient condition.

ANALYSIS

Determine appropriateness and relevancy of information.

OUTCOME IDENTIFICATION

Describe criteria for successful report.

PLAN

Prioritize information based on current patient status, change in condition, treatment, medications, and results of diagnostic tests.

IMPLEMENTATION

1. Provide a description of progress during shift using a systematic, logical approach.
2. Report status of identified outcomes.
3. Describe changes in patient condition.
4. Describe therapies or treatments and expected outcomes.
5. Describe consultations.
6. Review progress of discharge plan.

EVALUATION

Review report for organization, length, and thoroughness.

COMPETENCY VALIDATION #1: COMMUNICATION

Change-of-Shift Report

Competency Statement

The student will demonstrate ability to give organized, informative report.
The student demonstrated the ability to do the following:

1. Organize the demographic data from various sources.
2. Provide information in a clear, concise, and consistent manner.
3. Communicate patient status and note change in condition, treatments, medications, and results of diagnostic tests.
4. Determine relevant and appropriate information to report.
5. Provide progress report on patient teaching, discharge plan, and consultation with other members of the health care team.
6. Provide report in organized, concise manner.

COMPETENT

- Understands reasons for task and is able to perform tasks independently
- Understands reasons for task but needs supervision
- Understands reasons for task and is able to perform task with assistance

NOT COMPETENT

- Understands reason for task but performs task at provisional level
- Is unable to state reason for task and performs task at dependent level

SKILL CHECKLIST #1: CHANGE-OF-SHIFT REPORT

CHANGE-OF-SHIFT REPORT	SATISFACTORY	UNSATISFACTORY	NI/COMMENTS
ASSESSMENT			
1. Identify demographic data from Kardex or PCP (i.e., name, room number, diagnosis, age, and physician).			
2. Gather information from worksheets, multidisciplinary treatment plans, UAP report, and current patient condition.			
ANALYZE			
1. Determine appropriate and relevant information to be communicated.			
OUTCOME IDENTIFICATION			
1. Describe criteria for successful report.			
PLAN			
1. Prioritize information based on current patient status, change in condition, treatment, medications, and results of diagnostic tests.			
IMPLEMENTATION			
1. Provide a description of progress during shift using a systematic, logical approach to deliver information.			
2. Report status of identified outcomes.			
3. Describe changes in patient status.			
4. Describe therapies or treatments administered during the shift and expected outcomes.			
5. Describe consultations with interdisciplinary team members.			
6. Review progress of discharge plan.			
7. Detail progress in patient teaching plan.			
EVALUATION			
1. Review report for organization, length, and thoroughness.			

SCENARIO TO ACCOMPANY STUDENT WORKSHEETS

Giving Report

You are a nurse preparing for the completion of a 12-hour shift on a medical-surgical unit. A description of one of the patients follows:

Sam Brown, aged 65 years, has been admitted with heart failure and non–insulin-dependent diabetes mellitus (NIDDM). Dr. Hart has given the following orders: oxygen at 2 liters per minute per nasal cannula; 2-gram sodium diet; 1,800-calorie diabetic diet; saline lock; Accu-Chek (bedside blood sugar readings) before meals and at 2100 hours; up in the room as tolerated; weigh daily; chest x-ray; complete blood count (CBC); and cardiac profile. Appropriate medications were also ordered.

1. What information do you need to gather before report?

_____

_____

_____

_____

_____

_____

_____

_____

_____

2. Should all the information obtained with an assessment be communicated during report?

_____

_____

_____

3. In giving report, what things should be included?

_____

_____

_____

_____

_____

_____

_____

_____

4. After giving report, you think of items that you forgot. At times, you must call the unit after arriving home with additional information. What strategies could be used to decrease the incidence of this?

_____

_____

_____

_____

_____

_____

_____

_____

See the Answer Key in Appendix A for sample answers for this exercise.

SKILL SHEET #2: COMMUNICATION

Telephone Consultation

Purpose

To develop the student's skill in communicating important information to the physician.

Objectives

The student will demonstrate the ability to:

1. Determine necessity of call.
2. Identify significant data to report.
3. Identify desired outcome of call.
4. Place call in an organized, professional manner.
5. Write telephone orders accurately as given by the physician.
6. Document information regarding the phone call.

Steps: Telephone Consultation

ASSESSMENT

1. Determine necessity of call.
2. Obtain all diagnostic test results.
3. Write down which tests were performed.
4. Perform patient assessment.

ANALYSIS

Identify significant patient data related to problem.

OUTCOME IDENTIFICATION

Determine desired result of call.

PLAN

Inform others about call to avoid repeatedly calling physician and to minimize interruptions during call.

IMPLEMENTATION

1. Identify self, unit, and patient.
2. Identify purpose of call.
3. Identify actual and potential problems.
4. Provide clear, concise information.
5. Listen carefully.
6. Make recommendations when appropriate.
7. Answer questions appropriately.
8. Question inappropriate or ambiguous orders.

EVALUATION

1. Write orders on order sheet.
2. Document problems that led to phone call.
3. Chart the time the physician was contacted and the results of contact.

COMPETENCY VALIDATION #2: COMMUNICATION

TELEPHONE CONSULTATION

COMPETENCY STATEMENT

The student will demonstrate the ability to contact physician in a responsible manner and write telephone orders.

The student demonstrated the ability to do the following:

1. Verify that indicators for calling the physician are present.
2. Retrieve and interpret patient's diagnostic and laboratory data.
3. Conduct assessment of the patient and identify related abnormal results.
4. Collaborate in clear, concise manner by identification of the purpose of call and the actual and potential problems and by confirming tests available.
5. Question ambiguous or inappropriate orders.
6. Record accurately on the order sheet.
7. Verify and clarify the orders given by the physician.
8. Record order accurately with all pertinent data addressed.
9. Chart the transaction appropriately.

COMPETENT

- Understands reasons for task and is able to perform task independently
- Understands reasons for task but needs supervision
- Understands reasons for task and is able to perform task with assistance

NOT COMPETENT

- Understands reason for task but performs task at provisional level
- Is unable to state reason for task and performs task at dependent level

SKILLS CHECKLIST #2: TELEPHONE CONSULTATION

TELEPHONE CONSULTATION	SATISFACTORY	UNSATISFACTORY	NI/COMMENTS
ASSESSMENT			
1. Determine necessity of call.			
2. Obtain all diagnostic test results.			
3. Write down which tests were performed.			
4. Perform a patient assessment.			
ANALYSIS			
1. Identify significant patient data that are related to the problem and abnormal results.			
OUTCOME IDENTIFICATION			
1. Determine expected outcome of call.			
PLAN			
1. Inform others of impending call to avoid numerous phone calls and to minimize interruptions during call.			
IMPLEMENTATION			
1. Identify self, unit, and patient.			
2. Identify purpose of call.			
3. Identify actual and potential problems.			
4. Provide clear, concise information.			
5. Listen carefully.			
6. Make recommendations when appropriate.			
7. Answer questions appropriately.			
8. Question inappropriate and clarify ambiguous orders.			
EVALUATION			
1. Write orders on order sheet as given by physician and sign with T.O. (telephone order), the physician's name, and nurse's signature and title.			
2. Document the problem that led to the phone call.			
3. Chart the time the physician was contacted and results of contact.			

SCENARIO TO ACCOMPANY STUDENT WORKSHEETS

Calling the Physician

Use the following scenario to answer the questions at the end.

June Smith, aged 80 years, was admitted from a nursing home. She is dressed in a soiled hospital gown and is accompanied by her daughter. The transfer sheet says Ms. Smith has been vomiting bright red blood. She has a history of cerebral vascular accident (CVA) with expressive aphasia and Alzheimer's disease. She has no known allergies. Her skin is pale and cool. Her eyes are open, but she does not respond verbally. Her lungs are clear. Respirations are even and nonlabored. She moves all extremities well. Her abdomen is distended and tender on palpation. She has hyperactive bowel sounds. A reddened area approximately 1 × 2 cm is noted on her coccyx. Her vital signs are as follows: temperature, 94.7°F (34.8° C); pulse, 112 beats/min; respirations, 20 breaths/min; blood pressure, 106/74 mm Hg.

At the nursing home, she was taking the following medications:

Chewable aspirin (ASA), 64 mg orally per day
Cognex, 10 mg orally four times a day
Dulcolax suppository as needed

1. What are the steps in notifying the doctor?

_____

_____

_____

_____

_____

_____

_____

_____

_____

2. What would you tell the doctor?

_____

_____

_____

_____

_____

_____

_____

_____

_____

3. What orders might you receive?

_____

_____

_____

_____

_____

_____

4. What would you do if unable to contact the physician?

_____

_____

_____

_____

_____

_____

See the Answer Key in Appendix A for sample answers for this exercise.

PRACTICE EXERCISES: COMMUNICATION

ROLE PLAY: GIVING REPORT

Role-play a nurse giving report. You may use the following patients or make up your own. You have given care to the following three patients during your 12-hour shift. The details of their conditions are written incompletely to allow for creativity.

Anna Lopez 35-year-old female Diagnosis: left mastectomy yesterday Dr. Good	
IV:	Meds: Vicodin, 1 tablet orally every 4 hours as needed for pain
Treatments: Maintain left arm in elevated position. No blood pressures or venipunctures in left arm. Empty Jackson-Pratt drain every shift.	Diagnostic tests: Hemoglobin and hematocrit this AM
Patient education: teach patient drain care for discharge.	

Asa Chan Age: 82 years old Diagnosis: Right total-knee replacement 2 days ago Dr. Banes	

IV: D-5-W, 0.45% normal saline to
    infuse at 125 mL per hour
	Meds:
	Heparin, 5,000 units subcutaneously daily
	Morphine, patient-controlled analgesia (PCA) pump for
	    pain
	Vicodin, 1 tablet orally every 4 hours as needed for
	    moderate pain

Treatments:
Continuous passive motion machine (CPM)
    to be regulated by physical therapy (PT)
Sequential compression devices (SCD)
    to both lower extremities
Empty drainage device at least one time
    per shift.
	Diagnostic tests:
	Hemoglobin and hematocrit daily

Change dressing daily and as needed.	
Patient education: Quadricep exercises	

Sylvia Suarez Age: 88 years old Diagnosis: Left hip fracture with insertion of hip prosthesis yesterday Dr. Bones	
IV: Saline lock	Meds: Heparin, 5,000 units subcutaneously daily Rocephin, 1 gram IV daily Morphine, 2–4 mg IV every 2 hours as needed for pain

Treatments:
Physical therapy for pivot transfer
Sequential compression devices
   (SCD) to both lower extremities
Maintain lower extremities in good
   alignment with abductor pillow.
	Diagnostic tests:
	Hemoglobin and hematocrit daily

Change dressing daily and as needed. Patient education: Reinforce turn, cough, and deep-breathing instructions. Avoid acute flexion of hip.	

Answers will vary with student's experience.

CALLING THE PHYSICIAN

1. You are a staff nurse on a surgical unit. A patient has returned from knee replacement surgery 2 hours ago. The patient is complaining of incisional pain. Should you call the doctor?

   _____

   _____

   _____

   _____

   _____

2. You are a staff nurse at a long-term care facility. A new resident has been admitted to your wing. What should you do before contacting the physician?

   _____

   _____

   _____

   _____

   _____

   _____

   _____

3. What orders would you expect to receive from the call?

_____

_____

_____

_____

_____

_____

See the Answer Key in Appendix A for sample answers for this exercise.

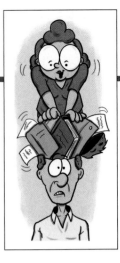

CHAPTER 8

PATIENT TEACHING

OBJECTIVES

1. Describe the four areas that must be assessed before beginning an educational presentation.

2. Differentiate between a goal and an objective.

3. List three methods of educational presentation.

4. Prepare a lesson plan.

5. Compare and contrast a lesson plan and a patient plan of care.

6. Discuss critical thinking concepts involved in patient teaching.

Patient teaching is a major nursing responsibility that affects the patient's recovery. In the current health care environment, patient teaching cannot be conducted in a haphazard manner. Patients are being discharged earlier and are performing more and more complicated treatments at home. A well-informed consumer is essential to obtain optimum health care results.

Before starting an educational presentation, it is important to determine what must be taught, what the learner must do, and how the learning will be evaluated. One way of accomplishing this goal is to apply the steps of the nursing process to patient teaching. Patient teaching is best approached as a problem-solving process involving critical thinking, decision making and priority setting.

APPLYING THE NURSING PROCESS

Patient teaching is goal directed and is based on rational thought processes. Therefore, it should involve critical thinking and is best approached by using analytical thinking. The steps to patient teaching parallel the nursing process, beginning with assessment. The nurse must assess the learning needs and characteristics of the learner. During analysis, the patient should be consulted regarding the selection of learning needs. This assists in prioritizing the needs. In the outcome identification step, the nurse establishes a goal and learning objectives and creates a lesson plan. When implementing the educational program, the nurse's goal should be to create an atmosphere of caring and concern. The process continues through evaluation of the educational program results and, if necessary, subsequent revisions. Following a procedure similar to the nursing process results in planned education with a higher success rate.

Learning Needs Assessment

Before beginning an educational presentation, four areas must be assessed. The teacher must know what the patient needs to learn, the characteristics of the learner, the patient's preferred learning style, and whether the patient is ready to learn. Many patient teaching programs are based on "canned" presentations that are expected to work well with all participants. This ignores the individuality of the patient. Bastable (2003) states, "Nursing assessment of needs, readiness, and styles of learning is the first and most important step in instructional design, but it is also the step most often neglected" (p.77).

The first step in patient teaching is to conduct a learning needs assessment. It is a waste of time to cover concepts a learner already thoroughly understands. A needs assessment must be performed to discover gaps in knowledge. Methods to accomplish this can vary from informal discussions or interviews to the more formal surveys or focus groups. It is important not to assume where knowledge gaps lie. A needs assessment is the educational base on which patient teaching is accomplished. The characteristics of the learner that must be considered in an assessment include the influences of culture, the learner's developmental stage and literacy level, and the presence of any disabilities.

The patient's cultural background has a profound effect on health care practices and beliefs. Therefore, it is important for the nurse to understand the health care practices of individual cultures before initiating patient education. However, possessing a complete knowledge of each culture's health practices is very difficult in today's diverse society. This makes a transcultural assessment of a culture's beliefs an essential step. A section of Andrews and Boyle's (2003) Transcultural Nursing Assessment Guide is presented in Box 8-1. The educator should consult a transcultural nursing text for generalizations concerning the beliefs of specific ethnic groups.

Another aspect that warrants consideration is the patient's developmental stage. As an individual progresses from infancy to senescence, changes occur in the person's knowledge base, ability to process information, and motivation to learn. Each learner is an individual, but generalizations can be

---

Box 8-1 Transcultural Assessment: Health-Related Beliefs and Practices

1. To what cause does the patient attribute illness and disease or what factors influence the acquisition of illness and disease (e.g., divine wrath, imbalance in hot/cold, yin/yang, punishment for moral transgressions, hex, soul loss, pathogenic organism, past behavior)?
2. What are the patient's cultural beliefs about ideal body size and shape? What is the patient's self image in relation to the ideal?
3. How does the patient describe his or her health-related condition? What names or terms are used? How does the patient express pain?
4. What does the patient believe promotes health (eating certain foods; wearing amulets to bring good luck; sleep; rest; good nutrition; reducing stress, exercise; prayer or rituals to ancestors, saints, or intermediate deities)?
5. What is the patient's religious affiliation? How is the patient actively involved in the practice of religion?
6. Does the patient rely on cultural healers (e.g., curandero, shaman, spiritualist, priest, minister)? Who determines when the patient is sick and when he or she is healthy? Who influences the choice or type of healer and treatment that should be sought?
7. In what types of cultural healing or health-promoting practices does the patient engage (use of herbal remedies; potions; massage; wearing of talismans, copper bracelets, or chains to discourage evil spirits; healing rituals; incantations; prayers)?
8. How are biomedical/scientific health care providers perceived? How do the patient and his or her family perceive nurses? What are the expectations of nurses and nursing care?
9. Who will care for the patient at home? What accommodations will be made by family members to provide caregiving?
10. How does the patient's cultural group view mental disorders? Are there differences in acceptable behaviors for physical versus psychological illnesses?

Adapted from Andrews, M., & Boyle, J. (2003). *Transcultural concepts in nursing care* (p. 536, Appendix A). Philadelphia: Lippincott Williams & Wilkins.

---

made regarding the progression that occurs with the maturation process. This process influences the educator's choice of instructional method. For example, peer groups are important for adolescents. Therefore, group sessions can be an effective teaching strategy. On the other hand, the young adult tends to be more self-directed. Young adults may function well with a teaching strategy that allows them to set their own pace, such as learning online or using programmed instruction. Table 8-1 contains a further discussion of this concept.

Literacy is an important consideration in health care education. Bastable (2003) claims, "at least *(text continues on page 177)*

TABLE 8-1 STAGE-APPROPRIATE TEACHING STRATEGIES

LEARNER	GENERAL CHARACTERISTICS	TEACHING STRATEGIES	NURSING INTERVENTIONS
INFANCY-TODDLERHOOD Approximate age: Birth–3 yr Cognitive stage: Sensorimotor Psychosocial stage: Trust vs. mistrust (Birth–12 mo) Autonomy vs. shame and doubt (1–3 yr)	Dependent on environment Needs security Explores self and environment Natural curiosity	Orient teaching to caregiver Use repetition and imitation of information Stimulate all senses Provide physical safety and emotional security Allow play and manipulation of objects	Welcome active involvement Forge alliances Encourage physical closeness Provide detailed information Answer questions and concerns Ask for information on child's strengths/ limitations and likes/dislikes
PRESCHOOLER Approximate age: 3–6 yr Cognitive stage: Preoperational Psychosocial stage: Initiative vs. guilt	Egocentric Thinking precausal, concrete, literal Believes illness self-caused and punitive Limited sense of time Fears bodily injury Cannot generalize Animistic thinking (objects possess life or human characteristics) Centration (focus is on one characteristic of an object) Separation anxiety Motivated by curiosity Active imagination, prone to fears Play is his/her work	Use warm, calm approach Build trust Use repetition of information Allow manipulation of objects and equipment Give care with explanation Reassure not to blame self Explain procedures simply and briefly Provide safe, secure environment Use positive reinforcement Encourage questions to reveal perceptions/feelings Use simple drawings and stories Use play therapy, with dolls and puppets Stimulate senses: visual, auditory, tactile, motor	Welcome active involvement Forge alliances Encourage physical closeness Provide detailed information Answer questions and concerns Ask for information on child's strengths/ limitations and likes/dislikes
SCHOOL-AGED CHILDHOOD Approximate age: 6–12 yr Cognitive stage: Concrete operations Psychosocial stage: Industry vs. inferiority	More realistic and objective Understands cause and effect Deductive/inductive reasoning Wants concrete information Able to compare objects and events Variable rates of physical growth Reasons syllogistically Understands seriousness and consequences of actions Subject-centered focus Immediate orientation	Encourage independence and active participation Be honest, allay fears Use logical explanation Allow time to ask questions Use analogies to make invisible processes real Establish role models Relate care to other children's experiences; compare procedures Use subject-centered focus Use play therapy Provide group activities Use drawings, models, dolls, painting, audiotapes, and videotapes	Encourage active involvement Forge alliances Encourage physical closeness Provide detailed information Answer questions and concerns Ask for information on child's strengths/ limitations and likes/dislikes

(continued)

TABLE 8-1 **STAGE-APPROPRIATE TEACHING STRATEGIES** (CONTINUED)

LEARNER	GENERAL CHARACTERISTICS	TEACHING STRATEGIES	NURSING INTERVENTIONS
ADOLESCENCE Approximate age: 12–18 yr Cognitive stage: Formal operations Psychosocial stage: Identity vs. role confusion	Abstract, hypothetical thinking Can build on past learning Reasons by logic and understands scientific principles Future orientation Motivated by desire for social acceptance Peer group important Intense personal preoccupation, appearance extremely important (imaginary audience) Feels invulnerable, invincible/immune to natural laws (personal fable)	Establish trust, authenticity Know their agenda Address fears/concerns about outcomes of illness Identify control focus Include in plan of care Use peers for support and influence Negotiate changes Focus on details Make information meaningful to life Ensure confidentiality and privacy Arrange group sessions Use audiovisuals, role-playing, contracts, reading materials Provide for experimentation and flexibility	Explore emotional and financial support Determine goals and expectations Assess stress levels Respect values and norms Determine role responsibilities and relationships Allow for 1:1 teaching without parents present, but with adolescent's permission, inform family of content covered
YOUNG ADULTHOOD Approximate age: 18–40 yr Cognitive stage: Formal operations Psychosocial stage: Intimacy vs. isolation	Autonomous Self-directed Uses personal experiences to enhance or interfere with learning Intrinsic motivation Able to analyze critically Makes decisions about personal, occupational, and social roles Competency-based learner	Use problem-centered focus Draw on meaningful experiences Focus on immediacy of application Encourage active participation Allow to set own pace, be self-directed Organize material Recognize social role Apply new knowledge through role-playing and hands-on practice	Explore emotional, financial, and physical support system Asses motivational level for involvement Identify potential obstacles and stressors
MIDDLE-AGED ADULTHOOD Approximate age: 40–65 yr Cognitive stage: Formal operations Psychosocial stage: Generativity vs. self-absorption and stagnation	Sense of self well-developed Concerned with physical changes At peak in career Explores alternative lifestyles Reflects on contributions to family and society Reexamines goals and values Questions achievements and successes Has confidence in abilities Desires to modify unsatisfactory aspects of life	Focus on maintaining independence and reestablishing normal life patterns Assess positive and negative past experiences with learning Assess potential sources of stress due to midlife crisis issues Provide information to coincide with life concerns and problems	Explore emotional, financial, and physical support system Assess motivational level for involvement Identify potential obstacles and stressors

OLDER ADULTHOOD

Approximate age: 65 yr and over
Cognitive stage: Formal operations
Psychosocial stage: Ego integrity vs. despair

Cognitive changes
Decreased ability to think abstractly, process information
Decreased short-term memory
Increased reaction time
Increased test anxiety
Stimulus persistence (afterimage)
Focuses on past life experiences

Use concrete examples
Build on past life experiences
Make information relevant and meaningful
Present one concept at a time
Allow time for processing/response (slow pace)
Use repetition and reinforcement of information
Avoid written exams
Use verbal exchange and coaching
Establish retrieval plan (use one or several clues)
Encourage active involvement
Keep explanations brief
Use analogies to illustrate abstract information

Sensory/motor deficits
Auditory changes
Hearing loss, especially high-pitched tones, consonants (S, Z, T, F, and G), and rapid speech
Visual changes
Farsighted (needs glasses to read)
Lenses become opaque (glare problem)
Smaller pupil size (decreased visual adaptation to darkness)
Decreased peripheral perception

Speak slowly, distinctly
Use low-pitched tones
Face patient when speaking
Minimize distractions
Avoid shouting
Use visual aids to supplement verbal instruction
Avoid glares, use soft white light
Provide sufficient light
Use white backgrounds and black print
Use large letters and well-spaced print
Avoid color coding with blues, greens, purples, and yellows
Increase safety precautions/provide safe environment

Involve principal caregivers
Encourage participation
Provide resources for support (respite care)
Assess coping mechanisms
Provide written instructions for reinforcement
Provide anticipatory problem solving (what happens if . . .)

(continued)

TABLE 8-1 **Stage-appropriate Teaching Strategies** (Continued)

LEARNER	GENERAL CHARACTERISTICS	TEACHING STRATEGIES	NURSING INTERVENTIONS
OLDER ADULTHOOD (CONTINUED)	Yellowing of lenses (distorts low-tone colors: blue, green, violet)	Ensure accessibility and fit of prostheses (i.e., glasses, hearing aid)	
	Distorted depth perception	Keep sessions short	
	Fatigue/decreased energy levels	Provide for frequent rest periods	
	Pathophysiology (chronic illness)	Allow for extra time to perform	
		Establish realistic short-term goals	
	Psychosocial changes	Give time to reminisce	
	Decreased risk taking	Identify and present pertinent material	
	Selective learning	Use informal teaching sessions	
	Intimidated by formal learning	Demonstrate relevance of information to daily life	
		Assess resources	
		Make learning positive	
		Identify past positive experiences	
		Integrate new behaviors with formerly established ones	

Adapted from Bastable, S. (2003). *Nurse as educator* (pp. 122–126). Sudbury, MA: Jones and Bartlett.

one out of every four to five Americans lack the literacy skills and knowledge to cope with the requirements of day-to-day living." (p. 195) Tasks that are sometimes taken for granted, such as reading the labels of over-the-counter medications or reading educational pamphlets, can present a challenge for many in our society. Individuals with poor reading skills may have higher medical costs as a result of decreased preventive care and higher rates of noncompliance. Box 8-2 presents suggestions for designing material for individuals with low literacy skills.

Educators must be aware of differences in learning styles. Many studies point to the fact that people have a preferred style of learning. (Brennan, 1984; Dunn, & Dunn, 1993; Van Wynen, 1997). Learners process information in different ways. One way is not better than another way, it is just different. An educator must be flexible in material presentation in order to accommodate the learner's particular style. The nurse also has a preferred learning style. A common error made by educators is to present material in their own preferred learning style. For example, a nurse who learns primarily through reading must guard against the trap of expecting all patients to grasp educational information presented in pamphlets.

Reese (2002) identified the following four basic learning styles and the preferred method of learning for each:

1. Visual-verbal learners prefer written language—textbooks, blackboards, and class notes.
2. Visual-nonverbal learners prefer pictures, videos, maps, charts, and diagrams.
3. Auditory-verbal learners prefer oral language—classroom lectures, group discussions, and audiotapes.
4. Tactile-kinesthetic learners prefer physical activity, movement, and hands-on activities.

An effective educator incorporates a variety of instructional methods and materials to accommodate differences in learning styles.

It is a common practice to ask a few questions concerning learning style while performing the

---

Box 8-2 SUMMARY OF GUIDELINES FOR DESIGNING EFFECTIVE LOW-LITERACY PRINTED MATERIALS

CONTENT

Clearly define the purpose of the material.
Decide when and how the information will be used.
Use behavioral objectives that cover the main points.
Verify the accuracy of content with experts.
Give "how to" information for the learner to achieve objectives.
Present only the most essential information (three to four main ideas: who, what, where, and when).
Relate new information to what the audience already knows.
Present content relevant to the audience and avoid cultural bias in writing and graphics.

ORGANIZATION

Keep titles short, yet use words that clearly convey the meaning of the content.
Provide a table of contents for lengthy material and a summary to review content presented.
Present the most important information first.
Use topic headings (advance organizers).
Make the first sentence of each paragraph the topic sentence.
Include only a few concepts per paragraph.
Use short, simple sentences that convey only one idea at a time; limit the length of the entire text.
Limit lists to no more than seven items.
Present each idea in logical sequence.

LAYOUT AND GRAPHICS

Select large, easily read print (minimum 12-point type) and use nonglossy paper.
Write headings and subheadings in both lowercase and uppercase letters; avoid fancy lettering.

Use bold type or underlining to emphasize important information.
Use lots of white space between segments of information.
Use generous margins and keep right-hand margins unjustified.
Provide a question-and answer format for patient–nurse interaction.
Select double spacing (between lines of type), type style (serif), and font (print size) for ease of reading.
Design a colorful eye-catching cover that suggests the message contained in the text.

LINGUISTICS

Keep sentences short (8–10 words)
Write in the active voice, using the present tense and the pronouns *you* and *your* to engage the reader.
Use one- to two-syllable words as much as possible, avoiding multisyllabic (polysyllabic) words.
Use words familiar and understandable to the target audience.
Avoid complex grammatical structures (i.e., multiple clauses).
Limit the number of concepts.
Focus content on what the audience should do as well as know.
Use positive statements; avoid negative messages.
Use questions throughout the text to encourage active learning.
Provide examples the audience can use to relate to personal experiences/circumstances.

Adapted from Bastable, S. (2003). *Nurse as educator* (p. 221). Sudbury, MA: Jones and Bartlett.

nursing admission assessment. For example, patients are often asked whether reading is a preferred style of processing information. For this reason, the assessment form should be consulted when preparing the educational material.

In many cases, time constraints may not allow the administration of a formal learning style instrument, but the nurse should still be aware that learning styles vary from patient to patient. Informal discussion with the patient can lead to information regarding his or her learning style and subsequently to changes in the presentation.

Admission forms can also provide insight into special learning needs. Frequently, patients are asked about personal information, such as their ability to hear and to read. This knowledge allows the educational facilitator to accommodate the patient's preferred method of presentation. For instance, commercially prepared handouts may be inappropriate for the visually impaired patient. Depending on the degree of disability, the nurse may elect to give instructions verbally or obtain pamphlets in extra-large type.

Another important aspect to consider in patient teaching is the patient's readiness to learn. Strong emotions may interfere with a patient's receptiveness to new concepts. The patient who is anxious about a medical condition or excited about discharge may experience an inability to focus. Imagine trying to listen intently to instructions after being given a diagnosis of cancer. Motivation to learn is also a part of readiness. Adult learners need to understand the applicability of the information. They need to know why the information is important to them. Learning is enhanced when it is "related to an immediate need, problem, or deficit" (Burgireno, 1985, pp. 20–21). Cultural beliefs and habits also affect readiness to learn. A patient may resist dietary education that conflicts with previous customs. This could result in the patient's refusal to listen and, consequently, may result in noncompliance. Familiarity with cultural beliefs assists the nurse in patient education.

Analyzing Needs

Once the nurse has identified a learning need, it should be validated with the patient. The patient may desire, for various reasons, to concentrate on certain aspects of the teaching. A more effective education will occur if the nurse discovers what material the patient would like to learn. This process is very similar to the development of an individualized care plan.

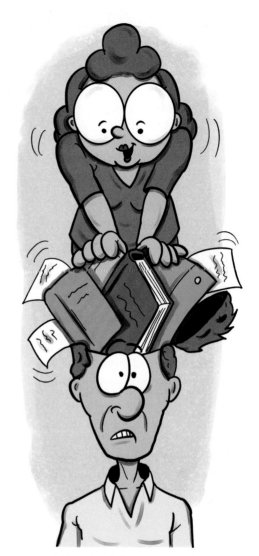

Avoid patient information overload.

When several educational needs have been identified, priorities should be established to ensure adequate time for teaching the essential material. For example, a newly diagnosed diabetic patient requires patient teaching. Within a limited timeframe, instructions for self-administration of insulin would take priority over the explanation of foot care. Both subjects are important, but often, judgments must be made regarding the most vital information that needs to be taught. Patient needs can be prioritized by using the categories of "must do," "should do," and "nice to do." "Must do" activities often concern safety or life-threatening issues. For example, education on self-administration of medication is a priority. Education related to patient well-being may fall in the "should do" category. Dietary instruction about low sodium foods could be a "should do" topic. Finally, "nice to do" educational topics are not essential. These include information concerning the fat content of selections from an area restaurant. Interested patients could obtain this from the business itself, and unless specifically requested by the patient, it would be low priority.

Outcome Identification

Goals should be identified before starting educational presentations, to ensure that the sessions are goal-directed. A goal is a general statement describing the desired destination of the teaching, or where the patient should end up. An example of a goal for the diabetic patient in the previous section would be: "Maintains control of blood glucose levels" (Doenges, Moorhouse, & Burley, 2000, p. 77). Because a goal is broad, there are a series of steps leading to the goal, which are called *objectives*. Objectives for the preceding goal might be: "Following a 15-minute discussion and demonstration, the patient will describe the proper technique for glucometer testing." Or, "The patient will demonstrate the proper technique for subcutaneous insulin administration by Friday." These main objectives can be further subdivided into enabling objectives. Enabling objectives are smaller steps leading to the main objective. In the previous main objective, the patient goal was to demonstrate the proper technique for insulin injection. Enabling objectives might be: "Given a vial of insulin, the patient will demonstrate the procedure for rolling the vial with 100% accuracy" and "The patient will list two reasons for site rotation." These two enabling objectives are written in slightly different formats. The first objective is written in the style recommended by Robert Mager. It includes performance, conditions, and criterion. Performance is "what a learner is expected to be able to do and/or produce to be considered competent" (Mager, 1997, p. 46). In the first example, the performance is to be able to roll insulin. The condition includes a description of circumstances under which the performance would happen, such as "given a vial of insulin." Finally, the criteria are standards for acceptable performance. In this case, it would be "with 100% accuracy." The second enabling objective is shorter. It frequently does not include the criteria for successful performance found in a Mager-style objective. Both methods of writing objectives are considered acceptable. One method of ensuring that an objective is properly worded is to make sure the action is measurable. This can be accomplished by using a measurable verb. See Box 8-3 for a sample list of measurable verbs.

Objectives can be written in the cognitive (thinking, knowledge), psychomotor (skills), or affective

Box 8-3 Verbs Frequently Used in Objectives	
Define	Summarize
Describe	Verbalize
State	Explain
Discuss	Assemble
Calculate	Operate
Compare	Demonstrate
Categorize	Create

(feeling, attitude, and values) domain (area). At times, objectives in the affective domain are ignored. However, the affective domain can be vital to the learning process. Bastable (2003) described some vital areas in the affective domain: "Patients and family members also are faced with making moral and ethical choices as well as learning to internalize the value of complying with prescribed treatment regimens and incorporating health promotion and disease prevention practices into their daily lives." (p. 247) A sample affective objective would be: "During a group discussion, the patient will verbalize any anxiety he has regarding discharge from the psychiatric facility." Psychomotor objectives normally involve action such as: "When provided with a glucometer and lancet device, the patient will correctly demonstrate the procedure for obtaining his own blood sugar." A cognitive, or thinking objective, might be: "The patient will describe four important concepts of diabetic foot care."

Clear objectives help the educator in several ways. They facilitate communication with the learner because both participants know the expected outcome. They also guide the instructor in the selection of proper instructional strategies. Complex objectives, such as those involving critical thinking, require different strategies than basic knowledge objectives. An example of a basic knowledge objective is: "The patient will name four side effects of Lanoxin by tomorrow with 80% accuracy." A more complex objective would be: "By tomorrow, the patient will design a workable plan to obtain assistance in the event of a medical emergency." The complexity of the objective also affects choosing the best method of evaluation. Therefore, objectives are essential to the teaching plan.

Planning the Lesson

Successful patient teaching doesn't just happen; it is carefully planned. One planning decision that must be made is the selection of the preferred in-

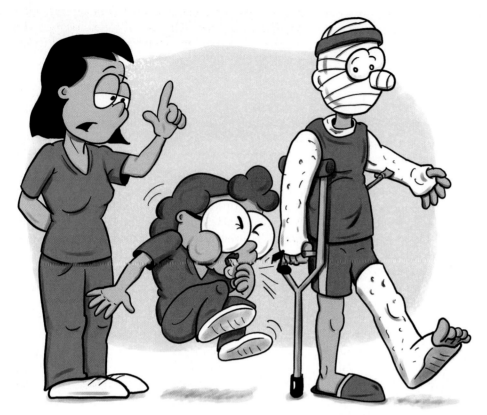

"Does the phrase 'Learn to walk before you run' mean anything to you?"

structional method. Obviously, the instructor wants to select an instructional method that leads to the accomplishment of the learning objective. However, there are many factors that can affect this decision. These factors include the availability of equipment, supplies, time, and finances. In today's tight economy, the educational budget may be reduced, resulting in a need for more creative planning. This may involve creativity in devising practice equipment or in scheduling time for education.

Instructional methods are usually divided into two large categories: traditional and nontraditional. Traditional methods are lecture, group discussion, one-to-one instruction, and demonstration. Nontraditional methods include role-playing, simulations, games, computer-assisted instruction (CAI), case studies, journals, and self-directed learning. Each method has advantages and disadvantages. For example, a lecture is a cost-effective way to present knowledge to a large group of people. However, in this method, the retention of the material does not tend to be high. It does not work well for the more complex objectives or those based on the

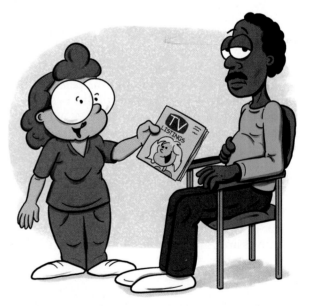

"I don't have any info about your treatment right now. I'll bet that eventually there'll be something about it on cable."

affective and psychomotor domains. Cost effectiveness is a consideration in teaching method selection. For example, asking the patient to perform the task immediately after the nurse demonstrates it works well when teaching psychomotor skills. However, it can be time consuming and therefore expensive in nursing time. The nurse might consider presenting the same material to small groups. The instructor would reach more learners, and, as an added bonus, the participants could share experiences. In planning a presentation, the nurse should always be open to new methods of instruction. Many instructors tend to concentrate only on traditional methods because of their familiarity with them. However, sometimes, nontraditional methods are the most effective teaching tool. For example, commercial or instructor-prepared games can enhance learning by making the experience more enjoyable. See Table 8-2 for a listing of the advantages and disadvantages of various teaching methods.

Another decision that needs to be made when planning patient teaching is choosing the most effective instructional material. These materials may include videotapes, computers and computer software (e.g., computer-generated presentations), handouts, displays, and models. The preferred patient learning style should be considered when choosing instructional material.

In facilitating the educational process, the nurse may prefer to use preprinted or computer-generated teaching tools. These help maintain focus and ensure that significant information is covered. However, using preprinted information does not eliminate the need to individualize the instruction.

After the resources are gathered, a lesson plan can be written. The lesson plan is similar to a written patient plan of care. Columns may be made for objectives, content to accompany the objectives, method of presentation, materials, time required, and type of evaluation. A typical form for a lesson plan can be found in Table 8-3. A completed example of a lesson plan can be found in the exercises at the end of this chapter.

Implementing the Educational Session

Before conducting the educational session, environmental factors must be considered. Rooms that are too hot or cold divert the learner's attention. The selection of a quiet area and the creation of an unhurried atmosphere will facilitate the learning process. For many patients, the stimulation of several senses enhances learning. Snacks may be a beneficial addition. The use of music or even the aroma of scented pens can provide an original touch without adding a great deal of expense.

An effective instructor strives to create a caring atmosphere throughout the educational process. The learners should be respected and should receive a great deal of positive reinforcement. The use of appropriate humor can also make a presentation more memorable.

As described in Chapter 5, Nursing Process Applications, the Nursing Interventions Classification (NIC) system presents some valuable activities related to patient education. Two that particularly relate to the process described above are Learning Facilitation (5520) and Learning Readiness Enhancement (5540) (McCloskey & Bulechek, 2000). See Box 8-4A and B for copies of these activities.

Evaluating the Educational Process

Evaluation of the educational process is another important aspect of patient education. As the demand for accountability continues to increase, outcomes measurement can only become more imperative. There are three basic categories of teaching evaluation: program evaluation, summative evaluation, and formative evaluation.

Program evaluation involves looking at the product and the expense of an educational program. Often, it is a requirement of various accrediting agencies that are concerned with overall program success. The necessity of a program may also need to be substantiated to receive reimbursement for it. An example of program evaluation would be the National League of Nursing Accrediting Commission review of nursing programs.

Summative evaluation examines the changes that occur as a result of the educational process. When the patient performs the activity following the course of lessons, summative evaluation determines whether the education truly altered patient behavior. For example, when medication instructions are given before discharge, a patient is asked to demonstrate knowledge of the medication regime. If during a home visit 6 months later, the nurse asks questions regarding the same regimen, a summative evaluation is being performed.

The major emphasis in this chapter is on formative evaluation. It is ongoing during the educational process. The instructor should periodically check with the learner regarding his or her assimilation of concepts. In educational settings, formative evalu-

TABLE 8-2 **Advantages and Disadvantages of Teaching Strategies**

STRATEGY	ADVANTAGES	DISADVANTAGES
TRADITIONAL		
1. Lecture	Works well with lower-level cognitive objectives	Low retention
	Cost-effective method to deliver instruction to large groups	Instructor centered
	Message reaches more in a timely manner	Does not engage learner
	Good for background material	Not individualized to learning style
		Not method of choice for affective or psychomotor objectives
2. Group discussion	Learner can actively participate	One member may dominate group
		Subject centered
		Shy members may feel left out
	Cost effective—more than one learner	Some people resist sharing experiences with groups of people
	Patients gain support from others with similar experience	Groups can wander off task
	Works well for cognitive and affective objectives	
3. One-to-one instruction	Works well with patients having low literacy skills	Isolates learner from others with similar concerns
	Can be individualized to the learner's needs	May be cost prohibitive due to instructor time required for delivery
	Allows patient to ask questions and clarify concepts	Patient may be uneasy regarding a test
4. Demonstration–return demonstration	Works well with psychomotor objectives	May be seen only by small group simultaneously
	Immediate feedback on performance	Labor intensive to view return demonstrations
	The step-by-step process works well with concrete sequential learners	
	Patient can observe exactly how the nurse wants the procedure performed	
NONTRADITIONAL		
1. Role-playing	Works well with the affective domain	Some are reluctant to participate
	Allows patient to rehearse desired behavior or coping skills	Some overdramatize
	Participants may examine attitudes and feelings	Requires a certain comfort level among participants
2. Simulation	Good technique for practicing decision-making and problem-solving skills	Expensive
	Situations resemble those encountered in real life but are presented in a safe learning environment	Labor intensive
3. Gaming	Works well for practice and review situations	Some participants are too competitive
	Makes repetitive subjects more enjoyable	Takes time
	Adds variety, increasing motivation and interest	Participants must possess background knowledge or skills
	Commercially made games and books describing games are often inexpensive	
	Games can be developed fairly easily by educators	
4. Self-directed	Good tool for adult learners	Requires literacy
	May be used to update knowledge and skills	Procrastination
		Decreased opportunity for questioning
	Self-paced	
	Instruction is consistent	
	Cost effective	

(continued)

STRATEGY	ADVANTAGES	DISADVANTAGES
5. Computer-assisted instruction	Works well with cognitive domain Accommodates various learning styles Self-paced Consistent instruction Can improve decision-making skills in a safe environment	Outdates quickly Some are intimidated by computers Technical difficulties Expensive Some health care programs are boring with poor graphics
6. Case studies	Works well for drill and practice learning Encourages application of knowledge Cost effective Encourages attainment of critical thinking skills	Requires literacy Can cause learner frustration if case is fully developed
7. Field trips	Content remains in memory longer when accompanied by visual image Heightens learner interest Useful for objectives in all three domains	Can be expensive Time consuming Some may not remain on task
8. Journals	Works well with affective objectives Useful for patient in tracking feelings and data Good mechanism for feedback Some communicate easier through writing	Time consuming Patient may resist

ation is often measured with a test. However, tests make many individuals nervous and may stall the educational process. Discussions with open-ended statements frequently obtain satisfactory evaluation results. Open-ended questions are those that cannot be answered with just a "yes" or "no." An example would be: "Tell me what you remember about foot care." Box 8-5 provides more examples of open and closed questions.

Conducting a formative evaluation allows the educator to make revisions in the plan as the patient teaching session progresses. Additional information may be obtained about the learner or learning needs. In this manner, continued knowledge gaps can be identified and corrected. Evaluation is an essential step in planning patient education.

SUMMARY

Patient teaching is an important aspect of nursing care. It should be an organized activity with specific goals. Careful planning is necessary to individualize the sessions to meet the patient's educational needs. The nurse must consider numerous aspects in developing the plan, including patient needs, learning style, learning readiness, motivation, emo-

tional status, cultural beliefs, and habits. Organization is enhanced by the use of a lesson plan. The steps in preparing a lesson plan parallel the steps in developing a plan of care. Priorities of patient needs should be established. Critical thinking is essential to the process. Instructional methods and materials must support the proposed objectives, and evaluation is vital to determine effectiveness and clarify any knowledge gaps.

KEY POINTS

- Patient teaching is a major nursing responsibility.
- Patient teaching is goal directed and involves critical thinking.
- Motivation, emotional aspects, cultural beliefs, and habits affect readiness to learn.
- Preparing a lesson plan closely parallels the steps of the nursing process. During the assessment phase, the educator must determine what the patient needs to learn, the patient's preferred learning style, and whether the patient is ready to learn.
- During the analysis step, learning needs should be validated with the patient. The priority learning needs are identified.

TABLE 8-3 Sample Lesson Plan

Goal:

OBJECTIVES	CONTENT	METHODS	ALLOTTED TIME	RESOURCES	EVALUATION

Box 8-4A LEARNING FACILITATION (5520)

Definition: Promoting the ability to process and comprehend information

ACTIVITIES:

Begin the instruction only after the patient demonstrates readiness to learn.

Set mutual, realistic learning goals with the patient.

Identify learning objectives clearly and in measurable/observable terms.

Adjust the instruction to the patient's level of knowledge and understanding.

Tailor the content to the patient's cognitive, psychomotor, and/or affective abilities/disabilities.

Provide information appropriate to developmental level.

Provide an environment conducive to learning.

Arrange the information in a logical sequence.

Arrange the information from simple to complex, known to unknown, or concrete to abstract, as appropriate.

Differentiate "critical" content from "desirable" content.

Adapt the information to comply with the patient's lifestyle/routines.

Relate the information to the patient's personal desires/needs.

Provide information that is consistent with the patient's values/beliefs.

Provide information that is compatible with the patient's locus of control.

Ensure that the material is current and up to date.

Provide educational materials to illustrate important and/or complex information.

Use multiple teaching modalities, as appropriate.

Use familiar language.

Define unfamiliar terminology.

Relate new content to previous knowledge, as appropriate.

Present the information in a stimulating manner.

Introduce the patient to persons who have undergone similar experiences.

Encourage the patient's active participation.

Use self-paced instruction, when possible.

Avoid setting time limits.

Provide adequate time for mastery of content, as appropriate.

Keep teaching sessions short, as appropriate.

Simplify instructions, as appropriate.

Repeat important information.

Provide verbal prompts/reminders, as appropriate.

Provide memory aids, as appropriate.

Avoid demands for abstract thinking, if patient can think only in concrete terms.

Ensure that consistent information is being provided by various members of the health care team.

Use demonstration and return demonstration, as appropriate.

Box 8-4B LEARNING READINESS ENHANCEMENT (5540)

Definition: Improving the ability and willingness to receive information

ACTIVITIES:

Provide a nonthreatening environment.

Establish rapport.

Establish teacher credibility, as appropriate.

Maximize the patient's hemodynamic status to facilitate brain oxygenation (e.g., positioning and medication adjustments), as appropriate.

Fulfill the patient's basic physiological needs (e.g., hunger, thirst, warmth, and oxygen).

Decrease the patient's level of fatigue, as appropriate.

Control the patient's pain, as appropriate.

Avoid the use of medications that may alter the patient's perception (e.g., narcotics and hypnotics), as appropriate.

Monitor the patient's level of orientation/confusion.

Increase the patient's orientation to reality, as appropriate.

Maximize sensory input by use of eyeglasses, hearing aids, and so on, as appropriate.

Minimize the degree of sensory overload/underload, as appropriate.

Satisfy the patient's safety needs (e.g., security, control, and familiarity), as appropriate.

Monitor the patient's emotional state.

Assist the patient to deal with intense emotions (e.g., anxiety, grief, and anger), as appropriate.

Encourage verbalization of feelings, perceptions, and concerns.

Provide time for the patient to ask questions and discuss concerns.

Address the patient's specific concerns, as appropriate.

Establish a learning environment as early in contact with patient as possible.

Facilitate the patient's acceptance of the situation, as appropriate.

Assist the patient to develop confidence in ability, as appropriate.

Enlist participation of family/significant others, as appropriate.

Explain how the information will help the patient meet goals, as appropriate.

Explain how the patient's past unpleasant experiences with health care differs from the current situation, as appropriate.

Assist the patient to realize the severity of the illness, as appropriate.

Assist the patient to realize susceptibility to complications, as appropriate.

Assist the patient to realize ability to control the progression of the illness, as appropriate.

Assist the patient to see alternative actions that are less risky to life-style, as appropriate.

Provide a trigger or cue (e.g., motivating comments/rationale and new information) toward appropriate action, as appropriate.

Box 8-5 Examples of Closed and Open Questions

CLOSED

Do you understand when to take your medication?
Did lack of money contribute to your decision not to take your medication?
Did you follow the 1,200-calorie diet?

OPEN

How does it feel to be on a diet restriction?
What did the doctor tell you about taking your medication?
What things contributed to your decision not to take your medication?

- Outcome identification, including both goals and objectives, is important before starting an educational presentation. Learning goals are broad in nature.
- Objectives are more specific and describe the desired result of instruction.
- In planning the educational presentation, the nurse chooses instructional methods and materials.
- Evaluation is necessary to determine the effectiveness of patient teaching.

REFERENCES

Andrews, M., & Boyle, J. (2003). *Transcultural concepts in nursing care.* Philadelphia: Lippincott Williams & Wilkins.

Bastable, S. B. (2003). *Nurse as educator.* Boston: Jones and Bartlett.

Brennan, P. K. (1984). An analysis of the relationships among hemispheric preference and analytic/global cognitive style, two elements of learning style, method of instruction, gender, and mathematics achievement of 10th-grade geometry students. Doctoral dissertation. St. John's University. *Dissertation Abstracts International, 45,* 3271A.

Burgireno, J. (1985). Maximizing learning in the adult with SCI. *Rehabilitation Nursing, 10*(5), 20–21.

Doenges, M. E., Moorhouse, M. F., & Burley, J. T. (2000). *Application of nursing process and nursing diagnosis: An interactive test for diagnostic reasoning.* Philadelphia: F. A. Davis.

Dunn, R., & Dunn, K. (1993). *Teaching secondary students through their individual learning styles.* Boston: Allyn & Bacon.

Mager, R. F. (1997). *Preparing instructional objectives.* Atlanta: Center for Effective Performance.

McCloskey, J. C., & Bulechek, G. M. (2000). *Nursing interventions classification (NIC).* St. Louis: Mosby.

Reese, S. (2002). Understanding our differences. *Techniques, 77*(1), 10–23.

Van Wynen, E. A. (1997). Information processing styles: One size doesn't fit all. *Nurse Educator, 22*(5), 22–50.

Student Worksheets

 SKILL SHEET: PATIENT TEACHING

Purpose

1. To provide a framework for planning and delivering patient education.
2. To facilitate formulation of a lesson plan.

Objectives

The student will demonstrate ability to do the following:

1. Perform a needs assessment.
2. Establish priority of the needs.
3. Compose a goal statement.
4. Write measurable objectives.
5. Prepare a lesson plan.
6. Evaluate effectiveness of patient teaching.

Steps: Patient Teaching

ASSESSMENT

1. Perform needs assessment.
2. Identify any patient special educational needs.
3. Determine preferred learning style.
4. Establish readiness to learn.

ANALYSIS

1. Validate educational needs.
2. Establish priorities among the needs.

OUTCOME IDENTIFICATION

1. Identify goal.
2. Compose measurable main and enabling objectives.

PLAN

1. Determine method of presentation.
2. Identify required teaching materials.
3. Formulate a lesson plan.

IMPLEMENTATION

1. Control distracting environmental factors.
2. Establish a caring, concerned atmosphere.

EVALUATION

1. Determine effectiveness of educational endeavors.
2. Revise lesson plan as needed.

COMPETENCY VALIDATION: PATIENT TEACHING

COMPETENCY STATEMENT

The student will demonstrate the ability to provide organized patient teaching, which meets the patient's educational needs.

The student demonstrated the ability to do the following:

1. Identify educational needs of the patient.
2. Assess patient special learning needs.
3. Establish priorities among the gaps in knowledge
4. Develop reasonable patient learning goals.
5. Develop measurable main and enabling objectives to reach the goals.
6. Create an effective lesson plan.
7. Establish an atmosphere conducive to learning.
8. Evaluate the extent to which educational goals have been achieved.
9. Revise and modify the lesson plan.

COMPETENT

- Understands reason for task and is able to perform task independently
- Understands reason for task but needs supervision
- Understands reason for task and is able to perform task with assistance

NOT COMPETENT

- Understands reason for task but performs task at provisional level
- Is unable to state reason for task and performs task at dependent level

SKILL CHECKLIST: PATIENT TEACHING

PATIENT TEACHING	SATISFACTORY	UNSATISFACTORY	NI/COMMENTS
ASSESSMENT 1. Perform needs assessment.			
2. Identify special needs.			
3. Determine preferred learning style.			
4. Establish readiness to learn.			
ANALYSIS 1. Validate needs.			
2. Establish priorities.			
OUTCOME IDENTIFICATION 1. Identify goal.			
2. Compose measurable objectives.			
PLAN 1. Determine method of presentation.			
2. Identify required materials.			
3. Formulate lesson plan.			
IMPLEMENTATION 1. Control distracting environmental factors.			
2. Establish a caring, concerned atmosphere.			
EVALUATION 1. Determine effectiveness of lesson plan.			
2. Revise plan as needed.			

SCENARIO TO ACCOMPANY STUDENT WORKSHEETS

Robert Smith, aged 69 years, has just been diagnosed with non–insulin-dependent diabetes mellitus (NIDDM). His initial fasting blood sugar was 385 mg/dL. Mr. Smith has experienced no significant health problems. He and his wife acknowledge a lack of understanding of the disease process. Upon assessment, the nurse discovers that Mr. Smith is literate and a visual learner. Motivation is supplied by the hope that he will "feel better." He is concerned about dietary restrictions due to his emphasis on food common to his cultural background.

A sample of part of the lesson plan follows.

LESSON PLAN

Goal: The patient will adequately manage his diabetes mellitus as evidenced by daily blood sugar levels of less than 170 mg/dL.

OBJECTIVES	CONTENT	METHODS	ALLOTTED TIME	RESOURCES	EVALUATION

The patient will be able to:
 	
1. Describe aspects involved in blood sugar control
 	
  a. List three factors that must be balanced to achieve blood sugar control.
 	
  b. List two physical problems that can result in reduced blood sugar control. (Cognitive)
	Review of disease process related to blood sugar control	One-to-one instruction	15 minutes	Handout
				Color posters
				Video
					Circle correct answers on an informal tool.

2. Demonstrate proper blood sugar testing with glucometer. (Psychomotor)	Discussion of theory behind testing Discussion and demonstration of proper technique	Demonstration	1 hour	Glucometer Lancet Alcohol Instruction booklet	Return demonstration
3. Express feelings regarding diagnosis of diabetes and their role in blood sugar control. (Affective)	Common feelings expressed by diabetic patients in dealing with disease	Group discussion Role-playing	30 minutes	Classroom	Participation in discussion

PRACTICE EXERCISES: PATIENT TEACHING

WRITING OBJECTIVES

1. Mr. Smith has been newly diagnosed with diabetes mellitus. Write an additional objective for the teaching plan.

_____

_____

_____

2. How would you evaluate successful attainment of this objective?

_____

_____

_____

See the Answer Key in Appendix A for sample answers for this exercise.

ESTABLISHING A TEACHING PLAN

1. Work though the skills assessment sheet. Focus on an educational gap you have identified in yourself.

   A. Discuss your preferred learning style. _____

   _____

   _____

   _____

   B. Do you feel motivated to learn this material? _____

   _____

   _____

   _____

   C. Is this a priority need?_____

   _____

   _____

   _____

   D. Write a goal statement. _____

   _____

   _____

   _____

E. Write one main and three enabling objectives for this educational need. _____

_____

_____

_____

_____

_____

F. What method of presentation would work best to attain the identified objectives? _____

_____

_____

_____

G. List the materials you would need to acquire for this method. _____

_____

_____

_____

_____

_____

H. Using the form below, establish a lesson plan for your own educational need. _____

_____

_____

_____

Goal:

OBJECTIVES	CONTENT	METHODS	ALLOTTED TIME	RESOURCES	EVALUATION

OBJECTIVES	CONTENT	METHODS	ALLOTTED TIME	RESOURCES	EVALUATION

OBJECTIVES	CONTENT	METHODS	ALLOTTED TIME	RESOURCES	EVALUATION

Answers will vary with student's experience.

UNIT THREE

APPLICATION OF COGNITIVE SKILLS

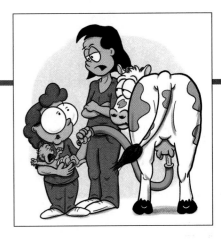

CHAPTER 9

Applying Clinical Reasoning to Various Practice Settings

OBJECTIVES

1. Define clinical reasoning.

2. Describe the role of the nursing process in clinical reasoning.

3. Explain the role of clinical reasoning in nursing practice.

4. Identify the criteria used to evaluate reasoning in nursing.

5. Discuss the integration of cognitive skills into the nursing process.

6. Describe the consequences of a nurse's failure to assess, monitor, and report.

7. Propose appropriate nursing actions based on interpretations of patient data.

8. Analyze circumstances and patient conditions that indicate a need to notify the physician.

9. Identify how to determine when lab values warrant physician notification.

10. Apply clinical reasoning for individual patient care decisions in a variety of settings.

This chapter focuses on the nurse's ability to apply consistent, competent reasoning skills when caring for the individual patient. Effective nursing judgment results from disciplined reasoning. The novice nurse must practice clinical reasoning to develop the mental skill necessary for making "reasoned judgments." This reasoning, referred to as clinical reasoning, provides the foundation for competent clinical practice. Chapter 11, Applying Nursing Judgment in Clinical Settings, concentrates on nursing judgment. Decision making for each patient in the clinical setting involves assessment, evaluation, and clinical reasoning. The three aspects of decision making occur simultaneously, but for the sake of simplicity, they are discussed separately in this chapter.

During the assessment phase, the nurse identifies the current level of patient condition and stability and interprets any variations in physical status, mental status, or the results of diagnostic tests. The nurse also performs an initial assessment to establish a baseline, and then continues to monitor the patient. Data are interpreted, noting deviations from normal, to measure variations and draw conclusions. When variations do occur, it is important to monitor the patient through reassessment in order to define the problem more clearly and to identify actions that will resolve the problem.

During the evaluation phase, the nurse compares current data with the previous data and with the normal progression of the disease process. For instance, interpreting lab data helps evaluate the patient's response to therapy. Throughout patient care, the nurse analyzes and evaluates patient responses. The plan of care and expected outcomes can then be changed, based on these judgments.

The skill of reasoning is essential in clinical decision making. The nurse must know what to look for, recognize a changing patient status, and decide what to do. For example, consider the following scenario: a patient is resting quietly, breath sounds clear, respirations easy and unlabored, skin color pink, and oxygen saturation (SpO_2) 98% with oxygen (O_2) per nasal cannula at 3 liters. After eating dinner, the patient rings for the nurse. Assessment reveals the patient sitting upright struggling to breathe, respirations labored, crackles bilaterally, color ashen, and SpO_2 82%. The first action the nurse should take is to determine whether the oxygen is in place and functional. The nurse should then increase the O_2 infusion rate, ensure that the head of the bed is in high position, and call the physician for further treatment orders.

DEFINITION

In the clinical setting, it is essential to determine the actual quality of the information presented and make a choice. The Foundation for Critical Thinking (1997) calls this skill "evaluative reasoning"; the goal of evaluative reasoning is to come to "reasoned judgment" (p. B5). This type of reasoning does not support knowledge for the sake of knowledge. The application of knowledge and judgment in the clinical setting is vital to competent practice.

REASONING

Consistent, competent reasoning skills are critical to obtaining optimum patient care outcomes. Being alert for unusual circumstances or deviations from normal and the ability to reason critically promote accuracy. Using evidence-based practice to make decisions in the clinical setting produces consistency. Standards of critical thinking used in the application of cognitive skills also yield greater consistency in outcomes. The cognitive skills are used as needed, unlike the nursing process, which is usually performed in a sequence of steps.

When processing data, it is important to continually evaluate reasoning. The criteria for evaluating reasoning in nursing practice include defining the problem clearly and precisely in your mind.

Next, examine the evidence to determine what other information is needed. Obtain and clarify additional data, discarding irrelevant facts to prevent distraction. Examine your logic, and give reasoned explanations for your conclusions. Identify the implications, consequences, and impact of both positive and negative outcomes, recognizing and assessing the validity of assumptions. Finally, review the consequences of possible actions and draw conclusions regarding the likelihood of achieving the desired outcome. To promote positive outcomes, the reasoning used in the processes of assessment, reassessment, data analysis, and modification of care must continually be evaluated. Box 9-1 contains a list of specific criteria for evaluating reasoning.

The scenarios portrayed in this chapter focus on using the clinical reasoning process to make decisions for individual patients in varied settings. The mental skills discussed in previous chapters of this book are combined in this chapter to form a reasoning process that can be used to monitor the unique needs of patients and determine what to do.

GUIDELINES FOR DECISION MAKING

Making clinical decisions can be very complicated because the knowledge derived from basic textbooks is not always sufficient to provide direction regarding "what to do" and " when to do it." It is essential to use professional standards as guidelines to decision making when evaluating individual patient circumstances, relevant textbook data, current diagnostic test findings, and the assessment findings of the nurse. The nurse must recognize that "All nurses are legally accountable for actions taken in the course of nursing practice, as well as for action delegated by the nurse to others assisting in the delivery of nursing care" (American Nurses Association [ANA], 2003b, p. 11)

Legal regulation is defined in nursing practice by legislative and regulatory agencies. One source of legal parameters to determine whether an action is within the scope of nursing practice is the state (provincial) Board of Nursing. This board is responsible for interpreting and enforcing rules. The state (provincial) Nurse Practice Act dictates the educational requirements for the licensure of nurses and defines what constitutes professional misconduct, negligence, the impaired nurse, and a violation of boundaries.

Professional standards define the practice base and are drawn from the scope of nursing practice. The ANA's (2003a) *Scope and Standards of Practice*

Good to know

---

1. **The purpose, goal, or end in nursing:** What is the purpose of the reasoning? Is the purpose clearly stated or clearly implied? Is the goal or end result justifiable? Is it a real problem?

2. **The question at issue for nursing problem to be solved:** Is the question at issue well stated? Is the question clearly understood? How does the question relate to basic purpose or goal? Does the expression of the question do justice to the complexity of the matter at issue? Are the question and purpose directly relevant to each other?

3. **The nursing point of view or frame of reference:** Is the point of view narrow or biased? Clarify or seek to clarify and obtain additional information as necessary. What data are irrelevant?

4. **The empirical dimension of nursing reasoning:** Is the evidence, experiences, or information essential to the issue? Is the information accurate? Does the reasoner address the complexities? Is there an adequate amount of pertinent data? What else do I need to know?

5. **The conceptual dimension of nursing reasoning:** Are the key concepts clarified when necessary? Are the concepts used justifiably? Is there a reasoned explanation for the conclusion?

6. **Nursing assumptions, the starting point of reasoning.** What are the assumptions? What am I taking for granted? Can anything else be assumed? What problems exist in assumptions made?

7. **Nursing inferences:** Were sound inferences made based on current knowledge and evidenced-based practice? If this is true, does that result follow? Is this conclusion a normal outcome of thought?

8. **Nursing implications and consequences where our reasoning takes us:** What are the consequences of the actions? What are the costs? What if the action results in a negative outcome? How will this action affect the outcome? How will it help? Were the desired outcomes reached? Should something have been done differently? Why?

9. **Implicit and explicit reasons in nursing:** Why are you defining your purpose in this way? Why did you state your question in this manner instead of in an alternative fashion? Why did you select this concept or theory instead of another? What implicit reasons led to the selection of your information interpretation, data selection, plan of care, and evaluation?

Adapted from Paul, R., & Elder, L. (2001). *The miniature guide to critical thinking: Concepts and tools* (p. 11). Dillon Beach, CA: Foundation for Critical Thinking; and Paul, R., & Heaslip, P. (1995). Critical thinking and intuitive nursing practice. *Journal of Advanced Nursing* 22(7), 40–47.

---

is the basic resource for defining the nurse's responsibilities to deliver quality care. The standards also provide resources for the identification of behaviors that constitute incompetent, unethical, or illegal practice. Every nurse should have a working knowledge of the ANA Code of Ethics (see Chapter 10, Box 10-3), the ANA Standards of Practice (see Chapter 5, Box 5-1), and the ANA Standards of Performance (Box 9-2).

The ANA Standards of Performance provide clarification and direction in nursing practice. Self-regulation is an essential skill necessary in the evaluation of ones' own practice. Standards I and II direct the nurse to evaluate the quality of his or her

---

STANDARD 1. QUALITY OF PRACTICE

The nurse systematically enhances the quality and effectiveness of nursing practice.

STANDARD 2. PRACTICE EVALUATION

The nurse evaluates one's own nursing practice in relation to professional practice standards and guidelines, relevant statutes, rules, and regulations.

STANDARD 3. EDUCATION

The nurse attains knowledge and competency that reflects current nursing practice.

STANDARD 4. COLLEGIALITY

The nurse interacts with and contributes to the professional development of peers and colleagues.

STANDARD 5. COLLABORATION

The nurse collaborates with patient, family, and others in the conduct of nursing practice.

STANDARD 6. ETHICS

The nurse integrates ethical provisions in all areas of practice.

STANDARD 7. RESEARCH

The nurse integrates research findings into practice.

STANDARD 8. RESOURCE UTILIZATION

The nurse considers factors related to safety, effectiveness, cost, and impact on practice in the planning and delivery of nursing services.

STANDARD 9. LEADERSHIP

The nurse provides leadership in the profession and the professional practice setting.

Adapted from American Nurses Association. (2003). *Nursing: Scope and standards of practice.* Washington, DC: Nursesbooks.org. Reproduced with the permission of the American Nurses Association.

---

own nursing practice. Quality is measured by the degree to which the care that is delivered consistently achieves the outcomes expected. Regulating one's own practice within the clinical environment based on standards, guidelines, statutes, and rules and regulations is essential. One example of this skill occurs when a nurse recognizes a lack of experience in handling a particular situation or problem and consults with a more experienced professional.

Standard III directs the nurse to maintain a current knowledge base and competency in his or her practice. The ability to identify learning needs and select appropriate activities to enhance clinical practice in the deficient area is essential to developing consistent and accurate clinical skills. For example, suppose an emergency room nurse has a knowledge deficit regarding the treatment protocol for anthrax exposure. The nurse can expand his or her knowledge to meet this need by attending a continuing education class provided by a local community college on issues affecting community bioterrorism preparedness. The nurse could also read articles in current nursing literature or review available information on the Internet. Continued self-improvement obtained by seeking out educational opportunities to correct weaknesses and de-

veloping lifelong learning habits facilitates the maintenance of a nurse's competency.

Standard V pertains to the integration of ethical provisions in all areas of practice. As a result of advances in medical technology, the nurse is increasingly exposed to situations that involve social and legal concerns. Public awareness concerning the nurse's unique relationship with, and responsibility to, patients and their families has focused more attention on accountability for nursing actions. Many decisions made by the nurse have ethical and legal ramifications.

Accountability dictates that the nurse is responsible for decisions made and actions initiated. Nurses should take credit for positive results achieved through good decision making as well as accepting responsibility for results of poor decisions. Chapter 10, Ethical Decision Making, presents a more in-depth view of health care ethics and legal issues regarding "how to think" in the workplace.

Standard VII instructs the nurse to use research-based findings to provide care to patients. Research-based evidence has been compiled into Nursing Interventions Classification (NIC), Nursing Outcomes Classification (NOC), and North Ameri-

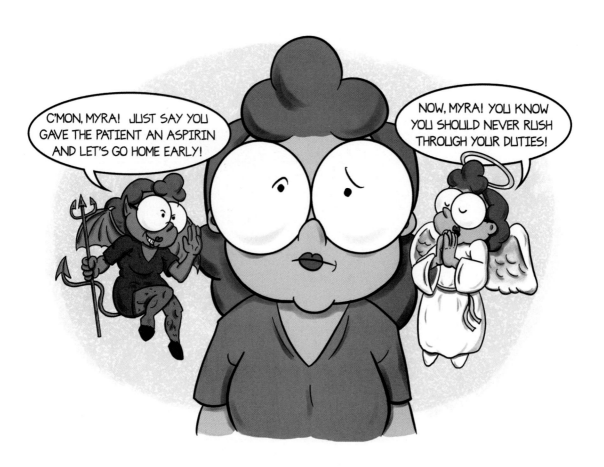

can Nursing Diagnosis Association (NANDA) guidelines and can be used in planning patient care. The Iowa Intervention Project identified NIC 6650 Surveillance as, "Purposeful and ongoing acquisition, interpretation, and synthesis of patient data for clinical decision making" (McCloskey & Bulechek, 2000, p. 629). Additionally, Craig and Smith (2002) identified the significance of evidence-based practice as, "Guidelines that can be used to reduce inappropriate variations in practice" (p. 187). Standards of care developed by individual institutions are used to direct nursing decisions related to specific equipment and certain procedures. These can be found in policy and procedure manuals within clinical facilities.

APPLICATION OF COGNITIVE SKILLS

The application of critical thinking to the cognitive skills is imperative to providing ongoing care.

At the onset, the nurse collects all the pertinent information and uses the skill of interpretation to define the meaning of the presenting patient information. For example, a nurse obtains the vital signs of a male patient and observes his respirations to be 30 breaths/min and labored. Recognizing that these are abnormal physical findings, the nurse then analyzes all the available data to define the problem or its cause. In this patient scenario, pertinent questions must be answered, such as: What additional assessment does the nurse need to make to explain the findings? What was the patient doing that could cause his symptoms? What does the nurse need to do first?

The nurse establishes desired or expected outcomes for the interventions to determine whether the identified problem will be resolved. After implementation of the intervention, the nurse conducts ongoing evaluation of progress toward the expected outcome. Again, pertinent questions must be asked: Is there evidence of lessening symptoms? Are there positive indicators of improvement?

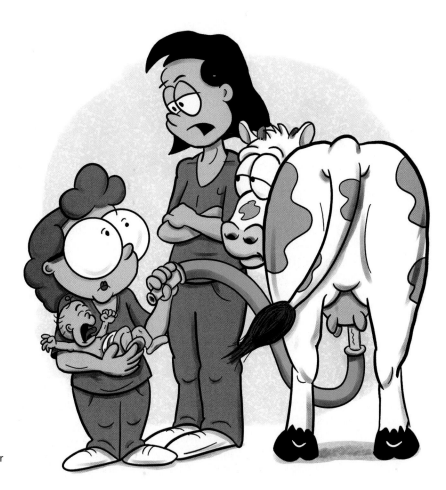

"Can you maybe think of a better way to feed milk to the baby?"

Does the patient have fewer complaints? Does he state, "I feel better"?

At this point, new factors need to be determined, such as: What are the respiratory rate and effort of the patient now? What is his oxygen saturation (SpO_2)? Based on new presenting information, such as patient symptoms or a lack thereof, the nurse uses the critical thinking skill of inference to draw a conclusion as to the meaning or implication of these new findings. For example, the patient's respirations had been 30 breaths/min and very labored, his skin color dusky, and the SpO_2 77%. The nurse intervened by elevating the head of the bed and applying prescribed O_2 through a non-rebreathing mask. Now, the patient's respirations are 22 breaths/min and less labored, his SpO_2 is 89%, and his color is improving. The nurse infers that the implemented interventions are appropriate.

After recognizing an effect, secondary to the intervention, the nurse must be able to provide a sound explanation or rationale for the result. For example, giving the patient O_2 through a non-rebreathing mask increased the O_2 available to body tissue, thereby causing a rise in the SpO_2 value and improvement in the patient's skin color. This critical thinking skill requires theoretical knowledge of cause and effect.

In the final step, the nurse uses the skill of self-regulation to continually question or reexamine his or her thinking. This involves self-examination: "Did I obtain all possible information"? "Did I base my conclusions on prior experience, and how might it have clouded my judgment?" What might have worked better?" A scenario presented in Box 9-3 provides an example of an application of the cognitive skills.

Another example of a clinical decision requiring reasoning is the delegation of tasks to health care workers in order to provide ongoing care. Whether the employment setting is acute care, long-term care, ambulatory care, or the home setting, dividing up the workload to achieve optimal care for all patients is essential. Making assignments based on the expertise and experience of available caregivers produces maximum productivity and cost-effective results.

When making assignments, the nurse should perform a brief assessment of each patient's needs and care requirements. During this process, certain questions need to be answered. For example: Are the assessment needs of the patient highly complex, or would a simple assessment be adequate without compromising the care? Is the stability of the patient expected to change? What are the risks for complications or change in status for this health state? What level of technology is required to com-

| Box 9-3 | Application of Cognitive Skills |

The nurse obtains a male patient's vital signs and observes his respirations to be 30 breaths/min and labored.

Interpretation: This is an abnormal physical finding.

Analysis: What additional assessment data do the nurse need to collect?

What was the patient doing that could cause his symptoms?

What does the nurse need to do first?

Evaluation: Is there evidence of lessening symptoms?

Are there positive indicators of improvement?

Does the patient have fewer complaints?

Does he state, "I feel better"?

What are the patient's respiratory rate and effort now?

What is his oxygen saturation (SpO_2)?

Inference: Because the patient's symptoms have resolved, the nurse can draw a conclusion that the interventions are appropriate.

Explanation: Giving oxygen (O_2) via nonrebreathing mask increases O_2 available to body tissue, thus causing a rise in the SpO_2 value and improvement in patient's skin color.

Self-regulation: "Did I obtain all of the facts?"

"Did I base my conclusions on prior experience, and how might this cloud my judgment?"

"What might have worked better?"

plete the care; for example, are the patient care needs routine, including such interventions as medication administration, sterile dressing changes, and Foley catheter insertion, or does the care require discharge planning, high-tech equipment, or in-depth assessment skills?

Next, the nurse should obtain a separate assessment of the skills and competencies of the caregivers. More questions must be answered. For example, if the assignment is given to an unlicensed assistive personnel (UAP) or a licensed practical nurse/licensed vocational nurse (LPN/LVN), is there adequate supervision available to ensure safe care? Does the staff have training for specialized procedures, such as electrocardiogram interpretation, disease-specific isolation precautions, or central lines that may be needed in the care of a specific group of patients?

Helpful resources for determining the delegation of tasks to available staff include job descriptions, staff member competency check sheets, and the personal input of the caregiver. Finally, the care requirements for the patients should be compared with human resources and tasks delegated accordingly. After delegation, the nurse must continue to monitor the progress of patients toward outcomes specified in their plan of care. The task of delegation is covered more thoroughly in Chapter 6, Delegation.

CLINICAL REASONING APPLICATIONS

Quality implies evaluation. Evaluation requires standards that define acceptable levels of care. The ANA Standards of Professional Practice identify nursing activities related to the quality of care. The nurse must compare his or her actions to these standards and evaluate the care rendered. As previously discussed, in the reality of health care, nurses are being asked to do more with fewer resources. Therefore, nurses must use their reasoning ability to make decisions that do not result in patient harm.

Evaluating the Workload

One potential area of concern for the nurse in maintaining quality nursing care is accepting patient assignments. A professional relationship with a patient is established when the nurse accepts a patient assignment. An impossible workload, in which the outcome fails to meet an appropriate standard of care, is unacceptable. Indicators that identify an unacceptable patient care assignment could be determined by the following results:

- Failure to monitor when indicated by patient's condition
- Inadequate treatment for the circumstance
- Excessive delay of treatments
- Failure to provide ongoing care for treatments and procedures
- Lack of time to provide patient teaching

Even if the work assignment results in the occurrence of only one of these indicators, the situation impairs the quality of patient care. Failure to meet the test for delivering nursing service at acceptable standards of quality places the nurse at risk for being held accountable for patient abandonment (negligence). "Knowing precisely what constitutes patient abandonment can help you fulfill your responsibilities as a nurse while protecting yourself against this serious charge" (Michael, 2002, p. 67).

Monitoring Patient Condition

Using clinical reasoning involves making a choice to monitor the status of a patient, to detect change, and to respond to the change with an appropriate intervention. It is essential to monitor the patient's response to the intervention by evaluating the outcomes of care. Giving meaning to the data as they are detected is vital to initiate a timely response for a changing status. Two specific examples of monitoring condition include calling the physician and interpreting lab data.

CALLING THE PHYSICIAN

Calling the physician involves an assessment of the patient situation and a decision regarding the necessity of the call. The specific steps of communication with the physician are covered in Chapter 7, Communication. The reasoning part of this event involves establishing the parameters regarding whether or not to place the call. The following guidelines to determine the need for calling the physician are designed to assist the nurse to make the correct decision:

- A changing patient status (e.g., critical findings needing immediate attention or assessments indicative of a worsening clinical situation, such as changing mental status or changing vital signs)
- Pain without ordered management options
- Acute elimination problems
- Significant medical problems requiring immediate attention that have no treatment orders (e.g., purulent drainage from wound without an order for an antibiotic)
- Lab values that require treatment orders
- Risk to safety

When in doubt as to what to do, the nurse should consult with a more experienced nurse or call the supervisor. If these resources are unavailable, the physician should be called.

INTERPRETING LAB VALUES

Another important area in which nurses must use reasoning is in the interpretation of lab data. Laboratory personnel report findings of the patient's lab data. The nurse must determine the meaning and the importance of the data. Knowing normal lab test values and being able to interpret normal and abnormal values correctly are essential. For example, the normal range for a prothrombin time is 11 to 12.5 seconds. When the patient is taking warfarin sodium (Coumadin), the therapeutic range is $1\frac{1}{2}$ to 2 times the normal (20 to 30 seconds). It is important for the nurse to focus on all of these parameters for the information to be useful in decision making.

The information presented here is not intended to replace information studied in medical and surgical nursing classes, but rather to provide guidelines for determining what to do with laboratory data once they are obtained. For example: Should you file the data in the chart and take no action? Should you call the physician immediately? Should you communicate the results to the next shift in report? Should you question a drug order or other treatment order?

Black, Hawks, and Keene (2001, p. 2301) identified the following analytic technique to determine when to call the physician regarding lab values:

- Is the value an expected abnormal finding? For example, creatinine is normally elevated in a patient with renal failure.
- Is the value an unexpected abnormal finding? For example, elevated blood sugar levels in a patient without diabetes may signal a disease.
- Is the value an unexpected normal finding? For example, a patient with angina and probable myocardial infarction would be expected to have elevated isoenzymes. Normal levels may mean that the patient has another cause of chest pain.
- Is the value an expected normal finding? For example, a healthy patient should have a normal complete blood count.

To determine whether to call the physician, the nurse should conduct the following steps. First, the data should be evaluated and the information compared to the clinical status of the patient. Lab values should not be considered in isolation from the patient. Next, the values should be compared to the age, medical diagnosis, assessment data, physical status, physician's orders, current treatment options, and previous lab values obtained. For example, the blood glucose level from the morning fasting lab draw was 369 mg/dL. The patient has a sliding scale insulin order prescribed for a glucose level up to 400. The nurse would administer the sliding scale insulin and take no further action. However, if the morning fasting blood glucose is 369 and the orders for the sliding scale coverage only extend to a level of 350, calling the physician is indicated. Also, if the circumstance of the elevated blood glucose level has occurred repeatedly in the mornings, even though the sliding scale covers the number, it should be discussed with the physician because this may be indicative of a need to change the routine insulin dosage. In conclusion, it is essential to consider the circumstances when making decisions about the lab values.

Knowledge and Ability for Varied Settings

Because of the increased use of highly sophisticated and complex equipment and the demand for the nurse's knowledge to encompass more complex illnesses, there is an increased expectation of responsibility and accountability in health care. Nursing care requirements, in many areas, involve a high level of autonomy in the delivery of safe and effective care. Specialized knowledge is required for each specialty area. Unique decisions are also frequently involved in various aspects of nursing care. The types of decisions nurses may face can vary from one clinical setting to another.

EMERGENCY ROOM NURSES

The emergency room nurse triages patients to determine who will receive immediate care and who can wait. An error in judgment can delay treatment, which may cause serious injury. The nurse must be knowledgeable about laws enacted that direct hospital personnel to delay discharge or transfer of patients until their condition is stable. These laws were intended to prevent "dumping patients" who have no insurance. The only exception to this rule is when the patient makes a written request to be transferred. Special training and ongoing inservice are required for critical care area nurses to ensure competence in advanced monitoring and management skills.

OBSTETRIC NURSES AND PEDIATRIC NURSES

In labor and delivery, the failure to use relevant, complex technological skills can produce injury or death to the newborn or mother. Nursing care for children requires special knowledge and skill in assessing for suspected child abuse or neglect as well as mandatory reporting of suspected cases. The potential for injury during nursing care is always increased when dealing with children. An understanding of the special guidelines for consent and of who can give permission for informed consent in the pediatric area is also critical.

MEDICAL-SURGICAL NURSES

The medical-surgical nurse must be knowledgeable about a wide range of medications, diagnostic tests, and various treatment modalities. He or she must also act as a patient advocate to support the patient's decisions and must provide self-care education to meet home care needs.

To provide competent care, medical-surgical nurses must be familiar with the safe use of restraints. The Patient Care Partnership provides guidelines for safety devices. These guidelines apply to many treatment options and include both physical and chemical restraints. It is imperative that the nurse be aware of these guiding principles in order to avoid the implications of negligence.

HOME HEALTH CARE NURSES

The use of home health care nursing has greatly increased in response to the demand for shorter hospital stays by managed care and the shrinking dollars allotted for in-hospital care. Because of the increase in outpatient procedures and earlier discharges, nursing procedures and care customarily delivered only in the hospital setting are now delivered in the home. The nurse in the home setting is not available at all times to monitor for ongoing change in status, however, so it is essential for the nurse to maintain high-level assessment skills and to know when to call the physician. The nurse must educate the patient and family about when and what should be reported to the physician. Nursing in the home setting covers a broad range of skills, including but not limited to personal care, mechanical ventilation, intravenous pain management, tube feedings, and patient and family teaching. The home health care nurse thus has enormous responsibility.

PSYCHIATRIC NURSES

Psychiatric nursing care has been influenced by the introduction of new categories of medications. Nurses must be alert for potential drug interactions and serious side effects. Patient safety is another area of concern in this specialty. Society has become increasingly violent, with progressively more cases of polysubstance abuse. This trend is reflected in the microcosm of the psychiatric unit. Additionally, the impact of managed care on the changes in the level of care provided (such as shorter length of stay) has forced the service provider to focus on increasing outpatient treatment modalities. The role of the nurse as patient advocate in the psychiatric setting can be crucial to the patient and the community.

PITFALLS IN CLINICAL REASONING

The failure to use appropriate decision-making skills in the clinical setting can result in charges of malpractice. One area of nursing practice that is frequently involved in malpractice claims is that of patient safety, which can be compromised either through failing to assess or monitor, failing to report, or omitting special needs from the plan of care. For example, consider a patient who presents in a confused state. The high risk for injury associated with this patient may result in a hip fracture if the nurse fails to monitor and implement appropriate strategies to prevent a fall.

Box 9-4 NEGLIGENT TORTS

Examples of negligent nursing actions include the following:

- Failing to monitor the patient
- Failing to report a change in patient status
- Failing to report another health care provider's incompetence
- Failing to provide for the patient's safety
- Restraining a patient improperly
- Improper medication administration
- Allowing a patient to be burned
- Failing to question an inappropriate medical order
- Using equipment incorrectly
- Failing to follow ordered treatments
- Failing to provide patient education and discharge instructions
- Giving the patient incorrect information

Adapted from Guido, G. W. (2001). *Legal and ethical issues in nursing* (p. 81). Upper Saddle River, NJ: Prentice Hall.

Failure to assess, to monitor for changing status, or to communicate (report) the change indicates lack of knowledge and judgment. Communication includes documenting trends in data.

The role of the nurse as patient advocate is a significant concern. When the nurse fails to perform duties appropriately, claims of negligence can occur. The nurse is expected to protect the patient from harm. Giving incorrect information, failing to question inappropriate orders, applying safety devices inappropriately, or failing to protect the patient from injury are only a few of the situations that breach the nursing duty to act as a patient advocate. Examples of nursing actions that frequently result in negligence claims can be found in Box 9-4.

Frequently, malpractice claims result from poor decisions. Common mistakes that are made in reasoning are described in Box 9-5. Nurses who

---

Box 9-5 Pitfalls in Clinical Reasoning

- Failure to identify the problem
- Faulty data gathering
- Lack of self-awareness (influenced by individual values)
- Failure to explore all options (usually related to pressures for immediate decision)
- Limitations in knowledge and experience (inhibits individual exploration of alternatives)
- Individual's inability to choose (or an inability to act on choices)

---

fail to reason skillfully are doing their patients a disservice.

SUMMARY

Clinical reasoning involves monitoring the patient's health care status through ongoing assessment and evaluation to detect variations. The cognitive skills are applied within the framework of the nursing process to give meaning to the data and to make decisions. Conclusions based on the data comparisons are used to evaluate response to prescribed treatments. Clinical reasoning is applied in a variety of settings to analyze circumstances and conditions in order to make treatment choices. The application of a sound knowledge base is critical to making consistently good decisions.

The appropriate use of human resources is essential in the health care industry to produce cost-effective care. It is very important that patient care not be compromised because cost cutting and productivity continue to be the driving force in health care delivery. For example, the use of the UAP is an emerging area of concern in nursing, along with short-staffing, which can compromise patient outcomes and lead to inadequate time for quality care delivery. A further area of concern involves early patient discharge without adequate preparation for self-care. To function in today's health care environment, the nurse must maintain proficient reasoning skills. Issues relating to staffing, quality care, and preparing patients for discharge are covered more thoroughly in Chapter 10, Ethical Decision Making.

Box 9-6 presents a scenario that demonstrates the evaluative reasoning process using the nursing process format. This process is the basis for clinical reasoning when making individual patient decisions.

KEY POINTS

- Effective reasoning skills are essential to obtaining optimal outcomes of patient care.
- Components of clinical reasoning include the standards of critical thinking, standards of practice, clinical competence, and effective communication skills.
- One example of a decision requiring clinical reasoning is the delegation of tasks to health care workers.
- Clinical reasoning should be used to make decisions that do not result in patient harm.
- Accepting an assignment that fails to meet appropriate standards of care may result in patient harm.
- Effective clinical reasoning skills involve monitoring the patient, detecting changes in status, and responding with appropriate interventions.
- The nurse uses clinical reasoning skills in the decision to contact the physician.

Box 9-6 Application of Reasoning Skill

Mike is a 56-year-old patient admitted with depression and alcohol abuse. His serum alcohol level was 0.16 on admission. No other drugs of abuse were noted in his lab results. On admission, Mike told the nurse he consumes about a fifth of vodka daily. The nurse starts the shift by administering Mike his daily vitamins. She notes a fine tremor of his hands as she hands him the medications.

1. **Assessment:** What areas of assessment would be important to perform immediately?
2. **Analysis:** What complication is the nurse most concerned about at this time?
3. **Outcome:** Identify an appropriate outcome for this need.
4. **Plan and implementation:** What nursing actions should be included in Mike's plan?
5. **Evaluation:** What follow-up measures would be important?

ANSWERS

1. **Assessment:** What areas of assessment would be important to perform immediately?

The nurse should obtain vital signs and compare them with Mike's baseline vitals. Elevated blood pressure and pulse would be significant. The nurse should complete an alcohol withdrawal tool such as the Clinical Institute Withdrawal Assessment for Alcohol (CIWA) scale.

2. **Analyses:** What complication is the nurse most concerned about at this time?
   Delirium tremens.
3. **Outcome:** Identify an appropriate outcome for this need.
   Example: Patient's CIWA scale will remain in normal range ongoing.
4. **Plan and implementation:** What nursing actions should be included in Mike's plan?
   Check medication administration record (MAR) for as needed medications for withdrawal symptoms. Increase fluids.
5. **Evaluation:** What follow-up measures would be important?
   Assessment of medication effectiveness, repeat CIWA scale.

- The nurse reasons when interpreting lab data and determining appropriate actions.
- Nursing decisions are often based on the knowledge required by a specialty area.
- The failure to make appropriate decisions can result in charges of malpractice.

REFERENCES

American Nurses Association (1998). *Standards of clinical practice.* Washington, DC: Author.

American Nurses Association. (2003a). *Nursing: Scope and standards of practice (public comment draft).* Washington, DC: American Nurses Publishing.

American Nurses Association. (2003b). *Nursing's social policy statement (public comment draft).* Washington, DC: American Nurses Publishing.

Anderson, M. A., & Braun, J. V. (1995). *Caring for the elderly patient.* Philadelphia: F. A. Davis.

Alfaro-LeFevre, R. (1999). *Critical thinking in nursing.* Philadelphia: W. B. Saunders.

Black, J. M., Hawks, J. H., & Keene, A. M. (2001). *Medical-surgical nursing: Clinical management for positive outcomes.* Philadelphia: W. B. Saunders.

Castillo, S. L. (1999). *Strategies, techniques, and approaches to thinking.* Philadelphia: W. B. Saunders.

Craig, J. V., & Smyth, R. L. (2002). *The evidence-based practice manual for nurses.* St. Louis: Churchill Livingstone.

Doenges, M. E., Moorhouse, M. F., & Geissler, A. C. (2002). *Nursing care plans: Guidelines for individualizing patient care.* Philadelphia: F. A. Davis.

Fishbach, F. (2002). *Common laboratory and diagnostic tests.* Philadelphia: Lippincott Williams & Wilkins.

Foundation for Critical Thinking. (1997). *Critical thinking: Basic theory and instructional structures.* Santa Rosa, CA: Author.

Guido, G. W. (2001). *Legal and ethical issues in nursing.* Upper Saddle River, NJ: Prentice Hall.

Huber, D. (2000). *Leadership and nursing care management.* Philadelphia: W. B. Saunders.

Jones, R., & Beck, S. (1996). *Decision making in nursing.* Albany: Delmar.

McCloskey, J. C., & Bulechek, G. M. (2000). *Nursing interventions classification (NIC).* St. Louis: Mosby.

Michael, J. (2002). Is it patient abandonment or not? *RN, 65*(8), 67–70.

Paul, R., & Elder, L. (2001). *The miniature guide to critical thinking: Concepts and tool.* Dillon Beach, CA: Foundation for Critical Thinking.

Paul, R., & Heaslip, P. (1995). Critical thinking and intuitive nursing practice. *Journal of Advanced Nursing, 22*(7), 40–47.

Tappen, R. M., Weiss, S. A., & Whitehead, D. K. (2001). *Essentials of nursing leadership and management.* Philadelphia: F. A. Davis.

Taylor, C., Lillis, C., & LeMone, P. (2001). *Fundamentals of nursing: The art and science of nursing care.* Philadelphia: Lippincott Williams & Wilkins.

Student Worksheets

 SKILL SHEET: APPLYING CLINICAL REASONING TO VARIOUS PRACTICE SETTINGS

Purpose

1. To develop skill in purposeful and ongoing acquisition, interpretation, and synthesis of patient data for making consistent competent clinical decisions.
2. To develop skill in identifying specific circumstances that indicate when to call the physician.

Objectives

The student will demonstrate the ability to:

1. Identify circumstances that warrant notification of physician.
2. Monitor and assess the patient's changing status.
3. Develop consistent and accurate clinical decision-making skills.
4. Modify and change interventions as indicated.

Steps: Clinical Reasoning

ASSESSMENT

1. Collect significant data related to patient status.
2. Assist in acquisition of diagnostic tests.
3. Retrieve diagnostic test results.
4. Assess patient to establish baseline data for the shift.
5. Compare assessment findings to baseline data.

ANALYSIS

1. Analyze the acuity level, needs, and stability of the patient.
2. Identify the most urgent needs.
3. Compare the urgency of the needs to the effect of delay in treatment.
4. Interpret results of diagnostic tests as warranted by patient status.
5. Evaluate physician orders in conjunction with patient status.

OUTCOME IDENTIFICATION

1. Identify expected outcome.
2. Prioritize actions based on patient status.
3. Establish goals.

PLAN

1. Select appropriate patient indices for ongoing monitoring.
2. Establish frequency of data collection and interpretation.
3. Identify patient's ability to perform self-care activities.
4. Review various treatment options.
5. Develop a plan of action to correct or minimize risk to patient's health.

IMPLEMENTATION

1. Initiate plan.
2. Explain diagnostic test results to patient as indicated.

3. Monitor appropriate patient indices for change in stability.
4. Collaborate with physician on changes in patient data indicating need for treatment changes.
5. Note type and amount of drainage from tubes and body orifices.
6. Troubleshoot equipment to ensure collection of reliable data.
7. Compare current status with previous status to detect change.
8. Initiate or change interventions to maintain specified parameters.
9. Collaborate with the interdisciplinary services as indicated.
10. Initiate ordered treatments in timely manner.

EVALUATION

1. Reassess the effectiveness of treatment.
2. Change interventions as indicated.
3. Revise plan of care as needed.
4. Document responses to interventions.

 COMPETENCY VALIDATION: APPLYING CLINICAL REASONING TO VARIOUS PRACTICE SETTINGS

COMPETENCY STATEMENT

The student will develop and demonstrate evaluative reasoning in response to the significance of individual pieces of data in the clinical setting.
The student demonstrated the ability to do the following:

1. Monitor appropriate indices for variation.
2. Compare data to the acuity, needs, and stability of the patient.
3. Prioritize care to meet patient needs based on circumstance.
4. Select appropriate treatment options based on indicators.
5. Collaborate with members of the health care team to achieve desired outcomes.
6. Assess, reassess, and evaluate the effectiveness of treatments.
7. Communicate outcomes of treatments and care.

COMPETENT

- Understands reason for task and is able to perform task independently
- Understands reason for task but needs supervision
- Understands reason for task and is able to perform task with assistance

NOT COMPETENT

- Understands reason for task but performs task at provisional level
- Is unable to state reason for task and performs task at a dependent level

 SKILL CHECKLIST: APPLYING CLINICAL REASONING TO VARIOUS PRACTICE SETTINGS

Clinical reasoning is applied within the framework of the nursing process. Therefore, this checklist is similar to the Nursing Process Checklist presented in Chapter 5, with the addition of areas where application of cognitive skills may be necessary to monitor the patient status, evaluate changes, and decide what to do.

In the practice world, not all components contained in the following Skill Checklist will be relevant to every patient situation. Sound clinical reasoning helps the nurse recognize those that are applicable to the specific patient situation and those that are not. Use only the steps that have relevance to your patient.

CLINICAL REASONING	SATISFACTORY	UNSATISFACTORY	NI/COMMENTS
ASSESSMENT			
1. Collect significant data related to patient status.			
2. Assist in acquisition of diagnostic tests.			
3. Retrieve diagnostic test results.			
4. Assess patient to establish baseline data.			
5. Compare assessment findings to baseline status.			
ANALYSIS			
1. Analyze the acuity level, needs, and stability of the patient.			
2. Identify the most urgent needs.			
3. Compare the urgency of the needs to the effect of delay in treatment.			
4. Interpret results of diagnostic tests as warranted by patient status.			
5. Evaluate physician orders in conjunction with patient status.			
OUTCOME IDENTIFICATION			
1. Identify the expected outcome.			
2. Prioritize actions based on patient status.			
3. Establish goals.			
PLAN			
1. Select appropriate patient indices for ongoing monitoring.			
2. Establish frequency of data collection and interpretation.			
3. Identify patient's ability to perform self-care activities.			
4. Review various treatment options.			
5. Develop a plan of action to correct or minimize risk to patient's health.			
IMPLEMENTATION			
1. Initiate plan.			
2. Explain diagnostic test results to patient as indicated.			
3. Monitor appropriate patient indices for change in stability.			
4. Collaborate with physician on changes in patient data indicating need for treatment changes.			

CLINICAL REASONING	SATISFACTORY	UNSATISFACTORY	NI/COMMENTS
5. Note type and amount of drainage from tubes and body orifices.			
6. Troubleshoot equipment to ensure collection of reliable data.			
7. Compare current status with previous status to detect change.			
8. Initiate or change interventions to maintain specified parameters.			
9. Collaborate with the interdisciplinary services as indicated.			
10. Initiate ordered treatments in timely manner.			
EVALUATION 1. Reassess the effectiveness of treatment.			
2. Change interventions as indicated.			
3. Revise plan of care as needed.			
4. Document responses to interventions.			

 ## SCENARIO TO ACCOMPANY STUDENT WORKSHEETS

Using Clinical Reasoning Skills

Return to the Nursing Process Scenario in Chapter 5; assessment needs have already been evaluated and a care plan developed. The focus now is to apply the clinical reasoning process to Jimmy Little.

Physical Data:

Jimmy Little, 61 years of age, presented in the emergency room (ER) with a temperature of 100.2°F (37.8°C) and complaints of abdominal pain. He rated the pain at 10 on a 1 to 10 scale and was admitted for urinary tract infection and urosepsis. Past medical history included cancer of the prostate.

Mr. Little reports incontinence related to a long-term indwelling catheter left in place during chemotherapy and removed last week. On catheterization in the ER, the nurse obtained only 30 mL of dark-brown urine with no visible blood noted. The 18-gauge Foley catheter was attached to a drainage bag after insertion. The patient verbalized that he had not been drinking fluids because it hurts when he voids. He reports no unintentional weight loss or gain of 10 pounds or greater. There is no visible or palpable edema noted. A saline lock was placed in the left forearm for antibiotic therapy while he was in the ER. The lock is patent and free of signs of infection.

Diagnostic Data

	PATIENT	NORMAL
Urine specific gravity	1.020	1.010
Blood	3+	Negative
Protein	1+	Negative
Ketones	Trace	Negative
pH	5	
Hemoglobin	16.6 g/dL	12–16 g/dL
Hematocrit	59%	42%–52%
Blood urea nitrogen	29 mg/dL	10–25 mg/dL
Creatinine	0.8 mg/dL	0.7–1.4 mg/dL
Potassium	3.4 mEq/L	3.5–5.3 mEq/L
Sodium	144 mEg/L	135–146 mEq/L
White blood cell count	11.5 mg/dL	5,000–10,000 mg/dL

Physical Assessment Data:

During the initial assessment, Mr. Little related that he is "dizzy" when he stands up. Vital signs reveal the following: temperature, 99.2°F (37.3°C); pulse, 98 beats/min; respirations, 20 breaths/min; sitting blood pressure, 98/60 mm Hg; reclining blood pressure, 118/72 mm Hg. His skin turgor is flaccid, mucous membranes are dry, and weakness is noted during movement.

1. What would you need to do about these findings?

_____

_____

_____

_____

_____

2. Is the current intravenous (IV) therapy consistent with the lab data and medical diagnosis?

_____

_____

_____

Unlike the nursing process, cognitive skills (critical thinking) can occur in any sequence. The nurse must decide when to apply these skills in clinical practice. Apply the skills to the following example:

While reviewing the chart to gather data, the nurse notes that the patient was given 500 mg of amoxicillin, and the doctor's order sheet was for 250 mg of amoxicillin three times daily.

Use your critical thinking skills to analyze this finding.

3. Use interpretation to describe what this means.

_____

_____

_____

4. Use analysis to determine the cause of the problem.

_____

_____

_____

_____

_____

5. Identify what questions need to be answered to contribute data regarding the situation.

_____

_____

_____

_____

_____

6. Evaluation: Identify the outcome expected from the administration of the drug and determine whether progress was made toward the outcome.

_____

_____

_____

7. Inferences: What conclusions can be drawn from the situation that will affect the nurse's decision?

_____

_____

_____

8. Explanation: Describe what to do. Why?

_____

_____

_____

9. Self-regulation: Describe what the nurse should do differently the next time to improve delivery of care (medication administration).

_____

_____

_____

See the Answer Key in Appendix A for sample answers for this exercise.

Practice Exercises: Clinical Reasoning in Various Practice Settings

APPLYING CLINICAL REASONING TO VARIOUS PRACTICE SETTINGS

Scenario 1: Mental Status Examination

Dan Bender, 67 years old, was admitted to the hospital following an episode of hyperglycemia related to diabetes mellitus. He has poor short-term memory but can recall things that happened in his childhood. His wife states that he has had this problem for some time but that lately it has become an increasing concern.

ASSESSMENT

1. To further assess the patient's mental status, what should the nurse do?

_____

_____

_____

2. Demonstrate application of the cognitive skills to the care needs related to Mr. Bender.

INTERPRETATION

_____

_____

_____

Analysis

_____

_____

_____

_____

_____

_____

_____

_____

Evaluation

_____
_____
_____
_____
_____
_____

Inference

_____
_____
_____
_____
_____
_____

Explanation

_____
_____
_____
_____
_____
_____
_____

Self-Regulation

_____
_____
_____
_____
_____
_____

ANALYSIS

1. Which cue needs further discussion with the patient's wife other and why?

_____
_____
_____
_____

2. Based on this information, the nurse should suspect what condition?

_____

_____

_____

3. Identify the priority nursing diagnosis for this patient at this time.

_____

_____

_____

OUTCOME IDENTIFICATION

1. Identify the goals appropriate to this patient's care.

_____

_____

_____

2. Which of these goals should receive priority in the care of the patient?

_____

_____

_____

3. List the indicators that should be recorded to indicate the goal has been met.

_____

_____

_____

_____

_____

_____

_____

_____

PLAN

1. Identify interventions appropriate for the hospital environment to prevent injuries.

_____

_____

_____

_____

_____

_____

_____

IMPLEMENTATION

1. Because the patient has altered mental status, how would instructions be different for a procedure?

_____

_____

_____

_____

_____

_____

EVALUATION

1. Describe the effectiveness in progressing toward the desired outcome.

_____

_____

_____

_____

_____

_____

See the Answer Key in Appendix A for sample answers for this exercise.

SCENARIO 2: CRITICAL CARE SETTING

An 83-year-old patient in the critical care unit (CCU) is alert and oriented and makes his own decisions about health care. The cardiac monitor is in complete heart block, rate 38 beats/min without ectopy. An order was given by the physician to obtain a signed consent form for insertion of a permanent pacemaker. The nurse prepared the permit for the patient to sign. The patient stated, "The doctor has not talked to me about this procedure" and refused to sign the permit until he can discuss it with the physician. The nurse notified the physician about the patient's request. The physician stated, "Just have him sign it and I will talk to him about it later!" and hangs up the phone.

1. What is the primary problem or issue?

_____

_____

_____

_____

_____

_____

2. What alternatives does the nurse have in planning interventions?

_____

_____

_____

_____

_____

_____

_____

Scenario 3: Critical Care Setting

A 43-year-old man was admitted to the CCU with a diagnosis of lower gastrointestinal (GI) bleeding. The surgeon has discussed the surgical intervention with the patient, and he agrees to have the surgery. The nurse takes the surgical permit into the patient's room for him to sign. This permit also contains a section for consent to Administration of Blood Products. The patient states that he is a Jehovah's Witness and cannot receive blood products. This section is crossed out per hospital policy, and the patient writes on the permit "I am a Jehovah's Witness and do not want any blood given to me."

1. What should the nurse do now?

_____

_____

_____

_____

_____

_____

_____

_____

2. After surgery, the patient returns to his room on a ventilator and is very drowsy. Postoperative orders include:

Type and cross-match 4 units of packed red blood cells (PRBCs) and transfuse 2 units when available.
Give 2 units fresh frozen plasma (FFP) when available.

The hemoglobin and hematocrit values are 4.9 g/dL and 15.3%, respectively. What should the nurse do?

_____

_____

_____

_____

_____

_____

_____

3. The surgeon cancels the order for the PRBCs and the FFP and talks to the patient's daughter about the situation and prognosis. An hour after the surgeon leaves, the patient's daughter, who is not a Jehovah's Witness, approaches the nurse and says she wants her father to have the blood. She further states that "if it is given while he is asleep, he will never know he got it." What should the nurse do now?

_____

_____

_____

_____

_____

_____

SCENARIO 4: CRITICAL CARE SETTING

A 67-year-old woman is in the telemetry unit with a diagnosis of congestive heart failure (CHF). She has slightly labored breathing at rest and fine crackles auscultated in the lower two thirds of both lung fields. Jugular vein distention is present, and 4+ pitting edema is evident in bilateral feet and lower legs. Oxygen is on at 3 liters per minute by nasal cannula (3L/NC), and pulse oximetry (SpO_2) reading is 91%.
  Doctor's orders include Lasix, 40 mg intravenous push (IVP) every 6 hours.

1. The nurse starts to give the Lasix, when the patient states, "I do not want that shot!" The nurse asks, "Why?" The patient states, "It makes me urinate so much, and I have such a hard time when I use the bedpan or commode. She further elaborates, "I get leg cramps that hurt so bad!" What alternative courses of action does the nurse have?

_____

_____

_____

_____

_____

_____

_____

SCENARIO 5: CRITICAL CARE SETTING

A 38-year-old man with a diagnosis of coronary artery disease (CAD) is a morning direct admit to the telemetry unit for a scheduled cardiac catheterization. Doctor's orders include routine cardiac catheter orders. The patient is very anxious and is accompanied by his wife. He is instructed to undress and put on a hospital gown. An IV solution of normal saline (NS) is started in the left hand, infusing at 50 mL/hr. The patient is given the Admission Data Sheet and is instructed to fill it out. When the electrocardiogram is performed, the patient becomes irritated, stating, "The doctor already did that in the office a month ago." While the nurse is preparing pain medicine for another patient, the laboratory phlebotomist comes to the nurse's station and informs the nurse that the patient is very upset and refuses to allow a blood draw because he had that done at the doctor's office. Upon entering the room, the nurse notes that the patient has removed the IV and is fully dressed in street clothes. He walks out of the room stating, "I'm not staying where people don't know what they are doing." As he and his wife are walking along the hallway, the wife turns to the nurse and states, "He really didn't want to do this anyway." The patient says, "Shut up Ethel!" and gets on the elevator.

1. What should the nurse do now?

_____

_____

_____

_____

_____

SCENARIO 6: OBSTETRIC AND PEDIATRIC CARE SETTING

Dr. Ludley's orders for a routine, active labor patient include:

IV fluids: 1,000 mL at 125 mL/hr
Clear liquid diet
Ambulate as tolerated
Catheterize as needed
Vital signs every 4 hours
Monitor fetal heart rate every 30 minutes

Angela, 25-year-old gravida 2 para 1, at 40 weeks' gestation, has been in labor for 7 hours. She is 70% effaced and dilated to 6 cm; the baby is at 0 station. The patient has not voided since admission and is complaining of feeling nauseated. For the past hour, she seems to have made little progress in her cervical changes. Her vital signs are normal, and the fetal heart rate (FHR) is within normal limits (WNL).

1. As her nurse, what will you do to help her with the present situation? Why?

_____

_____

_____

_____

_____

SCENARIO 7: OBSTETRIC AND PEDIATRIC CARE SETTING

The nursery room nurse is in charge of six babies for the day shift. A husband tells the nurse that Mrs. Mitchell would like to have her baby girl brought to her now so that she can feed her. Baby Mitchell's vital signs are as follows: temperature, 97.1°F (36.2°C); apical pulse, 130 beats/min; and respirations, 26 breaths/min. The baby is somewhat fussy.

1. What is the correct action to take at this time? Why?

_____

_____

_____

_____

_____

Scenario 8: Obstetric and Pediatric Care Setting

Debra, 22 years old, delivered her first child 2 hours ago. Now that the family has finally left, she is anxious to nurse her baby boy. Jeremy, however, does not seem at all interested in the breast-feeding experience. Debra is in tears and states she feels like a failure.

1. As her nurse, what would you do to help Debra remain positive about her ability to breast-feed her baby?

_____

_____

_____

_____

_____

Scenario 9: Acute Care Setting

Fred, 52 years old, was admitted with a diagnosis of type 2 diabetes mellitus, gangrenous right foot infection, and end-stage renal disease (ESRD). He is undergoing hemodialysis 3 days each week. His admitting orders include:

Bed rest
Labs in the morning: chemistry panel 16, glycohemoglobin level, complete blood count (CBC)
1,500-calorie carbohydrate-consistent diet
Fluid restrictions: 1,500 mL per 24 hours
Glucoscan 4 times per day
Sliding scale insulin coverage for Glucoscan per Dr. Sale's routine

The lab personnel called in the morning results:

	PATIENT VALUES	NORMAL VALUES
Potassium	5.5	(3.6–5.0)
Chloride	93	(98–107)
Creatinine	8	(0.7–1.5)
Blood urea nitrogen	53	(7–20)
Glucose	331	(70–110)

1. What should the nurse do about the labs?

_____

_____

_____

_____

_____

Scenario 10: Acute Care Setting

Catherine Blue, 80 years old, admitted from a local nursing home, was brought into the ER because she was vomiting bright red blood. Her skin is pale and cool, her abdomen is distended and tender to palpation, and hyperactive bowel sounds are present. A nasogastric tube, attached to low intermittent suction was inserted in the ER and has 200 mL of bright-red drainage in the container. IV fluids of 0.9 NS are infusing at 100 mL/hr into the right forearm with an 18-gauge catheter. The Foley catheter inserted in the ER has 50 mL of dark-amber urine in the drainage bag after 4 hours. The patient is moaning and restless. The nurse is unable to assess for pain because of the patient's history of earlier stroke, dementia, and aphasia. Laboratory results include hemoglobin 8.6 g/dL and hematocrit 24.9%.

1. What should the nurse do first?

_____

_____

_____

_____

Scenario 11: Acute Care Setting

Mrs. Blue's daughter, whose husband is the hospital administrator, insists that her mother be placed in a private room. The only private room available is on the pediatric unit, which the daughter refuses to consider. There is a private room close to the nurse's station that is currently occupied by a 92-year-old confused woman. The daughter wants the 92-year-old moved so that her mother can be placed in that room. The 92-year-old patient is severely confused and frequently attempts to climb out of bed. No family members are present.

1. What alternatives should the nurse consider?

_____

_____

_____

_____

_____

2. After all of the alternatives are explored, the nurse determines that Mrs. Blue must be placed in a semiprivate room. How should the nurse proceed?

_____

_____

_____

_____

_____

SCENARIO 12: ACUTE CARE SETTING

Mrs. Green had a partial gastrectomy with a gastrojejunostomy (Billroth II) and was placed in the critical care area for several days. During the surgical procedure, it was determined that metastatic cancer was present, and her prognosis for recovery is very poor. The family decides to sign for no code or resuscitation measures. Mrs. Green continues to require numerous treatments, close monitoring, IV fluids, frequent turning, and skin care to prevent breakdown. Her care could be managed on a surgical unit. The daughter wants her mother to be left in the critical care area because "she gets so much attention and a private room." However, there are limited critical care beds available, and the room may be needed for an admission during the night.

1. What are some alternatives the nurse can consider in providing for the care needs of this patient?

_____

_____

_____

_____

_____

_____

SCENARIO 13: HOME CARE SETTING

In preparing to schedule visits for the day, the nurse reviewed the written assignment. Four patients who live within 2 miles of each other are included. Patient information is as follows:

Patient 1. A 16-year-old girl, 3 days postpartum, who had a cesarian section at 35 weeks' gestation. The two times daily abdominal dressing change includes wound packing to a large abdominal wound. No signs of infection are evident.

Patient 2. A 63-year-old human immunodeficiency virus (HIV)-positive woman scheduled to receive an IV antibiotic for pneumonia.

Patient 3. A 45-year-old woman with a history of chronic renal failure. A nursing assessment and venipuncture are scheduled to determine the necessity for renal replacement therapy.

Patient 4. A 72-year-old man with an open, draining methicillin-resistant *Staphylococcus aureus*–positive wound to the right lower extremity. Orders include a whirlpool and complex dressing change at 11:00 AM. A hygiene alert is noted, meaning that his home is extremely unclean.

1. Outline the care needs of each patient. Identify what the nurse should do first.

Patient 1:

_____

_____

_____

Patient 2:

_____

_____

_____

Patient 3:

_____

_____

_____

Patient 4:

_____

_____

_____

SCENARIO 14: HOME CARE SETTING

The first home visit scheduled today is for a 72-year-old woman who requires a nursing assessment, venipuncture for prothrombin time, and evaluation of medication compliance. The patient performs a daily finger stick to monitor her blood sugar level. Her aseptic technique is poor; however, the procedure is otherwise performed correctly but without success. You offer to perform the finger stick and have difficulty obtaining an adequate blood sample. After venipuncture, bleeding stops almost immediately. No bruising or skin discoloration is noted upon physical assessment. Assessment is unremarkable other than a healing skin tear on the right forearm. The patient offers no complaints. However, the temperature in her home is noticeably cooler than comfortable because she is "trying to manage" on her fixed income. Evaluation of medication compliance reveals that the patient has a basic understanding of reason for taking medication and dosing schedule. When asked to look at medication bottles, the patient is reluctant and unable to produce all of the prescribed medications.

1. What is the primary problem or issue here?

_____

_____

_____

_____

_____

_____

SCENARIO 15: HOME CARE SETTING

The nurse has been assigned a 92-year-old hospice patient in the end stages of life with complaints of "more pain than she has ever been in before" as reported by her 72-year-old daughter. Upon arrival to the home, you discover that the patient is in a semi-comatose state. She is posturing to indicate abdominal discomfort and has a facial grimace, and her vital signs indicate that she is indeed in pain. Review of her medication schedule reveals appropriate administration of morphine through continuous pain pump and liquid morphine, 2 mg orally as needed or desired for breakthrough pain. The daughter has been encouraged to use as-needed medication when she is concerned that her mother is in pain. She has used this an average of six times in a 24-hour period. Physical findings include tenderness, guarding of abdomen, and distention. Urine is concentrated dark amber.

1. What should the nurse do?

_____

_____

_____

_____

_____

_____

_____

_____

_____

SCENARIO 16: PSYCHIATRIC CARE SETTING

Tim, a 34-year-old patient, was admitted to the acute psychiatric unit with a diagnosis of paranoid schizophrenia. Tim is unshaven and dressed in hospital scrubs. At the shift's beginning, the nurse observes that Tim isolating himself in his room. The nurse takes his vital signs and notes them to be as follows: temperature, 101°F (38.3°C); pulse, 80 beats/min; respirations, 32 breaths/min; blood pressure, 136/90 mm Hg.

1. What would be the first action of the nurse?

_____

_____

_____

2. What might the nurse interpret as the cause of any abnormal symptom?

_____

_____

_____

3. Write an appropriate nursing diagnosis for the patient need.

_____

_____

_____

4. Write an outcome statement that the nurse could use with this diagnosis.

_____

_____

_____

5. Following the initial assessment and action in question 1, what would be the appropriate nursing plan of care?

_____

_____

_____

Scenario 17: Psychiatric Care Setting

Mike was admitted to the acute psychiatric unit yesterday. He admits hearing command voices. This morning, he has been pacing and muttering. During breakfast in the lounge, he yells, jumps out of his seat, and begins throwing chairs at other patients. The nurse considers the following actions:

a. Call for help from unit staff.
b. Call for hospital security.
c. Enter lounge alone and attempt to quiet patient.
d. Go to supply room for restraining devices.

1. Analyze each option for the risks and benefits of choosing it.

   A. _____
   _____
   _____
   _____
   _____

   b. _____
   _____
   _____
   _____
   _____

   c. _____
   _____
   _____
   _____
   _____

   d. _____
   _____
   _____
   _____
   _____

Scenario 18: Psychiatric Care Setting

Ashley Smith has just finished nursing orientation on a medical unit of a hospital. One evening, Ashley observes another nurse obtain pain medication for a patient and then disappear into a conference room. About an hour later, Ashley talks with the patient as she assists with his turning. The patient states, "You know that pain injection I just got doesn't seem to be doing anything. It always worked before." Ashley does not want to anger the other nurse, who is a long-time employee. Therefore, she chooses to delay action and observe the nurse's behavior further. The next time she and the nurse work together, a similar incident occurs.

1. What should Ashley do?

_____

_____

_____

_____

_____

_____

See the Answer Key in Appendix A for sample answers for this exercise.

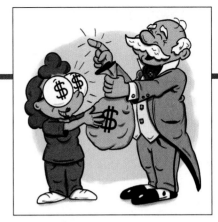

CHAPTER 10

Ethical Decision Making

OBJECTIVES

1. Describe the principles of ethics.

2. Identify the relationship of critical thinking to the ethical decision-making process.

3. Discuss how the American Nurses Association's Code of Ethics serves as a guideline to ethical decision making.

4. List the steps in ethical decision making.

5. Identify areas that are subject to frequent ethical dilemmas.

6. List the pitfalls involved in making ethical decisions.

In today's health care environment, nurses are faced with many important decisions. Some of them involve choices regarding what is the right or proper thing to do when two or more opposing alternatives are correct. These decisions fall in the realm of ethical decision making. The purpose of this chapter is to explore the process nurses undergo when faced with these dilemmas.

DEFINITION

Ethics is a branch of philosophy. It is concerned with the principles of right and wrong. Harkness and Dincher (1999) state that ethics includes "how people should act and what sort of character they should have" (p. 24). Standards of conduct and moral judgment form a foundation for ethics. An individual's ethical philosophy is influenced by values, past experiences, and moral training. Value refers to the personal worth given an idea

or activity. Values are learned in childhood but are adapted with the addition of new information and experiences. To deliver quality care, the nurse must be aware of his or her own values along with those of the patient. Clarification of one's own value system is important in understanding why one option is more appealing than another. The nurse's own value system affects decisions made in nursing practice. Nurses who understand the effect of their own beliefs and values on the nurse–patient interaction are better prepared to meet the needs of patients. Values clarification is a method of identifying both the nurse's and the patient's beliefs. Raths, Simon, and Harmin (1978) described a three-step model with seven substeps, to help clarify individual values. The first step in the model is choosing, which allows free choice, identifying alternatives, and selecting an alternative. The second step, prizing, involves individual satisfaction with the choice and verbalization of this to others. Internalization and repetition of the choice is the third step. Examples of these steps applied to a significant situation are presented below.

- *Choosing:* After choosing nursing as a career option, an individual makes the decision to pursue a nursing education. Consequently, the individual may reduce work hours to part-time, declining additional shifts when requested. This is more likely to provide adequate study time, leading to the acquisition of the knowledge and skill required for a nursing career.
- *Prizing:* After the choice is made, the nursing student expresses satisfaction with the chosen career and proudly shares the decision with family and friends.
- *Acting:* While working as an unlicensed assistive personnel (UAP), the nursing student consistently schedules time for study to support the choice. The student may also limit activities that detract from learning, such as attending parties.

Understanding values and how they develop can better prepare the nurse to prevent and resolve ethical conflicts. Following the common principles of ethics increases the nurses' ability to recognize and select the best action for each situation.

ETHICAL GUIDES

Nurses may be guided in ethical decision making by several sources. Two important foundations for practice are the list of ethical principles prepared by Beauchamp and Childress (1989) and the American Nurses Association (ANA) Code of Ethics.

Ethical Principles

Beauchamp and Childress are philosophers who identified four ethical principles. These principles include autonomy, nonmaleficence, beneficence, and justice (Taylor, Lillis, & LeMone, 2001). At times, fidelity and veracity are added to the list because of their important role in bioethics.

AUTONOMY

The nurse should strive to protect patient autonomy. Autonomy is the right to self-determination. The patient, through active participation, can work with the health care team to make decisions, select treatment goals, and develop a treatment plan. Even if the medical staff disagrees with the choice, legally competent adults have the power to choose. The Patient's Bill of Rights enacted in 1973 em-

phasizes patients making choices to direct their own care. In today's health care environment, focus is on the rights as well as the responsibilities of both hospital and patient. The Patient Care Partnership (2003) embraces shared responsibility and therefore accountability by both the provider and the patient for the outcomes. The primary concept of partnering is focused on the patient being at the center of his or her health care team to make decisions. It is a collaborative model that empowers the patient and embraces informed and shared decision making and self-management. A copy of the Patient Care Partnership can be found in Box 10-1. Nursing activities that support patient rights are listed in the Nursing Intervention Classification (NIC) 7460, which is appropriately named Patient Rights Protection (McCloskey & Bulechek, 2000).

Making decisions for the patient is known as *paternalism.* This practice is a restriction of the patient's autonomy. Any time the nurse forces a patient to submit to a treatment against his or her will, the nurse is guilty of paternalism. If the patient is deceived or threatened into cooperation, paternalism has occurred, even if the activity is therapeutic. Patients also have the right to refuse medication. For example, the nurse who threatens a patient with an injection following noncompliance with an oral medication administration has impinged on the rights of the patient.

NONMALEFICENCE AND BENEFICENCE

Nonmaleficence directs the nurse to do no harm. Beneficence involves doing good on the patient's behalf. The four components of these principles are to prevent harm, remove harm, cause no harm, and bring about a positive effect with nursing actions. To accomplish this, the nurse should use the ANA Standards of Practice for guidelines on decision making (see Chapter 5, Box 5-1). The standards are used to measure acceptable levels of care that a reasonable, prudent nurse would deliver. The nurse must also practice within the legal constraints identified in the state (provincial) Nurse Practice Act.

To avoid patient harm, the prudent nurse must maintain competency. The health care field is changing rapidly. Nurses must commit to becoming lifelong learners and seeking learning opportunities. Failure to maintain competency and perform as a reasonable, prudent nurse could result in charges of negligence.

Proper delegation of nursing duties is another nonmaleficence issue. To delegate, the nurse should assess the delegate's experience and competencies. The Nurse Practice Act and institutional policies should also be reviewed. Failure to follow these

Box 10-1 The Patient Care Partnership

A Patient's Bill of Rights was first adopted by the American Hospital Association (AHA) in 1973. This revision was approved by the AHA Board of Trustees in April 2003.

The Patient Care Partnership: Understanding Expectations, Rights, and Responsibilities

When you need hospital care, your doctor and the nurses and other professionals at our hospital are committed to working with you and your family to meet your health care needs. Our dedicated doctors and staff serve the community in all its ethnic, religious, and economic diversity. Our goal is for you and your family to have the same care and attention we would want for our families and ourselves.

The sections below explain some of the basics about how you can expect to be treated during your hospital stay. They also cover what we will need from you to care for you better. If you have questions at any time, please ask them. Unasked or unanswered questions can add to the stress of being in the hospital. Your comfort and confidence in your care are very important to us.

What to Expect During Your Hospital Stay

- **High-quality hospital care.** Our first priority is to provide you the care you need, when you need it, with skill, compassion, and respect. Tell your caregivers if you have concerns about your care or if you have pain. You have the right to know the identity of doctors, nurses, and others involved in your care, as well as when they are students, residents, or other trainees.
- **A clean and safe environment.** Our hospital works hard to keep you safe. We use special policies and procedures to avoid mistakes in your care and keep you free from abuse or neglect. If anything unexpected and significant happens during your hospital stay, you will be told what happened, and any resulting changes in your care will be discussed with you.
- **Involvement in your care.** You and your doctor often make decisions about your care before you go to the hospital. Other times, especially in emergencies, those decisions are made during your hospital stay. When they take place, making decisions should include:
  - *Discussing your medical condition and information about medically appropriate treatment choices.* To make informed decisions with your doctor, you need to understand several things:
    - The benefits and risks of each treatment
    - Whether it is experimental or part of a research study
    - What you can reasonably expect from your treatment and any long-term effects it might have on your quality of life
    - What you and your family will need to do after you leave the hospital
    - The financial consequences of using uncovered services or out-of-network providers

  Please tell your caregivers if you need more information about treatment choices.
  - *Discussing your treatment plan.* When you enter the hospital, you sign a general consent to treatment. In some cases, such as surgery or experimental treatment, you may be asked to confirm in writing that you understand what is planned and agree to it. This process protects your right to consent to or refuse a treatment.

Your doctor will explain the medical consequences of refusing recommended treatment. It also protects your right to decide if you want to participate in a research study.
  - *Getting information from you.* Your caregivers need complete and correct information about your health and coverage so that they can make good decisions about your care. That includes:
    - Past illnesses, surgeries, or hospital stays
    - Past allergic reactions
    - Any medicines or diet supplements (such as vitamins and herbs) that you are taking
    - Any network or admission requirements under your health plan
  - *Understanding your health care goals and values.* You may have health care goals and values or spiritual beliefs that are important to your well-being. They will be taken into account as much as possible throughout your hospital stay. Make sure your doctor, your family, and your care team know your wishes.
  - *Understanding who should make decisions when you cannot.* If you have signed a health care power of attorney stating who should speak for you if you become unable to make health care decisions for yourself, or a "living will" or "advance directive" that states your wishes about end-of-life care, give copies to your doctor, your family, and your care team. If you or your family need help making difficult decisions, counselors, chaplains, and others are available to help.
- **Protection of your privacy.** We respect the confidentiality of your relationship with your doctor and other caregivers and the sensitive information about your health and health care that are part of that relationship. State and federal laws and hospital operating policies protect the privacy of your medical information. You will receive a Notice of Privacy Practices that describes the ways that we use, disclose, and safeguard patient information, and that explains how you can obtain a copy of information from our records about your care.
- **Help in preparing you and your family for when you leave the hospital.** Your doctor works with hospital staff and professionals in your community. You and your family also play an important role. The success of your treatment often depends on your efforts to follow medication, diet, and therapy plans. Your family may need to help care for you at home.

  You can expect us to help you identify sources of follow-up care and to let you know if our hospital has a financial interest in any referrals. As long as you agree that we can share information about your care with them, we will coordinate our activities with your caregivers outside the hospital. You can also expect to receive information and, where possible, training about the self-care you will need when you go home.
- **Help with your bill and filing insurance claims.** Our staff will file claims for you with health care insurers or other programs such as Medicare and Medicaid. They will also help your doctor with needed documentation. Hospital bills and insurance coverage are often confusing. If you have questions about your bill, contact our

(continued)

guidelines could result in patient harm. For example, delegating a treatment considered a registered nurse (RN) responsibility to a UAP, owing to lack of nursing time, could lead to patient injury.

JUSTICE

The principle of justice is the moral obligation to treat people fairly and equally. Issues concerning the distribution of social benefits and equitable patient treatment arise in this principle. Justice can become an issue when there is a limited supply of a medication, beds, or nursing staff. All patients should receive the same level of care regardless of social status, financial status, race, or sexual orientation. A dilemma in this area could be the decision whether or not to expend limited resources on a terminally ill patient.

FIDELITY

Fidelity includes keeping one's promises and acting in the patient's best interest. As the old saying goes, "don't make promises you can't keep." Telling the patient, "Everything will be all right" may seem reassuring, but the nurse does not have the power to guarantee that everything will be all right. Issues included in this principle are confidentiality and functioning as a patient advocate.

Because of the nature of the profession, the nurse is often privy to confidential patient information. Sharing information with others, who do not have the right to know, is unethical. Even casual remarks made in the cafeteria or elevator can result in legal action against the nurse.

Operating as a patient advocate is also an important nursing role. As an advocate, the nurse informs the patient about the health care plan and then supports the patient in his or her decision to accept or reject the plan. This decision may not be the one preferred by the family or the health care workers. However, the patient has the right to decide his or her own health care issues.

To act in the patient's best interest, the nurse should complete accepted assignments. A nurse

who becomes angry and leaves in the middle of a shift has abandoned the patients. Being charged with patient abandonment can result in legal consequences (criminal penalties) as well as loss of professional licensure.

VERACITY

Veracity means telling the truth. It involves giving as much information as possible and informing the patient if information is not available. "Being honest or telling the truth means relating the facts as one knows and understands them" (Rumbold, 2000, p. 164). Telling an individual about his or her disease may cause anxiety, but the patient has a right to know. Guidelines for appropriate nursing activity choices related to veracity are included in NIC (5470) Truth Telling (Box 10-2) (McCloskey & Bulechek, 2000).

A clean and safe environment involves special policies and procedures to avoid mistakes and prevent abuse or neglect. The Patient Care Partnership places the responsibility on the hospital to provide a clean and safe environment. This involves special policies and procedures to avoid mistakes and provide appropriate care. If there is an error, the hospital should be forthcoming in discussing the event and any resulting changes in the plan of care with the patient. The novice nurse may need to consult with a more experienced nurse or supervisor for direction when the situation occurs.

AMERICAN NURSES ASSOCIATION CODE OF ETHICS

As a profession, nursing is committed to the ethical behavior of its practitioners. The ANA has developed a Code of Ethics, which provides a framework for decision making. This code is listed in Box 10-3. A Code of Ethics is a written list of the

Definition: Use of whole truth, partial truth, or decision delay to promote the patient's self-determination and well-being

Activities:

Clarify own values about the particular situation

Clarify the values of the patient, family, health care team, and institution about the particular situation

Clarify own knowledge base and communication skills about the situation

Determine patient's desire for truth in the situation

Point out discrepancies between the patient's expressed beliefs and behaviors, as appropriate

Collaborate with other health care providers about the choice of options (i.e., whole truth, partial truth, or decision delay) and their needed participation in the options

Determine risks to patient and self associated with each option

Choose one of the options, based on the ethics of the situation and leaning more favorably toward the use of truth or partial truth

Establish a trusting relationship

Deliver the truth with sensitivity, warmth, and directness

Make the time to deal with the consequences of the truth

Refer to another if that person has better rapport, better knowledge and skills to deliver the truth, or more time and ability to deal with the consequences of telling the truth

Remain with the patient to whom you have told the truth and be prepared to clarify, give support to, and receive disapproval from

Be physically present to communicate caring and support, if decision to withhold information has been made

Choose decision delay when there is missing information, lack of knowledge, and lack of rapport

Attend to verbal and nonverbal cues during the communication process

Monitor the patient's responses to the interaction, including alterations in pain, restlessness, anxiety, mood change, involvement in care, ability to synthesize new information, ability to verbalize feelings, and reported satisfaction with care, as appropriate

Document the patient's responses at various stages of the intervention

Adapted from McCloskey, J. C. & Bulechek, G. M. (2000). *Nursing interventions classification (NIC)* (p. 676). St. Louis: Mosby.

---

values and standards of conduct within a profession. The nine statements of the ANA code provide direction in making ethical decisions. The following sections examine the ANA code in more detail.

Standard 1

Standard 1: The nurse, in all professional relationships, practices with compassion and respect for the inherent dignity, worth, and uniqueness of every individual, unrestricted by considerations of social or economic status, personal attributes, or the nature of health problems.

Adherence to this principle is vital to ethical practice. The provision directs the goals and values of nursing as a profession. Nurses must respect individual patients and deliver care with compassion. No exceptions should be made based on a patient's economic status or ability to pay for

Approved June 30, 2001

1. The nurse, in all professional relationships, practices with compassion and respect for the inherent dignity, worth, and uniqueness of every individual, unrestricted by considerations of social or economic status, personal attributes, or the nature of health problems.

2. The nurse's primary commitment is to the patient, whether an individual, family, group, or community.

3. The nurse promotes, advocates for, and strives to protect the health, safety, and rights of the patient.

4. The nurse is responsible and accountable for individual nursing practice and determines the appropriate delegation of tasks consistent with the nurse's obligation to provide optimum patient care.

5. The nurse owes the same duties to self as to others, including the responsibility to preserve integrity and safety, to maintain competence, and to continue personal and professional growth.

6. The nurse participates in establishing, maintaining, and improving health care environments and conditions of employment conducive to the provision of quality health care and consistent with the values of the profession through individual and collective action.

7. The nurse participates in the advancement of the profession through contributions to practice, education, administration, and knowledge development.

8. The nurse collaborates with other health professionals and the public in promoting community, national, and international efforts to meet health needs.

9. The profession of nursing, as represented by associations and their members, is responsible for articulating nursing values, for maintaining the integrity of the profession and its practice, and for shaping social policy.

Reprinted with permission from American Nurses Association Code of Ethics for Nurses with Interpretive Statements, © 2001 American Nurses Publishers, American Nurses Association, Washington, D.C.

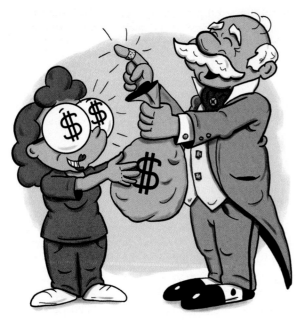

"Dear lady, please accept this obscenely large amount of money for bandaging my paper cut!"

services. Respect is conveyed when referring to a patient by name instead of "the gallbladder in Room 328."

Standards 2 and 3

Standard 2: The nurse's primary commitment is to the patient, whether an individual, family, group, or community.
Standard 3: The nurse promotes, advocates for, and strives to protect the health, safety, and rights of the patient.

The code's second provision affirms a commitment to patient advocacy. Violations occur when a nurse fails to respect a patient's wishes. For example, an alert patient informs the surgical nurse that he has changed his mind regarding scheduled surgery. The permit has already been signed. The nurse, acting as a patient advocate, should clarify the reason and inform the physician. A violation would occur if the nurse offered false reassurances but took no further action. In another example, the patient is unable to make his wishes known. However, a properly executed advance directive with a no cardiopulmonary resuscitation (CPR) exists. The family is upset with the do not resuscitate (DNR) status. It is the nurse's job to support the advance directive as

designated by the patient. The nurse has a right to possess a set of values and beliefs but does not have the right to expect others to share the same values.

Patient issues are also promoted in the third provision. This standard refers to patient rights. Some rights, such as confidentiality, have become a challenge in the present health care environment owing to the growing popularity of computerized charting and other technologies such as fax machines. As a result of carelessness, confidential information may be left unattended, allowing access by unauthorized individuals.

Standards 4 and 5

Standard 4: The nurse is responsible and accountable for individual nursing practice and determines the appropriate delegation of tasks consistent with the nurse's obligation to provide optimum patient care.
Standard 5: The nurse owes the same duties to self as to others, including the responsibility to preserve integrity and safety, to maintain competence, and to continue personal and professional growth.

The fourth and fifth provisions emphasize responsibility, accountability, and competence. Nurses have an obligation to maintain competency in their practice. Nursing care should be based on current practice knowledge because the field of nursing is always changing. To remain current, the nurse must seek knowledge and apply it to practice.

The nurse is also accountable for proper delegation. For example, unstable patients with unpredictable outcomes should only be the responsibility of the RN. If the patient is injured as a result of care being delegated to a licensed practical nurse/licensed vocational nurse (LPN/LVN), the RN is accountable. The nurse must be aware of the skills of her co-workers in order to delegate appropriately. Tasks delegated to a UAP may be appropriate by practice, but not for the individual who has no experience with the task.

Standard 6

Standard 6: The nurse participates in establishing, maintaining, and improving health care environments and conditions of employment conducive to the provision of quality health care and consistent with the values of the profession through individual and collective action.

The nurse must take responsibility for contributing to ethical practice within the organizational structure of employment. This can be accomplished by refusing to work for institutions that routinely violate human rights and require nurses to compromise their integrity. Nurses can also become change agents by joining quality control committees and mentoring new nurses. For example, consider the nurse who is unhappy with the discharge process in her institution. Being an active member of a team working on patient discharge issues can result in positive changes. On the other hand, constantly complaining about the problem does not tend to bring about such changes.

Standard 7

> Standard 7: The nurse participates in the advancement of the profession through contributions to practice, education, administration, and knowledge development.

This provision ensures continued learning. Nurses have a responsibility to contribute to the profession's body of knowledge. Participating in research, applying research findings, and initiating policies to promote change can accomplish this. For example, a nursing unit is conducting a trial of a new blood pressure device. The nurse in charge takes time to participate in a study and document findings regarding the new equipment.

Standard 8

> The nurse collaborates with other health professionals and the public in promoting community, national, and international efforts to meet health needs.

Health needs are worldwide. The nurse participates in activities that support health care for all underserved people. An example of this standard is a nurse who becomes politically active to promote a bill for child heath care. A nurse may also choose to volunteer in an underdeveloped country.

Standard 9

> The profession of nursing, as represented by associations and their members, is responsible for

articulating nursing values, for maintaining the integrity of the profession and its practice, and for shaping social policy.

All nurses are charged with the responsibility of promoting the nursing profession. Nurses should lobby for measures that enhance nursing as a profession. This is usually best accomplished by membership in a professional association.

CRITICAL THINKING

Ethical decision making in health care is necessary when moral issues arise during the delivery of nursing care. Nurses must make decisions regarding what is the right thing to do. These decisions are aided by the use of critical thinking skills. Alfaro-LeFevre (1999) cited a correlation between moral development and critical thinking ability. She stated, "People with a mature level of moral development—those with a clear, carefully reasoned sense of what's right, wrong, and fair—are more likely to think critically" (p. 31). The critical thinker can see situations from the patient point of view and considers all options.

Many decisions will involve a dilemma. "An ethical dilemma is a difficult moral problem that involves two or more mutually exclusive, morally correct courses of action" (Chally & Loriz, 1998, p. 17). The nurse must choose when there is no

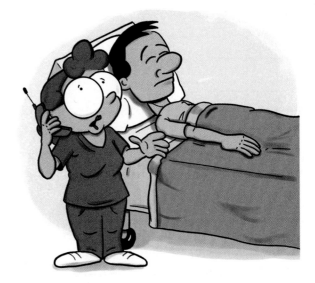

"Where did I get my cell phone? I kinda borrowed it from a patient. He's been in a month-long coma so I don't think he'll mind."

obvious best answer. Ruggiero (1991, p. 30–31) presents the following advice on dilemmas:

- Relationships with other people create obligations of various kinds, and these should be honored unless there is a compelling reason not to.
- Certain ideals enhance human life and assist people in fulfilling their obligations to one another. These ideals should be served whenever possible.
- Where two or more obligations are in conflict, decide which is the most serious obligation or which existed first.
- Where two or more ideals are in conflict, ask which is the highest or most important ideal.

It is important to use standards and other available tools in the process of making decisions. A useful tool for guiding the decision-making process is a tree developed by Catalano, which is depicted in Figure 10-1.

PROCESS OF ETHICAL DECISION MAKING

ASSESSMENT

Decision making starts with an assessment phase. The decision maker must gather all appropriate information to determine those facts that have the most bearing on the situation—for example, who is affected most by the decision and what obligation is owed to this individual. Developing the sensitivity to recognize an ethical situation is essential in nursing practice. Occasionally, gathering more facts will provide the answer. For example, short-staffing may be a problem on a nursing unit. In this case, data regarding the staff situation should be obtained. If the problem occurs regularly, the decision maker should gather all facts that affect the situation, including the acuity level of the patients. Risks to patients should be identified, and factors

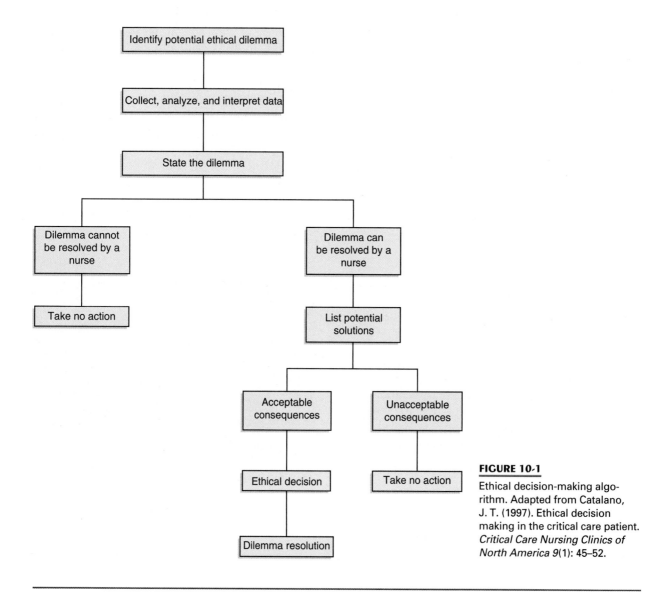

FIGURE 10-1

Ethical decision-making algorithm. Adapted from Catalano, J. T. (1997). Ethical decision making in the critical care patient. *Critical Care Nursing Clinics of North America 9*(1): 45–52.

that contribute to poor quality of care and staffing concerns should be described. A meeting with both management and staff should be held to submit the involved concerns through discussion and in writing.

When a choice relates to delivery of nursing service, the decision maker should consult appropriate resources to determine what should be done and who should do it. Helpful resources may include the nursing supervisor, the institutional policy and procedure manuals, the Ethics Committee of the institution, the ANA Standards of Practice (see Chapter 5, Box 5-1), and the state (provincial) Board of Nursing regulations governing practice.

The issue must also be clarified. The following questions should be asked: Who will be affected? What commitment or obligation is owed to each individual involved? When the issue is patient centered: What is the mental capacity of the patient? Are there prearranged requests such as a living will or DNR order? In these cases, the decision maker should organize the pertinent facts, listing potential economic, social, and political pressures that will affect the decision. Validating what the affected parties would prefer can be helpful when developing courses of action for consideration.

Analysis

During the analysis phase, the decision maker determines the values that are in conflict. Analysis of the dilemma will increase awareness of relevant information to consider in developing alternatives. When the conflict involves patient choices,

using NIC (5480) Values Clarification can help the decision maker explore personal values to get a clearer picture of his or her preferences. Box 10-4 outlines nursing activities presented in NIC that assist the nurse in values clarification.

In some cases, the situation will resolve itself. For example, consider the patient who refuses to give consent for a procedure. This decision could have very negative effects on the patient. After careful consideration and some time to contemplate the information, however, the patient chooses to sign the consent.

During the analysis phase, the decision maker should generate multiple alternatives, which should be analyzed and ranked based on right and wrong and the consequences of the choices. Also, the resolutions recommended by parties on both sides of the issue should be identified. These will be highly influenced by personal values, professional values and ideals, bias, and patient preference and needs. It is also important to determine whether the options fit with religious views, values, and personal beliefs. There may be other issues affecting desirability, such as lack of equipment, lack of available staff, lack of time, or lack of clinical competency.

An ideal alternative would have a high degree of probability—that is, a high likelihood of leading to the outcome with few undesirable effects or consequences. The amount of risk involved with each alternative is also a factor to be considered. In the field of nursing, decisions are made under conditions of uncertainty and change. Every decision carries some risk because it brings about change. It is important to explore emotional, social, and physical risk to both patient and staff.

Box 10-4 VALUES CLARIFICATION (5480)

Definition: Assisting another to clarify her/his own values in order to facilitate effective decision making

ACTIVITIES

Think through the ethical and legal aspects of free choice, given the particular situation, before beginning the intervention.

Create an accepting, nonjudgmental atmosphere.

Use appropriate questions to assist the patient in reflecting on the situation and what is important personally.

Use a value sheet clarifying technique (written situation and questions), as appropriate.

Pose reflective, clarifying questions that give the patient something to think about.

Encourage patient to make a list of what is important and not important in life and the time spent on each.

Encourage patient to list values that guide behavior in various settings and types of situations.

Help patient define alternatives and their advantages and disadvantages.

Encourage consideration of the issues and consequences of behavior.

Help patient to evaluate how values are in agreement with or conflict with those of family members/significant others.

Support patient's decision, as appropriate.

Use multiple sessions, as directed by the specific situation.

Avoid use of the intervention with persons with serious emotional problems.

Avoid use of cross-examining questions.

Adapted from McCloskey, J. C., & Bulechek, G. M. (2000). *Nursing interventions classification (NIC)* (p. 693). St. Louis: Mosby.

Outcome Identification

Providing safe nursing care is always the desired outcome. The expected outcome should serve as a guide in making decisions.

Often, decision makers sacrifice what is really important to achieve a goal that does not really matter. For example, on a short-staffed unit, a nurse may focus on personal care for patients when patient safety is the primary concern.

By using clearly stated outcomes, success becomes measurable. A poor-quality decision is likely without prior consideration of all possible choices or if the goal is inconsistent with the values of the affected individual.

Plan

During the planning stage, the decision maker should choose the best option or combination of options that provides for priority needs and achieves the desired outcome. Information should be organized and alternatives developed that represent various moral points of view. Development of alternatives that will resolve the dilemma while minimizing the consequences is important. The decision maker must be prepared to defend his or her choice. Awareness and understanding of different perspectives better prepares the nurse to justify actions.

Sometimes, keeping a unit staffed consumes so much energy that the nurse fails to recognize the underlying problem. In many cases, the frequent call-ins are actually a symptom of poor management, low morale, or staff exhaustion, secondary to working many extra shifts. Until the real problem is identified, remediation efforts will be counterproductive. By staying focused on the outcome, the decision maker remains focused on the real problem.

Implementation

Implementation involves implementing the moral action selected to resolve the dilemma. In the decision-making process, follow-up through the chain of command is essential when a dilemma presents itself. It is also important to support a blame-free environment and monitor side effects of the decision.

Evaluation

The results of the decision should be evaluated. The nurse should always ask questions and monitor responses. For example: Were the actions eth-

ical? Does the solution generate the desired outcome? Can the consequences be justified? Do the benefits outweigh the risks?

ETHICAL DILEMMA

The scenario presented in Box 10-5 demonstrates ethical reasoning using the nursing process format. This process is the basis for ethical reasoning in making patient decisions.

Consider the following scenario and how you would respond to the ethical dilemma: During a home health visit, the nurse notices many visitors coming and going in the home. During one of the home visits, the nurse overhears the patient on the telephone discussing selling methamphetamines. The nurse realizes that the patient is selling drugs from his home. This information was discovered during the privileged professional relationship with the patient. If the nurse reports these suspicions to the police, will he or she violate the patient's confidentiality?

An ethical decision needs to be made: In this case, truth telling supports our system of justice. Breaking the law does not fall under the patient confidentiality umbrella.

ETHICS COMMITTEES

In hospitals and long-term care facilities, groups of individuals convene to discuss, clarify, and make decisions resolving issues related to patient welfare. To support objectivity in making difficult patient care decisions, these groups are composed of people with varied backgrounds and beliefs. The committee should consist of individuals who are knowledgeable about legal and ethical issues. Discussion is a vital part of the committee's moral decision-making process because all members should agree with the decision. When the whole team, including the patient and family, are involved in the decision-making process, members feel better about following through with the chosen alternative.

FREQUENT AREAS OF DILEMMA

Self-Determination

The Patient Self-Determination Act of 1990 outlines specific legal and ethical obligations related to safe care. These include informed consent and patient's rights. "Consent is the voluntary authorization by a patient or the patient's legal repre-

SCENARIO

Linda Allen, a 62-year-old patient, has a history of right breast cancer with metastasis to the liver. During the admission procedure, her physical status is noted to be frail and emaciated, with a weight of 72 pounds. Her vitals are: blood pressure, 82/40 mm Hg; pulse, 64 beats/min and irregular; respirations, 32 breaths/min. When asked about a code status, she states, "Oh, I don't want to die, I'm not a quitter." The patient's vitals are unstable, and death is imminent.

ASSESSMENT

What areas of assessment would be important to perform immediately?

Verify your information. Review the patient's medical diagnosis, illness, and present plan of care. Clarify with the patient her understanding of a code. She said, "I don't want to die." Not that she wants everything done. This is a futile situation. Clarify her understanding of the disease process and its effect on the body.

Coding the patient in a futile situation causes unnecessary pain and suffering. The nursing obligation to protect the patient, preserve dignity, and avoid needless suffering and procedures is also present. Use of resources that could better be used to serve patients with some chance of recovery is also another consideration.

ANALYSIS

What complication is the nurse most concerned about at this time?

What is in the patient's best interest?
What constitutes professional duty?

OUTCOME IDENTIFICATION

The patient will receive the medical care she requires to maintain dignity and respect for her wishes while minimizing unnecessary pain and suffering.

PLAN AND IMPLEMENTATION

An ethics consult can be very effective, but her condition is unstable. She has a low blood pressure, irregular pulse, and a terminal diagnosis.

OPTIONS

1. Do nothing because the patient has stated what she wants. This may result in coding the patient and causing unnecessary suffering.
2. Clarify with the patient her understanding of a code. She said, "I don't want to die." Not that she wants everything done. This is a futile situation. Education about her disease process and its effect on the body are indicated.
3. Call the physician and ask him/her to have the conversation with the patient.

EVALUATION

Was progress toward the patient's desired outcome achieved?
Does the decision support ethical principles?
Are there universal applications of this outcome for future situations?

---

sentative to do something for the patient" (Guido, 2001, p. 129). The patient has a right to be informed about his care and to make decisions about that care. Informed consent is an important part of that process. The nurse must explain the treatment or procedure in a manner that the patient can understand. Elements that must be included in the explanation are as follows:

- A brief explanation of the procedure
- The qualifications and names of people performing and assisting with any treatment or procedure
- The possibility of harm, pain, discomfort, or death, relative to the procedure
- Any alternative therapy available for the condition
- The identification of the outcome without intervention
- The knowledge that the patient has a right to refuse treatment, even after treatment has begun

The physician should seek and obtain informed consent for medical treatment, procedures, and research or experimental treatments. The nurse should seek and obtain informed consent for the delivery of nursing care. These boundaries sometimes become unclear when the patient discusses his or her experiences with the nurse and the nurse fills in gaps to answer the patient's questions.

The physician frequently delegates the task of obtaining informed patient consent to the nurse. Responsibility for educating the patient regarding the procedure is the legal responsibility of the physician. The nurse is responsible for helping patients understand information presented by the physician. However, the nurse should not use his or her knowledge and relationship with the patient to persuade the patient to choose one option over another. "The nurse is well advised to contact the physician immediately, rather than attempt to talk a reluctant patient into a proposed procedure" (Guido, 2001, p. 135).

In addition to the right to be informed and to make decisions, the patient has a right to complain about his or her care or any other aspects of the nursing plan. Moreover, he or she has a right to be free of pain, to be free of abuse, and to retain privacy. Finally, the patient has a right to receive care in a safe setting, to ask questions about charges, and to be free of restraints and drugs that are not medically necessary.

Living wills are directives regarding treatment choices, given by competent individuals to health care providers, should they no longer be able to direct those choices for themselves. Patients have a right to prepare a written document regarding refusing treatments or ending life-prolonging treatments. The patient may also initiate a DNR directive after learning of a specific diagnosis or prognosis of a disease process (Guido, 2001, p. 158).

Other death and dying issues that pose problems include euthanasia, DNR mandates, and the withdrawal of life-sustaining treatment. Advance directives cover many of these areas of concern. It would seem that not initiating every effort in the first place would resolve many of these problems. That, however, is not the norm. The question at issue is: if the situation becomes futile, when does one stop active intervention or withdraw life support?

Professional Caregiver Issues

RISK FOR INJURY

Appropriate interventions to manage the confused individual include an assessment to determine whether the cause of the problem is delirium, dementia, or depression. A patient with signs of delirium usually demonstrates symptoms of rapid change in behavior and thinking ability. Assessment is also done to identify a potential physical cause for the patient's confusion. Relevant interventions might include using mittens or elbow splints to prevent pulling out tubes, asking the family to sit with the patient, and discussing with the physician the discontinuation of a medication that may be a contributing factor.

For the patient with dementia, validation therapy is used to stimulate pleasant thoughts and memories. This can be accomplished with the use of touch, picture books, or other familiar objects. Calling by name and maintaining eye contact can also be helpful.

The depressed patient will benefit from the use of therapeutic communication and planning ways to decrease feelings of loneliness and isolation. For the patient with a new diagnosis, helpful alternatives include teaching management of the disease process through education, enhancing coping skills, and involving the patient in support groups.

INADEQUATE STAFFING

The increased nursing shortage in the marketplace brings a new set of problems to the health care environment. These issues of concern include providing adequate staffing appropriate to the complexity and acuity level of patient needs, floating nurses who may not possess the specialty knowledge and skill necessary to provide safe nursing care, and using temporary or agency staff nurses to supplement staff on nursing units.

When the nurse does not have the abilities to perform the tasks or procedures that a particular patient population may need, patient safety becomes a concern. Competency is a management responsibility. Nursing management must evaluate the nurse's skills to ensure safe, appropriate nursing care delivery.

The nurse who is asked to float to an unfamiliar unit must clarify his or her own personal qualifications by asking the following questions:

- Do I possess the knowledge and skill needed to provide safe nursing care?
- What resources are available? Are there experienced nurses with whom I can collaborate?
- Will an orientation be provided to ensure that I can safely administer medications, perform procedures, and provide a safe level of care in an unfamiliar environment?
- Will the deficits between the skill needed and the knowledge available lead to harm or potential harm to patients involved?

Personnel shortages present serious concerns for patient safety. When there are inadequate supplies, equipment, staff, or available beds for the acuity level of the patients on the unit, decisions must be made relative to the distribution of services and supplies.

The nurse must clarify the situation. The nurse's responsibility to the patient includes the following:

- The nurse owes a duty to the patient to provide safe, professional care, performing activities within the scope of nursing practice.
- The nurse has a responsibility to the patient to use and distribute scarce resources in an appropriate manner without abandoning or neglecting the patient.
- The nurse has a responsibility to the patient to provide adequate supervision to persons providing care in the health care environment.

Nursing skills that are emphasized vary with the practice setting. Therefore, nurses practicing outside their area of expertise must be especially careful. It is critical to request orientation, cross-training, or other measures that enhance existing skills, so that no harm comes to patients. Nurses may request restricted duty, such as passing medications, providing personal care, assessing vital signs, and other familiar tasks. Unit-specific staff may be assigned to care for the central line, manage chemotherapy, or monitor the progress of labor patients. Chapter 11, Applying Nursing Judgment in Clinical Settings, explores this topic in more detail.

BIOMEDICAL ADVANCES

Society has changed from revolving around communities with a common set of beliefs and values to a world of multicultural and multifaith beliefs. Bioethical issues such as transplantation, in vitro fertilization, and genetic engineering have created controversy and focused attention on different belief systems. In the past, the health care system operated on a paternalistic system, in which the doctor knew best, nurses implemented the orders of the doctor, and the patient complied with what the doctor recommended. The focus was on the disease process and its treatment. Today, the treatment is directed toward the patient. This enables the patient to make appropriate choices that will help prevent disease instead of just treating it. The role of the nurse is focused on teaching, in order to encourage patient autonomy. The nurse's role as patient advocate is essential to safeguard the rights of individual patients because "without the advocacy and protection of rights, there are no rights" (Bandman & Bandman, 1990, cited in Rumbold, 2000, p. 8).

PITFALLS IN ETHICAL DECISION MAKING

The following are common pitfalls to avoid when making an ethical decision:

- *Disregard for others: using another individual to achieve an end, without consideration for his or her integrity.* An example of this would be assigning less difficult patients to a long-term UAP and assigning more difficult patients to the new UAP. The more difficult patient would not receive the benefits of the more experienced UAP. The new UAP may suffer burnout and leave.
- *Inappropriate application of standards: making decisions that others would not make, given similar circumstances.* An example would be continuing to accomplish the task based on "that's the way it's always been done" instead of using newly accepted standards.
- *Personal gain: having a vested interest, ulterior motive, or seeking personal gain by mak-*

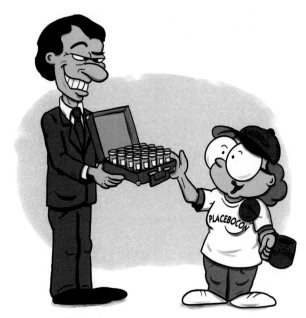

"You mean, if I push your company's new drug I get all this free stuff? Sure!"

ing a given decision. An example of this pitfall is the nurse who always seeks the role of shift charge, then assigns herself one easy patient and divides the remaining workload among a limited number of staff members.
- *Conflict of values: responding to a need without genuine concern for those affected by the decision.* An example would be when the patient has asked for an analgesic, but the nurse takes a coffee break before meeting the patient's needs for pain management.

SUMMARY

The principles of ethics describe how people should and should not act. In nursing, these principles are guided by the ANA Code of Ethics. Critical thinking skills are used when two or more options will produce the same effect to determine the better choice from the patient's perspective. Ethical decision making incorporates the use of the nursing process framework. Areas that are subject to frequent ethical dilemmas include self-determination, ongoing care, inadequate staffing, and bioethical issues. Pitfalls in ethical decision making often involve disregard for others, inappropriate application of standards, personal gain, and conflicting values.

- Ethics is concerned with the principles of right and wrong.
- Standards of conduct and moral judgment form a foundation for ethics.
- Ethical principles include autonomy, non-maleficence, beneficence, justice, fidelity, and veracity.
- Autonomy, or the right to self-determination, is embraced by the Patient Care Partnership.
- The ethical concept of nonmaleficence proposes that nurses do no harm. Beneficence is doing good on the patient's behalf.
- Beneficence and nonmaleficence are accomplished by maintaining competency, practicing within the scope of practice identified in the state (provincial) Nurse Practice Act, and relying on the ANA Standards of Practice for decision-making guidelines.
- Justice mandates that people be treated fairly and equally.
- Fidelity means loyalty or allegiance. The nurse should act as the patient advocate.
- Ethical decision making uses critical thinking. It can be approached in a nursing process format.
- When a conflict involves patient choices, values clarification can facilitate a clearer picture of the dilemma.
- In health care organizations, Ethics Committees convene to discuss, clarify, and resolve issues related to the welfare of the patient.
- Ethical dilemmas frequently occur with issues involving self-determination, professional caregiver issues, and safety devices. Biomedical advances have added new ethical dilemmas.
- The Patient Self-Determination Act of 1990 outlines specific legal and ethical obligations related to safe care, including informed consent and patient rights.

REFERENCES

Alfaro-LeFevre, R. (1999). *Critical thinking in nursing.* Philadelphia: W. B. Saunders.

American Hospital Association. (2003). *The patient care partnership: Understanding expectations, rights, and responsibilities.* Chicago: Author.

American Nurses Association. (2001). *Code of ethics for nurses with interpretive statements.* Washington, DC: Author.

American Nurses Association Code of Ethics Project Task Force. (2000). A new code of ethics for nurses. *American Journal of Nursing, 100*(7), 69–72.

Anderson, M. A., & Braun, J. V. (1995). *Caring for the elderly patient.* Philadelphia: F. A. Davis.

Bandman, E. I., & Bandman, D. (1990). *Nursing ethics through the life span.* Englewood Cliffs, NJ: Prentice-Hall.

Beauchamp, T. L., & Childress, J. F. (1994). *Principles of biomedical ethics.* New York: Oxford University Press.

Catalano, J. T. (2000). *Nursing now: Today's issues, tomorrow's trends.* Philadelphia: F. A. Davis.

Chally, P. S., & Loriz, L. (1998). Ethics in the trenches: Decision making in practice. *American Journal of Nursing, 98*(6), 17–20.

Deloughery, G. (1998). *Issues and trends in nursing.* St. Louis: Mosby.

Guido, G. W. (2001). *Legal and ethical issues in nursing.* Upper Saddle River, NJ: Prentice-Hall.

Harkness, G. A., and Dincher, J. R. (1999). *Medical surgical nursing: total patient care.* St. Louis: Mosby.

Husted, G. L., & Husted, J. H. (2001). *Ethical decision making in nursing and healthcare.* New York: Springer Publishing.

Marquis, B. L., & Huston, C. J. (2003). *Leadership and management functions in nursing.* Philadelphia: Lippincott Williams & Wilkins.

McCloskey, J. C., & Bulechek, G. M. (2000). *Nursing interventions classification (NIC).* St. Louis: Mosby.

McCloskey, J. C., & Grace, H. K. (1997). *Current issues in nursing.* St. Louis: Mosby.

Purtilo, R. (1993). *Ethical dimensions in the health care profession.* Philadelphia: W. B. Saunders.

Raths, L. E., Simon, S. B., & Harmin, M. (1978). *Values and teaching.* Columbus, OH: Charles E. Merrill.

Ringsven, M. K., & Bond, D. (1991). *Gerontology and leadership skills for nurses.* Boston: Delmar.

Rocchiccioli, J. T., & Tilbury, M. S. (1998). *Clinical leadership in nursing.* Philadelphia: W. B. Saunders.

Ruggiero, V. (1991). *The art of thinking: A guide to critical and creative thought.* New York: Harper Collins.

Rumbold, G. (2000). *Ethics in nursing practice.* New York: Royal College of Nursing, Bailliere Tindale.

Tappen, R. M., Weiss, S. A., & Whitehead, D. K. (2001). *Essentials of nursing leadership and management.* Philadelphia: F. A. Davis.

Taylor, C., Lillis, C., & LeMone, P. (2001). *Fundamentals of nursing: The art and science of nursing care.* Philadelphia: Lippincott Williams & Wilkins.

Zerwekh, J., & Claborn, J. C. (2000). *Nursing today: Transitions and trends.* Philadelphia: W. B. Saunders.

Student Worksheets

 ## SKILL SHEET: ETHICAL DECISION MAKING

Purpose

To facilitate the student's ability to problem solve in a logical and sequential manner in situations in which no clear choice is readily apparent.

Objectives

1. To assist the student's development of an organized process in the application of judgment and reasoning skills in the resolution of ethical issues.
2. To increase the student's knowledge base of appropriate references to use as a resource in resolving unclear issues (e.g., ANA Code of Ethics, Standards of Practice, Institutional Policy and Procedures).

Steps: Ethical Decision Making

ASSESSMENT

1. Identify the problem in the situation.
2. Collect information about facts that have the most bearing.
3. Identify mental competency of the patient, family input, any prearranged requests set forth in a written document about the patient's wishes and family's wishes, and any psychosocial factors potentially affecting the situation.
4. List everyone affected by the decision and the nurse's obligation to each.
5. Sort and organize pertinent facts.
6. Validate the preferences of affected parties.

ANALYSIS

1. Use critical thinking skills to interpret values in conflict.
2. State the ethical issue clearly.
3. Examine own value system and its effect on decision.
4. Integrate existing knowledge gained in previous experiences in similar situations.
5. Determine consequences of decision in terms of right and wrong.

OUTCOME IDENTIFICATION

Identify desired outcome of the decision.

PLAN

1. Generate courses of action that are capable of producing desired outcome.
2. Evaluate appropriateness of each strategy based on acceptable consequences, desirability, and unacceptable consequences.
3. Analyze and rank alternatives based on desirability and personal risk.
4. Compare each alternative in terms of priorities and acceptability of potential outcome.
5. Choose the alternative with the best chance of success and that has the least undesirable outcome.

IMPLEMENTATION

1. Initiate and complete the appropriate course of action necessary to intervene in the dilemma.
2. Deliver safe and effective nursing care based on Standards of Practice.
3. Identify areas not within the scope of nursing and refer to the appropriate health care member.

EVALUATION

1. Determine whether the decision resolves the dilemma.
2. Establish whether the desired outcome was achieved.
3. Take responsibility for own actions.
4. Communicate outcomes when appropriate.

COMPETENCY VALIDATION: ETHICAL DECISION MAKING

COMPETENCY STATEMENT

Demonstrate ability to make decisions, which are appropriate to the situation and based on relevant data.

The student demonstrated the ability to:

1. Identify the dilemma clearly and precisely.
2. Establish the purpose of the decision to be made and the desired outcome.
3. Generate multiple alternatives capable of producing the desired outcome.
4. Use scientific principles and rationale to support the decision.
5. Select the decision that best correlated with priorities and demonstrated an acceptable consequence.
6. Select the action that could achieve resolution of the dilemma in an ethical manner.
7. Evaluate and reevaluate the effect of the decision after implementation and make needed adjustments.

COMPETENT

- Understands reasons for task and is able to perform tasks independently
- Understands reasons for task but needs supervision
- Understands reasons for task and is able to perform task with assistance

NOT COMPETENT

- Understands reasons for task but performs task at provisional level
- Is unable to state reasons for task and performs task at dependent level

SKILL CHECKLIST: ETHICAL DECISION MAKING

ETHICAL DECISION MAKING	SATISFACTORY	UNSATISFACTORY	NI/COMMENTS
ASSESSMENT			
1. Identify the problem in the situation.			
2. Collect information about facts that have the most bearing.			
3. Clarify the issue.			
4. List those affected by the decision and nurse's obligation to each.			
5. Sort and organize pertinent facts.			
6. Validate preferences of affected parties.			
ANALYSIS			
1. Use critical thinking skills to interpret values in conflict.			
2. Identify the ethical issue.			
3. Examine own value system and its effect on decision.			
4. Integrate existing knowledge gained in previous experiences.			
5. Determine consequences of decision in terms of right and wrong.			
OUTCOME IDENTIFICATION			
1. Identify desired outcome of the decision.			
PLAN			
1. Generate courses of action that are capable of producing desired outcome.			
2. Evaluate appropriateness of each strategy based on acceptable consequences, desirability, and unacceptable consequences.			
3. Analyze and rank alternatives based on desirability and personal risk.			
4. Compare each alternative in terms of priorities and acceptability of potential outcomes.			
5. Choose the alternative that best correlates with priorities and demonstrates the least undesirable outcome.			

ETHICAL DECISION MAKING	SATISFACTORY	UNSATISFACTORY	NI/COMMENTS
IMPLEMENTATION			
1. Initiate and complete the appropriate course of action to intervene in the dilemma.			
2. Deliver safe and effective nursing care based on Standards of Practice.			
3. Identify areas not within the scope of nursing and refer to the appropriate health care member.			
EVALUATION			
1. Determine whether the decision resolves the ethical dilemma.			
2. Establish whether the desired outcome was achieved.			
3. Take responsibility for own actions.			
4. Communicate outcomes when appropriate.			

 SCENARIO TO ACCOMPANY STUDENT WORKSHEETS

Raymond Long, 73 years old, has expressed to his family numerous times that he does not want a ventilator or CPR to prolong his life. He has no advance directives written. However, the patient has been brought to the emergency room (ER) with a possible pulmonary embolus. He is experiencing chest pain and arrhythmias on the monitor. The family verbalizes the patient's request, but the physician informs them that this is a new situation unrelated to his previous problems. The physician further states, "This is a treatable condition, and your father could have several good years left in him." The patient's physical status is very shaky, and the physician has not yet agreed to the DNR order. It is evident that the family is being pressured by the physician to agree to extraordinary measures. What should the nurse do next? Discuss the consequences of each option.

ASSESSMENT

Problem

The patient is very unstable and has verbalized a choice for "no CPR" and "no mechanical ventilation," but the physician is still insisting on using extraordinary measures to sustain life.

The patient and family have requested a DNR status.

The physician is applying pressure for the use of extraordinary measures against the wishes of the patient and family.

The patient is very unstable and at high risk for a code being required to sustain life.

ANALYSIS

The patient's has a right to choose; the physician's desire is to preserve life.

The patient's has a right to advance directives.

The physician should respect the patient's right to choose.

OUTCOME IDENTIFICATION

The desired outcome should reflect the patient's right to choose. An informed, autonomous patient, whose wishes are respected, is the goal.

PLAN

_____

_____

_____

_____

_____

IMPLEMENTATION

_____

_____

_____

_____

_____

_____

_____

_____

_____

_____

EVALUATION

_____

_____

_____

_____

See the Answer Key in Appendix A for sample answers for this exercise.

Practice Exercises: Ethical Decision Making

USE OF ANA CODE OF ETHICS

Scenarios: Using the Code of Ethics

Use the ANA Code of Ethics to determine what the patient could reasonably expect from the nurse in the following situations.

1. A 23-year-old man was admitted with a fever, constant diarrhea, nausea and vomiting, and weight loss. The patient has recently been diagnosed with human immunodeficiency virus (HIV) infection. He has not been taking his medication. The nurse in charge of the patient's care refuses to answer the call light. During medication pass, the charge nurse notes that the patient's nurse placed his medication on the bedside table and said, "Here, take these," and walked away. How should the charge nurse intervene?

_____

_____

_____

_____

_____

_____

_____

_____

_____

_____

2. An 89-year-old woman was admitted to the medical unit with respiratory distress, secondary to lung cancer. The patient wants to sign a DNR order, but the daughter is unwilling to allow this to happen, stating, "Mother is not in the proper mental state to decide." The nursing evaluation indicates that the patient is alert and understands the risks. What should the nurse do?

_____

_____

_____

_____

_____

_____

_____

_____

_____

3. With the patient in bed, the new nurse changes the bed linens while the bed is in a high-Fowler's position. After the bed is made, the nurse leaves the side rails down and leaves the room. About 5 minutes later, the family arrives. They immediately ring the call light because the patient is lying on the floor. The patient has a nosebleed and a large raised area on the side of his head. How should the charge nurse intervene?

_____

_____

_____

_____

_____

_____

_____

_____

_____

4. During change of shift in a busy ER, the charge nurse begins to notice a staff nurse who is slurring words and making inappropriate decisions. The charge nurse questions the nurse and asks if he is all right. She detects the odor of alcohol on his breath. How should the nurse intervene?

_____

_____

_____

_____

_____

_____

_____

_____

_____

5. The home health nurse notes that a 37-year-old patient with tuberculosis (TB) failed to keep appointments with the department and to fill his medication prescription at the local pharmacy. The home health nurse failed to follow up with a report to the health department. How should the nurse director of the home health department intervene?

_____

_____

_____

_____

_____

_____

_____

6. The nursing unit had four sick call-ins from staff today as a result of a terrible snowstorm. Central staffing has no replacements. The on-duty RN and UAP have both worked on this unit for 20 years. The UAP's son recently died after a long struggle with cancer. During his illness, the UAP managed his pain at home with injections. The RN has a patient load of 18 patients. After the RN delegated a morphine sulfate (MS) injection to the UAP, the patient admitted for a bilateral radical mastectomy is found unconscious, respirations of 6 breaths/min. What should not have occurred in this situation? What needs to change? How should the nurse supervisor intervene for this patient?

_____

_____

_____

_____

_____

_____

_____

_____

7. The skilled care unit has had several deaths that have been "unexpected." In each case, a certain nurse was responsible for the patient's care. Later, it was proved that the nurse intentionally caused these deaths. What should the nurse have done?

_____

_____

_____

_____

_____

_____

_____

8. The medical surgical unit is using a new type of intravenous (IV) catheter. The nurse using the new equipment has found that the catheter sheath tends to break during insertion. The nurse fails to share this information with the team, reasoning, "the paper work is too much bother." What should the nurse have done?

_____

_____

_____

_____

_____

_____

_____

_____

9. The nurse refuses to delegate because he or she wants to ensure that his or her patients are receiving optimum care. A new patient was admitted with end-stage renal disease and has a sudden rise in blood pressure. The nurse fails to observe this vital sign change because he or she is busy with so much work to do. What should the nurse have done?

_____

_____

_____

_____

_____

_____

_____

_____

10. The 89-year-old terminally ill patient assigned to the nurse is alert and oriented. The patient's husband wants to admit her into the hospice program. He states that he doesn't want his wife to know that she is terminal or being placed in the hospice program because he doesn't want her to worry. What should the nurse do?

_____

_____

_____

_____

_____

_____

_____

_____

11. A newly admitted 28-year-old patient confides to the nurse that he has recently been diagnosed as having human immunodeficiency virus (HIV). A few hours after admission, the nurse receives a phone call from a female stating that she is his wife. She asks why the patient was admitted and requests a report on the patient's health status. What should the nurse do?

_____

_____

_____

_____

_____

_____

_____

12. The 32-year-old patient with an admitting diagnosis of pancreatitis frequently has a significant other of the same gender in his room. The nurse assigned to him today refuses to touch the patient to provide personal care and ignores him when he asks questions. The nurse remarks to a co-worker, "How can a person sleep with the same sex?" What should the nurse do for this and all patients?

_____

_____

_____

_____

_____

_____

_____

_____

_____

See the Answer Key in Appendix A for sample answers for this exercise.

 # SCENARIOS: MAKING ETHICAL DECISIONS

SCENARIO 1

Edna Green, a 50-year-old patient with type 1 diabetes, has been receiving dialysis for the past 4 years. She is under the medical care of Dr. Jones and has revealed to him during conversations in the office that she does not want to be resuscitated or placed on a ventilator. During dialysis this morning, she developed respiratory failure, was resuscitated, and was placed in the intensive coronary care unit (ICCU). At present, the physician is considering a DNR order when the family arrives. The physician verbalizes that during his professional relationship with Edna, she confided that she did not want extraordinary measures to prolong her life. The daughter states, "We have discussed this several times, and Mom wanted everything possible done." The patient's daughter further states, "Our daughter is getting married next month and Mom said wild horses couldn't keep her away." What should the nurse in charge of her care do next? Discuss the consequences of each decision.

OPTIONS
1. Ethics consult is the only viable option. This will facilitate discussion of quality of life and gather input from family, physician, and other experienced professionals.
2. Do nothing. Respect family's opinion because they are now the decision makers. This leaves everybody in crisis.

SCENARIO 2

Nurse Joan arrived on duty at 7:00 PM. Gregory Brand, a 62-year-old patient 2 days after fractured hip repair, had a temperature of 100.8°F (38.2°C). At 11:00 PM, his face was flushed, and he was perspiring heavily. Nurse Joan inspected the wound dressing, and no drainage was noted. A review of the chart reveals no antibiotic order. She placed a call to the physician and received the following orders:

Deep breathe and cough every hour
Tylenol, 10 grains orally every 4 hours as needed

At 10:00 PM, the temperature is 102°F (38.8°C). A review of the medication administration record (MAR) reveals that only pain medications and Tylenol have been ordered. Nurse Joan places another call to the physician. He states, "Just have him deep breathe and cough like I told you the first time and don't call me again." He hangs up on the nurse. At 1:00 AM, the patient's temperature is 102.8°F (39.3°C). What should the nurse do? Discuss the consequences of each option.

OPTIONS

1. Do nothing and just accept the physician's order.
2. Call the physician back and get reprimanded.
3. Review the chart to determine whether there is another physician that can be called.
4. Notify the nursing supervisor.

Scenario 3

Angela Lane, a 78-year-old patient with a history of congestive heart failure (CHF) and degenerative arthritis, arrived in the ER complaining of acute epigastric pain and vomiting blood. After the initial assessment, she was transported to the gastroenterology lab and treated for a bleeding ulcer. During the procedure, Mrs. Long arrested, and a code was initiated per family instructions. The patient was transported to the ICCU after resuscitation and placed on a ventilator. The next day, different family members requested that the ventilator and all treatment be stopped; however, the physician believes the patient will make a full recovery to the previous health status and refused to comply. What should the nurse do?

OPTIONS

1. Do nothing. Leaves everybody in crisis.
2. Ethics consult is an option for all to express views and come to an understanding and agreement. If the patient clearly lacks decision-making capacity, and the family can't agree after the consult, the Healthcare Surrogate Act compels that someone be appointed. This requires time to have a court-appointed decision maker thoroughly assess the patient's situation.
3. Obtain social services consultation to discuss power of attorney (POA) and advance directives with the patient.

Scenario 4

Donna Lay, a 42-year-old patient admitted for cholelithiasis, developed intractable vomiting at 2:00 AM. Nurse Clara called the physician for an antiemetic order. The doctor's wife answered the phone and asked what the problem is. The wife is a nurse that works in the ICCU at the same hospital. The wife listens to the nurse explain the situation, and then without hesitation states, "Give her Compazine, 5 mg IV push, now." Nurse Clara knew the wife didn't wake the doctor. Identify the confidentiality issue related to Nurse Clara's interaction with the physician's wife.

Discussing the patient's concerns with the physician's wife is a violation of confidentiality. The information should only be discussed with someone who has a need to know.

What should Nurse Clara do?

OPTIONS

1. Do nothing about the concern. Give the drug.
2. Call the nursing supervisor and ask him or her to intervene. Do not give the drug because this is an invalid order.

Scenario 5

Fred Green, a 52-year-old patient, was admitted from the ER in third-degree heart block with a heart rate of 32 to 44 beats/min on the cardiac monitor. His chief complaints included weakness, fatigue, and syncopal episodes during the past 3 weeks. The physician explained the need for a pacemaker and answered all of the patient's questions. He wrote an order to obtain a surgical consent for insertion of a permanent transvenous pacemaker and prepare for surgery. After preparations were complete and Mr. Green was transported to the holding area in the operating room (OR), he stated, "I don't want a pacemaker in my chest, I just want to get out of here." The nurse called the physician and informed him of the problems. The physician came to the holding area and told the patient, "We can discuss this after the procedure." The physician went into the OR. What should the nurse do next? Discuss the consequences of each option.

OPTIONS

1. Do nothing. The patient has already signed an informed consent. Proceed with the procedure because further delay may cause harm to the patient.
2. Call the nursing supervisor and ask him or her to intervene.
3. Assess the patient's reason for refusal. It may be a misunderstanding or anxiety. The nurse is the patient advocate. Clarify with the patient his understanding of a pacemaker. A patient has a right to informed consent and may rescind that consent at any time. He has a right to refuse treatment options as long as he fully understands the risks involved and is willing to accept the consequences. The health care provider's role involves helping the individual with life decisions. Call the physician out of the OR and ask him or her to discuss this issue further.

Scenario 6

Melinda Green, RN, a new nurse, is assigned to work on the postcritical care unit (PCU) tonight. Three RNs, as well as the unit secretary for this shift, have called in sick. The unit is typically short-staffed without people calling in. At present, each RN has nine high-acuity patients each for primary care, must process their own orders, and must answer the phones. Staffing has been very similar for several days. Loretta Gray, a 72-year-old patient, is confused and disoriented. As a result of repeatedly climbing out of bed over the side rails, the nurses have placed her in a vest restraint safety device to prevent a patient fall. When Melinda enters the room, the patient is begging to be untied. After a discussion with the patient, Melinda believes that she would not climb out of bed if staff responded to the patient promptly. She does demonstrate the ability to ring the call light correctly. What should Nurse Melinda do next?

OPTIONS

1. Indirect intervention. Use distraction, determine whether family can come sit or whether a sitter is available to stay.
2. Assess the patient for mentation; assess the physician's order and the chart to determine the reason for the device. If the restraints have been placed because of staffing issues, remove them. Put the bed in low position and explore the use of a lap tray with a chair while observing behavior. Consult with the nurse manager to discuss staffing issues. Complete an occurrence report to avoid further incidents.
3. Do nothing. Leave restraints on and assume that she needs them because you have an order.

Scenario 7

Irene Carter, a 44-year-old patient admitted for liver cancer, is receiving large doses of morphine sulfate through a patient-controlled analgesia (PCA) pump. Death is imminent, and hospice nurses are following up in the home setting for her nursing assessments. Irene's pain is increasing, and the morphine has been increased to the extent that the nurses fear any further increase in dosage may hasten her death. When the nurse arrives today, Irene rates her pain at 10 on a 1 to 10 scale. What should the nurse do next?

OPTIONS

1. Do nothing. This violates the patient's right to appropriate pain management.
2. Call the physician for breakthrough pain medication that does not affect the respiratory system. Assess the description of the pain. Discuss with Irene the level of pain that is acceptable to her. Review the medication sheet to determine whether there are other supplemental drugs that might cover the breakthrough pain episodes. Consult with the pharmacist or other hospice nurses for options that have been effective in similar situations with other patients. Discuss the risks and benefits of various pain management drugs with the patient and family members. Determine an acceptable pain management regimen with the patient, taking into consideration the risks and benefits.

Scenario 8

Kay Stack, a 29-year-old patient, was admitted for new onset of diabetes mellitus, type 1. She is divorced with two small children, 4 and 5 years of age. All three are currently living in the home of Kay's retired mother. The mother is on a limited income and unable to assist with the medical expenses. Kay works at a fast-food restaurant and has no insurance. The physician wrote a discharge order for today. The nurse informed the physician about a concern for Kay's inability to perform the Glucoscan. Additionally, the nurse discussed the lack of funds to purchase equipment for insulin injections with the physician. The physician continued to dictate the discharge note and then left the unit. What factors should the nurse assess next?

ANSWER

_____

_____

_____

_____

_____

_____

What options should the nurse consider?

OPTIONS

1. Refuse to discharge the patient until she is able to perform skills for diabetic management independently.
   Outcome: Reimbursement issues for the hospital and a delay does not change the fact that the patient does not have the resources to buy supplies and medication.
2. Do nothing. Discharge the patient.
   Outcome: The nurse has failed to protect the patient from harm. This is an unsafe discharge. The diabetic patient must have insulin, syringes, and supplies to control the blood sugar and maintain diabetic control.
3. Collaborate with social services and ask for an ethics consult. The patient has a right to a transition plan, and this is an unsafe discharge.
   Outcome: Delaying the discharge until appropriate arrangements can be made through social services to help the patient find resources to obtain needed medical care and home care to arrange further patient teaching to ensure that she is able to perform needed skills independently are essential for this patient to have a safe discharge.

Scenario 9

Andrea Glen, a 43-year-old patient, was admitted for small cell carcinoma in the lung with metastasis to the brain. Death is imminent. She has seven children; two children want everything done including a code, and the other five want a palliation-only status for their mother. The Ethics Committee has already had a conference with them, and still no decision can be reached. What should the nurse do?

ANSWER

_____

_____

_____

_____

_____

Scenario 10

Mary Louise Long is a 67-year-old patient who has been a resident in a long-term care facility for the past 10 years. During the past 4 years, she has gradually become nonambulatory as a result of pressure caused by a large ovarian cyst. The cyst has been determined to weigh about 32 pounds and is probably benign based on multiple diagnostics tests performed to evaluate the decreased activity level. The patient refuses surgery because she is convinced she will die. What should the nurse do?

OPTIONS

1. Do nothing. Abide by the patient wishes. Patient will most likely continue to deteriorate.
2. Call an ethics consult to ensure that family can be involved. This will ensure that everyone understands that the patient could be ambulatory if the surgical intervention were successful. If the patient continues to refuse, the patient's choice must be honored.
3. Patient teaching. Evaluate her understanding of surgery risks and benefits. After 4 years, it is unlikely that this will be effective, but it is important to at least try.

Scenario 11

David Martin, a 22-year-old patient, had a brain tumor on the right side. As a result of surgery, chemotherapy, and radiation, the tumor was eradicated during a 2-year period. Six months after the physicians informed the family that the tumor was eradicated, a new primary tumor developed on the left side of the brain. The patient has already reached the maximum lifetime dose of chemotherapy agents deemed effective for this type of cancer cell. The physician refused to prescribe the continuation of chemotherapy because the side effects of the drugs are multiple myocardial arrhythmias and cardiac arrest. The wife insists that it worked before and requests to use the same drugs because they were effective in the past. The patient demands to continue the chemotherapy. What should the nurse do?

OPTIONS

1. There are no options for active treatment. Palliative treatment is the only alternative. Call social services and work with the patient to gain some insight and develop realistic expectations. The focus should be redirected to quality time and putting affairs in order.
2. A psychiatric consult may be indicated if the situation continues, and the nurse should also ask the physician to explain the side effects of the drugs further.
3. Do nothing. Leaves everybody in a crisis.

Scenario 12

John Jones, a 22-year-old admitted to the oncology unit for active acquired immunodeficiency syndrome (AIDS), has a 3 year-old child and a pregnant wife. During the admission interview, he openly discussed illegal drug use and described a lifestyle that included multiple sexual partners and long-term substance abuse. However, he also related that his wife is unaware of his sexual indiscretions. What should the nurse do?

OPTIONS

1. Encourage the patient to discuss these issues with his wife. Educate him about the consequences of his behavior to the unborn child and wife. Encourage him to disclose this information to his wife so that testing can be performed and treatment if indicated. Confidentiality prevents telling. Consult with social services to discuss these issues with the patient.
2. Do nothing. This maintains confidentiality but denies wife and unborn child treatment if indicated.

See the Answer Key in Appendix A for sample answers for this exercise.

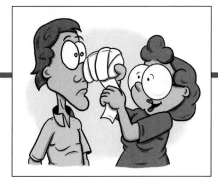

CHAPTER 11

Applying Nursing Judgment in Clinical Settings

OBJECTIVES

1. Define nursing judgment.

2. Analyze the individual needs of multiple patients to determine expected outcomes.

3. Assess the individual needs of multiple patients to determine the most urgent needs.

4. Identify the need for further assessment in situations where data gaps exist.

5. Evaluate data in situations that require a nursing judgment (clinical judgment) to be made.

6. Determine priority with multiple patients by comparing the effects of treatment delay.

7. Compare the competency and skills of nurses with experience in various specialty areas.

8. Compare desired outcomes among multiple patients to guide actions.

9. Demonstrate the ability to make the best patient care assignment.

10. Demonstrate the ability to make room assignments.

This chapter focuses on nursing judgment, a skill required in choosing how to meet the needs of a group of patients. Frequently, a care assignment includes taking care of multiple patients simultaneously. Decision making among groups of patients can be complicated. The nurse must deal with the varied needs and problems involved with delivering care for 10 to 15 patients, as opposed to choosing among the alternative needs of one or two patients. Important factors to consider when making group decisions include the physical status and stability of each patient, the implications of delaying care, the priorities of care for each patient, the expertise and experience of available personnel, and the individual needs of the total group.

It is critical to develop strong skills in problem solving, priority setting, and decision making, coupled with a good working application of the nursing process, before attempting to cultivate the group decision-making skill. Another skill essential to this process involves the ability to identify variations in physical and mental status and diagnostic test results. The combination of a strong knowledge base with the effective application of cognitive skills enhances the ability to make comparisons of expected outcomes, followed by sound nursing care decisions.

Throughout this chapter, patient scenarios are supplied to practice analysis of each individual in a group, evaluate the significance of the circumstances, and compare the effect of various courses of action on the outcomes. These patient scenarios will help the reader develop the ability to evaluate decisions affecting multiple patients more realistically.

DEFINITION

Decision-making for groups of patients requires the use of nursing judgment (clinical judgment). According to Ringsven and Bond (1997), "Judgment is the ability to make comparisons and then decisions." (p. 324) The process of critical thinking is inherent to nursing judgment. In nursing, data are gathered through the application of the nursing process. After the data are generated, the nurse must evaluate and compare the information to be able to draw conclusions. The critical thinker is able to make sound judgments using the available data, by giving each piece of evidence the appropriate weight or significance in the overall situation. This is called *analytical thinking*.

"Analytical thinking occurs when we take (some whole) and use our thinking to take that whole apart, to divide it up in some manner, in order to understand the whole better from the perspective of its parts" (Foundation for Critical Thinking, 1997, p. B6). Therefore, analytical thinking avoids jumping to inappropriate conclusions.

The competent nurse uses analytical thinking in making clinical judgments. Hall (1996) states,

"Competence is the advance assessment of ability; performance is the ongoing assessment of ability" (p. 212). The complexity within the health care system demands much more than just being able to perform a procedure step by step. Decisions made by nurses today must be based on evidence and applied in a competent manner. Components of competency are frequently assessed through the observation of actual performance. A measure of expertise usually relates to actual performance and is rated with specific criteria. In clinical practice, it is measured by the patient outcome. The competency skills necessary for critical thinking that leads to sound reasoning include interpretation, analysis, evaluation, inference, explanation, and self regulation.

Competency, as defined by Benner (1982), is "the ability to perform the task with desirable outcomes under the varied circumstances of the real world" (p. 303). It implies being able to make decisions about immediate versus delayed interventions within a group of assigned patients. The competent nurse decides which patient has priority need, identifies the problem requiring immediate attention and the appropriate interventions, and acts accordingly. Detailed specifics concerning decision making within groups are not frequently addressed in textbooks because of the varied and unique needs of the individual patients. Unlike the educational setting, where a typical assignment usually includes 2 or 3 patients, the real-world work assignment may include 15 to 20 patients. Additionally, actual clinical practice includes the use of

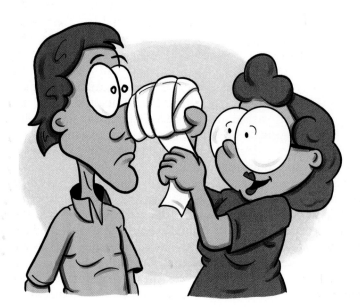

"There we go! If that nasty pollen can't get in your nose, you can't sneeze, right?"

assistive personnel, who possess varied skills and competencies.

Nursing judgment is the ability to analyze and interpret the individual needs of a group, evaluate the significance of each circumstance, compare the effect on the outcome of each action or alternative, and draw conclusions to make a decision that achieves the best outcome for everyone affected. Multiple factors must be considered when making decisions regarding care for groups of patients. The physical status and stability of each patient, the implications of delaying care, the priorities of care for each patient, the expertise and experience of available personnel, and the needs of each patient can significantly alter the decision.

THE DECISION-MAKING PROCESS

Evaluating Condition and Multiple Circumstances

As previously stated, decision making in groups is the process of making choices for multiple patients while achieving optimal care for each patient. One of the most complex skills in the practice of nursing is evaluating the needs of groups of patients, comparing these needs to events at hand, and choosing the best fit for that situation. Practicing the skill of comparing the needs of individual patients to achieve the desired outcomes for each will improve the beginner's competency. Critical thinking is inherent in the process of rational, purposeful decision making because individual patients bring different variables to a situation.

The following is a practice exercise to enable the reader to use critical thinking skills to evaluate the circumstances of four patients presented on a typical 3-to-11 shift. After report, it must be decided which of the four patients described below should be attended to first.

A. A 36-year-old woman, 2 days after hysterectomy. She has not voided since a Foley catheter was removed 8 hours ago. Current vitals are as follows: blood pressure, 167/88 mm Hg; pulse, 102 beats/min; respirations, 28 breaths/min. Complaints include abdominal pain and tenderness on palpation.

B. A 72-year-old man admitted for nausea, vomiting, and flu-like symptoms. Intravenous (IV) fluids of 5% dextrose in 0.9 normal saline (D-5 NS) are infusing at 100 mL/hr, the cardiac monitor shows sinus rhythm, heart rate is 98 beats/min, and the patient has not voided since admission 8 hours ago.

C. A 31-year-old man admitted for pneumonia 3 days ago with intravenous antibiotic (IVAB) therapy. The IV is infiltrated, and the next antibiotic will be due soon.

D. A 72-year-old man admitted for a fractured right hip, scheduled for surgery in the morning. He has refused to sign the operative permit until the physician comes and discusses the procedure with him.

After assessing the four patients, the nurse determines the following: Patient A is in acute distress and should be catheterized immediately. Patient B is probably dehydrated but just needs more fluid onboard to void. Patient C is urgent, but the antibiotic is not overdue yet; therefore, the situation is less urgent than that of Patient A. Patient D is also urgent but there is time to resolve the issue before morning. Therefore, Patient A is the most urgent in this circumstance. At the end of this chapter, more four-patient scenarios are provided for further practice of the group decision-making skill. In the clinical component of the nursing curriculum, the student should practice this skill by applying the guidelines presented in the next sections.

Monitoring Change and Multiple Patient Issues

The first step in monitoring change in group situations is to gather information about each patient. Sources of information may include change-of-shift report, the patient's chart, the patient's history, and a physical examination. It is important to distinguish different features of the individual patients in the group. The disease process, courses of illness, and plans of care of each individual patient should be reviewed. The ability to recognize variations, interpret findings, and draw conclusions through application of a strong knowledge base helps the nurse recognize when something needs to be changed or fixed. Additionally, the pathophysiology of the disease processes, the signs and symptoms of pathology, complications, the therapeutic and nontherapeutic effects of medications, and the evidence-based rationales for specific interventions must be considered. To facilitate a better understanding of this concept, the following exercise reviews the same patient scenarios presented above, while noting additional circumstances. In this case, following report, which patient should the nurse attend to first?

    A. A 36-year-old woman, 2 days after hysterectomy. She has not voided since a Foley catheter was removed 8 hours ago. Current vitals signs are as follows: blood pressure, 167/88 mm Hg; pulse, 102 beats/min; respirations, 28 breaths/min. Complaints include abdominal pain and tenderness on palpation.

    B. A 72-year-old man admitted for nausea, vomiting, and flu-like symptoms. IV fluids of D-5 NS are infusing at 100 mL/hr, the cardiac monitor shows sinus rhythm, the heart rate is 98 beats/min, and the patient has not voided since admission 8 hours ago.

    C. A 31-year-old man admitted for pneumonia 3 days ago with IVAB therapy. The IV is infiltrated, and the next antibiotic will be due soon.

    D. A 72-year-old man admitted for a fractured right hip, who had surgery this morning. Baseline vitals are as follows: blood pressure, 128/74 mm Hg; pulse, 78 beats/min; respirations, 24 breaths/min. Assessment of vitals after report taken by the unlicensed assistive personnel (UAP): blood pressure, 112/68 mm Hg; pulse, 98 beats/min; respirations, 28 breaths/min. Report revealed petechiae on the chest and arms and a large hematoma on the right hip.

The nurse determines that Patient A is still very urgent, however, Patient D is an orthopedic patient. Postoperative orthopedic patients routinely receive anticoagulants to prevent blood clots, and the petechiae and hematoma are obvious signs of an active bleed. The airway, breathing, and circulation (ABCs) take priority; therefore, Patient D is most urgent.

Establishing What to Do First

The next step in making group decisions is to identify the problems of each patient involved and develop a list. The individual needs of all the patients should be evaluated to determine expected outcomes and to establish similarities and differences. The patient conditions should then be analyzed to determine the significance of the information. Immediate needs should be determined by analyzing the urgency of each patient need. The most urgent needs for the individuals in the group should be identified, and the effect of a delay in treatment should be determined, to decide which patient takes priority.

FIRST-LEVEL CARE PRIORITIES

First level priority problems include problems that are immediately life threatening, an unstable or changing physical status, or findings that indicate a worsening condition. Untreated medical problems can pose a threat to the stability of the patient. Some examples include a diabetic patient with a high blood sugar and no orders for insulin or treatment, abnormal lab findings that require treatment, a large fluid deficit or excess during a shift, pain without management options, or an acute change in vital signs. Additionally, administration of intravenous medications is a primary priority in caregiving.

SECOND-LEVEL CARE PRIORITIES

Second-level care priorities must be addressed because delay may result in untoward effects. However, these are nonemergent problems (not life threatening). This level would include scheduled medications by oral, intramuscular, and subcutaneous routes, imminent discharge with incomplete teaching, and personal care issues that pose threat of harm, such as an incontinent patient with the potential for developing skin breakdown. Needs that fit into this level include mental status changes, acute pain relief, acute urinary elimination problems, untreated medical problems requiring immediate attention, risks for infection, and threats to safety and security.

THIRD-LEVEL CARE PRIORITIES

Third-level needs involve deficits that can be resolved easily or present minimal disruption of normal function. These include personal care issues, comfort, and health-related problems secondary to deficits in areas such as knowledge, activity, rest, and family coping. Third-level needs, such as bathing, grooming, physical mobility, and general emotional support, are important to the patient's well-being. However, the effect of a delay in providing for these has less impact on the outcome for recovery. It is always essential to evaluate the presenting circumstances before drawing this conclusion.

Measuring Progress Toward Desired Outcomes

Specific interventions will cause a predictable or expected effect. Outcomes are changes that will occur as a result of the interventions that are selected. The combination of the actions (interventions) should achieve the goals for the plan of care. The individualized plan of care for each patient should be the first consideration in the evaluation. It should outline what is expected and identify when care can be terminated. For example, the following questions should be answered: Do the objectives specify what problems need to be alleviated before discontinuing the plan of care? What specific knowledge is required for meeting the individualized needs of each patient in the group? What are the skill and competency requirements of the available caregivers?

The following practice scenario focuses on the outcome of the intervention:

The schedule of the community health nurse includes four patients (described below) that need to be seen today. Which patient should the nurse see first?

A. A 19-year-old patient, 18 weeks' gestation, who has not felt the baby move yet
B. A 28-year-old patient, 24 weeks' gestation, whose job requires her to travel extensively
C. An 18-year-old patient, 36 weeks' gestation, who has missed numerous appointments and is scheduled for a checkup tomorrow
D. A 32-year-old patient, 28 weeks' gestation, who works night shift and has 5 children that are cared for by her disabled husband

In this circumstance, the outcome is the determining factor. The nurse visit to Patient A will not affect the outcome, and although it is important, it is not the priority. Patient B and Patient D describe normal circumstances without evidence of factors suggesting potential complications. Patient C is in urgent need of prenatal care, and the nurse visit could affect the outcome of the pregnancy. Therefore, Patient C should be visited first.

Determining What Needs to Be Done

The nurse must determine what is urgent and what can wait. Each patient must be reviewed for the implications of a delay in treatment. For example, will the delay in treatment or care cause harmful or adverse effects? Consider the new postoperative patient who has a potential for a major complication or the patient scheduled for a cholecystectomy who experiences chills. These are examples of patients for whom a delay in care may cause adverse effects in outcome or recovery.

When comparing the needs of patients in a group, individual acuity level, stability, and needs should be considered. The skills and competencies of available caregivers should be compared. Also, the needs of the patients must be compared to the abilities of the workers. A working plan for the entire shift should be developed, and it must be ascertained that the priorities are accomplished. The plan that best correlates with priorities and demonstrates the least likelihood of causing the undesirable side effects should be chosen. The skill for developing a plan, which is presented in Chapter 6, Delegation, must be applied simultaneously with the skill of priority setting to determine urgency.

Developing an Action Plan

Scheduled activities should be a primary consideration in developing the working plan for a shift. Nonscheduled activities can then be added to the plan. When the working plan is not identified early in the shift, time is wasted (e.g., the waste of time that occurs when the nurse is forced to spend time "putting out fires"). This wasted effort takes away from time available to deal with major problems. It is necessary to have an organized system (working plan) before optimal care and outcomes can be achieved.

Determining Who Can Do It

Before delegation, consider the roles of available UAP, licensed practical nurse/licensed vocational nurse (LPN/LVN), and registered nurse (RN) staff members and the tasks that can be legally delegated. The nurse's level of expertise, the nurse's past experience, and guidelines established by individual states, professional organizations, and institutions should be used when assessing the abilities of available staff members and comparing them to the care needs of each patient.

Delegation involves the evaluation of the competency level of skills possessed by available staff. For example, are there RNs who have demonstrated consistent, competent clinical judgment in the past? The skills and competencies manual on the unit should be used to assist in determining the appropriate assignment for unfamiliar staff members.

Tasks that do not require the expertise of an RN can be delegated. Activities that involve stan-

TABLE 11-1 How to Determine Individual Assignments Based on Ability

RN	LPN/LVN	UAP
Complex procedures	Technical skills	Standard, routine care with predictable outcomes
Application of nursing process in situations requiring nursing judgment	Selected treatments and some medications	Activities specified in the job description
Activities of coordination and collaboration to determine care	Care of stable patients with predictable outcomes	Assistance to the nurse
	Provision of patient teaching	
Provision and evaluation of patient and family teaching	Data gathering during patient assessment	Tasks and nonnursing duties
Supervision of care delivered by others	Therapeutic and preventative nursing activities	
Role of as patient advocate		
Care for unstable patients with unpredictable outcomes	Documentation and evaluation of care provided	
Complex assessment and evaluation of patient status	Contribution of data to the plan of care	
Nursing judgment–required assessment of delegate's capabilities and competency	Actions within the job description and Nurse Practice Act	
Determining which staff member to assign to specific tasks		
Delegation of tasks and activities		

dard, unchanging procedures for patients can also be delegated. These include frequently occurring activities in a patient's daily care, such as bathing, feeding, dressing, and transferring activities. Activities that are complex or complicated should not be delegated. Table 11-1 depicts a list of assignments appropriate for different levels of health care staff. Assessment, evaluation, and nursing judgment are the responsibilities of the RN. The RN cannot delegate these skills to a less qualified staff member. Stable patients with predictable outcomes can be assigned to a qualified team member. The care of an unstable patient or an activity for which the outcome is uncertain cannot be delegated. It is important that the nurse does not accept assignments that he or she is not capable of performing. Examples of factors influencing delegation are depicted in Box 11-1.

FLOAT NURSE

When call-ins or inadequate staffing cause a shortage on one unit, and extra staff members are available on another unit, "floating" a nurse becomes necessary. As the current nursing shortage increases, this practice can be expected to be prevalent. When nurses are required to float into a setting where their skill level and qualifications do not meet the requirements for caregiving, solutions must be developed to ensure that patient care is not compromised.

Nurses should not refuse assignments to areas just because they lack some specific skill. Instead, they should focus on what they are able to do in a shared partnership or other type of arrangement.

Box 11-1 Factors Influencing Delegation

Can Delegate:
- Stable patients
- Requirements within caregiver's job description and legal constraints
- Adequate supervision available
- Within skill and competencies of individual caregiver

Cannot Delegate:
- Unstable patient with unpredictable outcome
- Condition requires complex assessment
- Problem solving and critical thinking required
- Nursing judgment required
- Potential for harm exists

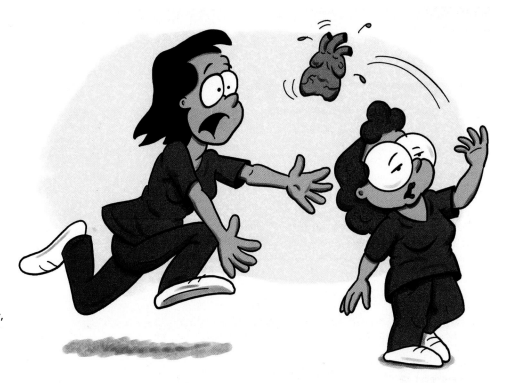

"Welcome to Cardiology, Floaty. Here, I think they're using this in surgery or something down the hall."

However, if appropriate supervision or assistance is lacking, then a more careful consideration is in order.

Skills common to all areas of acute care include assessment, documentation, risk management, medication administration (including monitoring for drug interactions and therapeutic effects; however, knowledge base used to monitor various drugs may differ), telephone communications, and taking telephone orders from physicians. Skills used in various areas but applied in unique, unit-specific ways include delegation; directing and supervising LPN/LVNs, UAP, and other staff members; patient and family teaching; coordinating patient care activities with other departments; multitasking with groups; discharge planning; developing care plans; and intervening as the patient advocate. These are considered standard skills for all nurses.

Potential sources of weakness among staff may develop as a result of unclear expectations, which may occur when nurses float to an unfamiliar unit. Educational preparation may be inadequate for certain skills such as advanced cardiac life support (ACLS) or interpreting electrocardiograms. When work involves unfamiliar or inadequate skills, supervision and direction must be adequate to compensate for the deficiencies. An evaluation of past experiences, level of motivation, and personal characteristics of the staff may be necessary before making a decision about patient assignments. Box 11-2 identifies standard and specialized skills involved in professional nursing practice.

Considerations When Accepting Assignments

Guido (2001) developed a guideline for float nurses accepting assignments when temporarily assigned to another unit and for the nurse assigning the tasks (Box 11-3). This tool contains helpful considerations concerning the responsibilities of both the float nurse and charge nurse.

It is critical that the nurse performing outside of his or her area of expertise request orientation, cross-training, or other measures to enhance existing skills. This is necessary in order to ensure patient safety. The float nurse could also request restricted duty, such as passing medications, providing personal care, obtaining vital signs, and other more familiar tasks. Regular staff members would then be responsible for performing the unit-specific care, such as central line management, administration of chemotherapy, or monitoring of labor patients. With the demands for cost cutting and downsizing emerging as a priority in the health

Box 11-2 Standard Skills and Specialized Skills

STANDARD SKILLS

- Documentation
- Therapeutic communication
- Cardiopulmonary resuscitation
- Unit-specific medication administration
- Monitoring of drug interactions and therapeutic effects
- Telephone communication
- Delegation and supervision of staff
- Patient and family education
- Coordinating patient care activities
- Multitasking with groups
- Discharge planning
- Developing plans of care
- Acting as patient advocate
- Physical assessment skill

SPECIALIZED SKILLS

- Interpretation of electrocardiograms (ECGs)
- Specialty area certification skills
- ACLS and PALS
- Titrating drugs based on body weight
- Unit-specific diagnostic test interpretation
- Management of patient with ventilator care
- Management of PCA pumps
- Epidural analgesic administration
- Monitoring and care of unit-specific needs (e.g., labor, premature infant, psychiatric patients)
- Use of complex equipment (e.g., fetal monitor, central line management)
- Hemodynamic monitoring

Box 11-3 Guidelines: Float Nurses

THE RESPONSIBILITIES OF A NURSE TEMPORARILY ASSIGNED TO ANOTHER UNIT INCLUDE:

1. Before accepting a patient assignment, state any hesitancy that you might have about it to appropriate persons (direct supervisor, nurse-manager, or team leader). Make your objections clear and specific. Follow your verbal hesitancies with a written memo to your supervisor, and make a photocopy of the memo for your records. In the written memo, state ways in which you would feel more comfortable in the reassignment, for example, a formal orientation period or more specific knowledge of the nursing routine for the new unit.
2. State your qualifications and skills concerning assessment skills, performance of routine procedures, and the like to the appropriate charge person. Thoroughly understand the patient assignment before accepting it because, once accepted, you are legally accountable for the nursing care of the patients and could be charged with abandonment if you choose to leave before the next shift of nurses arrives.
3. Identify your immediate resource person, and ask any questions you might have about the assignment, orders, routine procedures, and the like. Resource persons might be the charge nurse, a physician, a team member, or an interdisciplinary staff person.
4. Recognize and give yourself credit for your strengths as well as enumerating your weaknesses. Ask for help only if truly needed, remembering that you are capable of routine nursing procedures and assessments.
5. Remember that much of the case law concerning float nurses concerns the broad area of medications. Double-check references, call the pharmacist, or contact your direct supervisor before administering any medication about which you are unsure. If there are numerous unfamiliar medications to be given to several patients, arrange to perform more routine nursing procedures for the patients while another nurse who is familiar with the medications, unit, and patients administers all the medications.

THE RESPONSIBILITIES OF THE CHARGE NURSE TO WHOSE UNIT A NURSE IS TEMPORARILY REASSIGNED INCLUDE:

1. Thoroughly assess the qualifications of the reassigned nurse. Ask specific questions so that you may compe-

tently make patient assignments. Offer to orient the assigned nurse to the unit, and start with the more critical policies and procedures first.
2. Make the patient assignments carefully. Refrain from taking advantage of the float nurse by overloading the float nurse or by assigning difficult patients merely because this nurse is not a permanent member of your staff. The float nurse may later decide to ask for permanent assignment to your unit based on your fairness and management style.
3. Continue to reassess the reassigned nurse. Offer assistance as needed, and follow behind the float nurse as much as possible to reassure yourself that competent patient care is being delivered.
4. Keep your immediate supervisor apprised of changes within the unit or in patient status. Whether additional help is available or not, you may escape potential liability as you correctly assess the situation and ask for help when it is needed.
5. Reassign patients as dictated by changes in their status or in the number of patients because of admissions to the unit.
6. Run interference as much as possible to assure all the nurses on the unit that you are continually balancing the needs of the patients with the individual demands and needs of the nursing staff.
7. Be aware that much of the case law in this area involves medication errors. Be constantly available as a resource person, and ask questions to ascertain that the float person understands proper dosages, administration routes, and potential side effects. Alternately, give the medications yourself, and allow the float nurse to assume other responsibilities of direct and indirect patient care.
8. Nurses who feel appreciated often perform to higher expectations. Give float nurses reassurance that they are doing a good or great job, how much they are appreciated, and how much the staff appreciates the extra hands.

Adapted from Guido, G. W. (2001). *Legal and ethical issues in nursing.* Upper Saddle River, NJ: Prentice Hall.

care setting, the nursing role continues to change while the use of UAP increases. At the same time, the complexity and acuity level of the patient population have increased dramatically. These changes continue to affect how nurses manage the care of their patients. As the roles and responsibilities change, the nurse must be able to identify the knowledge and skill needed to adapt to the changes. Additionally, the nurse must develop a plan to fill the gaps, in order to maintain the competency and skill necessary to compete in the job market.

It is essential that patient care not be compromised despite the fact that cost cutting and productivity continue to be the driving force in health care. Other issues that are of major concern include early patient discharge without adequate preparation for self-care, compromised patient outcomes due to short-staffing, and inadequate time to assess and deliver patient care according to the standards of care established by the profession and licensing bodies. Every nurse should have a working knowledge of the American Nurses Association (ANA) Code of Ethics (see Chapter 10, Box 10-3), the ANA Standards of Practice (see Chapter 5, Box 5-1), and the ANA Standards of Performance (see Chapter 9, Box 9-2).

Questioning Assignments

If an assignment is within the scope of nursing practice, but the nurse has little experience or lack of training for it, the nurse should submit an occurrence report acknowledging acceptance of the assignment under protest. Additionally, the nurse should describe the cross-training that would be necessary to raise his or her competency to a level that would facilitate the handling of the assignment in the future. See Box 11-4 for a general rule for accepting assignments.

Specialty Nurse Skills and Competencies

Table 11-2 identifies some of the skills and competencies necessary for delivering care in specialty areas. This list is a representative sample and not intended to be all-inclusive.

Box 11-4 General Rule for Accepting or Refusing an Assignment

When to accept an assignment: when refusing the assignment could lead to charges of patient abandonment.
When to refuse an assignment: when lack of knowledge or training would compromise the safety of the patient.

EMERGENCY ROOM NURSES

The emergency room (ER) provides a unique opportunity to expand the role of the nurse beyond that of caregiver, to include collaborative practice with many disciplines. The ER nurse must be skilled in triaging patients based on priority needs, performing initial assessments, and initiating emergency interventions. Credentials for the ER nurse include, but are not limited to, ACLS, pediatric advanced life support (PALS), trauma classes, and emergency nursing pediatric classes. The ER nurse should demonstrate high-level skill in initiating venipuncture, titrating drugs, correlating laboratory results with patient status, giving discharge instructions, and collaborating with the physician. When the ER nurse floats to an unfamiliar clinical unit, potential practice concerns may include the standard medication administration record (MAR), documentation, organization, and the ability to use specialty equipment, such as a patient-controlled analgesia (PCA) pump, feeding tubes, or total parenteral nutrition (TPN) equipment.

CORONARY INTENSIVE CARE NURSES

The intensive coronary care unit (ICCU) nurse must maintain high-level skill in the same areas as the ER nurse. The ICCU nurse requires additional training and skill consistent with the use of high-level equipment. Specific skills required of the ICCU nurse include, but are not limited to, the management of patients with ventilators, chest tube drainage, mediastinal and other intrathoracic drainage, central lines, hemodynamic monitoring, cardiac monitors, multiple intravenous infusions, intraaortic balloon pumps, and hypothermia and hyperthermia blankets, in addition to providing for primary nursing care needs. Because of the acuity level of patients, the nurse-to-patient ratio is much lower in the ICCU than in other clinical units. When comparing the critical care nurse to the medical-surgical nurse, the ICCU nurse may experience practice concerns related to multitasking with large groups, delegation, and the supervision of UAP and LPN/LVNs.

PEDIATRIC NURSES

The pediatric nursing role has changed enormously as a result of innovations in technology and managed care. Research-based practice and care pathways have replaced a status quo practice. Pediatric nurses assist children and their families by educating them to manage chronic diseases. The strengths of the pediatric nurse include implementing age-specific skills and procedures, performing dual child and parent care, using age-appropriate

NURSING AREA	ASSUMPTIONS OF STRENGTHS	ASSUMPTIONS OF WEAKNESSES
Emergency room	Multitasking groups of clients Electrocardiogram (ECG) interpretation ACLS and PALS certification Titrating drugs to symptoms Complex physical assessments	Unit-specific documentation PCA Unit-specific medication administration record
Critical care areas	Complex physical assessment Titrating drugs to symptoms Parenteral therapy Patient-controlled analgesic (PCA) and epidural analgesic administration Management of central lines Management of parenteral nutrition ECG interpretation Management of complex high-tech equipment ACLS and PALS certification Primary care Management of patients with ventilator Preoperative and postoperative care	Multitasking with groups Unit-specific medication administration Delegation and supervision
Pediatric	Sterile dressings Management of parenteral therapy Nonverbal communication Category-specific precautions Dual patient care Low-dose drug administration	Decubitus care Adult assessment Adult drug administration Titrating drugs to symptoms PCA pumps Epidural analgesics Adult drug dosages Communications
Obstetrical	Sterile dressings Management of parenteral therapy Dual patient care Admission assessments Postoperative care for abdominal surgery Management of epidural analgesics Pain management Using complex equipment Care of infants and adolescents Multitasking Monitoring and care of labor patient Postpartum care	Disease-specific isolation Unit-specific medication administration Death and dying care Critical and cardiac care PCA pump Diagnostic test preparation Neurologically impaired Disease processes Develop plan of care for disease processes
Psychiatric	Communication Psychosocial assessment Therapeutic relationships Psychotropic drug administration Care of substance abuser Cognitive disorders	Parenteral therapy Unit-specific medication Physical assessment Cardiac and critical care Sterile technique
Oncology	Central line management Communication Physical assessment Psychosocial management Death and dying Pain management and PCA pumps Wound care Management of parenteral therapy and blood Chemotherapy administration	Critical care Titrating drugs to symptoms Category-specific isolation

(continued)

NURSING AREA	ASSUMPTIONS OF STRENGTHS	ASSUMPTIONS OF WEAKNESSES
Medical-surgical	Sterile technique Preoperative and postoperative care Wound drainage devices Diagnostic test preparations Care of the cognitively impaired Category-specific precautions Managing parenteral therapy Manage blood infusions Pain management PCA pumps Delegation and supervision Medication administration Multitasking with groups Patient and family education Death and dying Development of plans of care Admission assessments	Monitoring and care of labor patients Managing infants and children Use of fetal monitor Postpartum care Dual patient care Psychotropic medications Titrate drugs to symptoms Management of ventilator patient ECG interpretation Management of chemotherapy ACLS and PALS certification

*This chart is meant to be a representative sample and not a comprehensive list. It is designed to be a place for the novice nurse to begin analyzing the roles of nurses in the various areas.

communication skills, using age- and weight-appropriate drug dosages, and using micropumps. Advances in treatment modalities and diagnostic methods have greatly affected pediatric nursing. As the trend shifts away from the acute care setting, complex care is being provided in the home. Complex treatments such as pediatric intravenous therapy, central line management, parenteral and enteral nutrition, and ventilator maintenance are being provided in the home of the pediatric patient.

In addition to surveillance and health promotion, emphasis has expanded to include home care of the acute and chronically ill pediatric patient. It is critical that nurses continue to be creative and design new models of care that meet the needs of today's pediatric population, which is shifting to ambulatory and outpatient services.

When the pediatric nurse floats to an unfamiliar clinical unit, potential practice concerns may include age-specific care issues and knowledge of disease processes, such as drug dosages, illness assessments, decubitus care, and care of the dying patient.

OBSTETRIC NURSES

Obstetric nursing previously focused on the hospitalized patient. In the past, patients with complicated pregnancies were hospitalized in order to monitor the pregnancy. Currently, because of decreased lengths of stay in the hospital, these patients are managed by electronic monitoring and home visits by the nurse. The skills of the hospital-based obstetric nurse include, but are not limited to, monitoring and caring for patients in labor, using complex equipment such as fetal monitors, caring for newborns, caring for postpartum patients, caring for adolescents, caring for abdominal surgical patients, and multitasking.

Compared with the medical-surgical nurse, the obstetric nurse may experience practice deficits when floating to another clinical unit. These deficits may include knowledge of the disease processes, knowledge of disease-specific diagnostic findings and of their implications, the ability to care for cognitively impaired adults, the delivery of postmortem care, and the ability to develop disease-specific nursing care plans.

ONCOLOGY NURSES

The oncology nurse would characteristically demonstrate strong skills in managing patients with central lines, TPN, chemotherapy, PCA pumps, and pain and nausea, and in providing psychosocial and compassionate care.

When the oncology nurse floats to an unfamiliar clinical unit, potential practice concerns may include category-specific isolation, ACLS support protocol, hemodynamic monitoring, and care of obstetric patients.

PSYCHIATRIC NURSES

The psychiatric nurse's strengths include, but are not limited to, communication, psychosocial and therapeutic relationship skills, and knowledge of psychotropic medications, substance abuse, and cognitive disorders.

Potential practice concerns when the psychiatric nurse floats to an unfamiliar clinical area may include age-specific care (including obstetric and infant), hemodynamic monitoring, ventilator care, and chemotherapy.

MEDICAL-SURGICAL NURSES

The medical-surgical nurse has strong skills in performing assessments, diagnostic test preparations, patient teaching, preoperative and postoperative care, wound care, and care of cognitively impaired patients. Their strengths also include delegating and supervising, collaborating with personnel from other departments, and multitasking.

Performance concerns, when floating to another unit, will most likely be in areas such as infant and child care, monitoring and care of labor patients, fetal monitoring, postpartum care, psychotropic medication knowledge, chemotherapy administration, and pediatric advanced life support.

ROOM ASSIGNMENT PROCESS

Making room assignments is a nursing responsibility. It is essential to consider the circumstances and compare the varied needs and problems of all the patients affected in the decision-making process. This process requires the nurse to make a clinical judgment regarding room assignments to ensure the best outcome.

Admission to a hospital room occurs in one of three ways. The patient was admitted from the ER or from a direct admit or transferred from one unit to another. The process begins when the admitting department is notified that a patient needs a room. Then, the admitting clerk notifies the nursing unit of an admission and provides limited information. This information usually includes the patient's age, gender, admitting medical diagnosis, and attending physician. The RN on the unit processes the information and evaluates all factors. If more information is needed, the RN contacts the ER or referring agency directly, to fill in the data gaps. The RN, then, makes the room assignment and notifies the

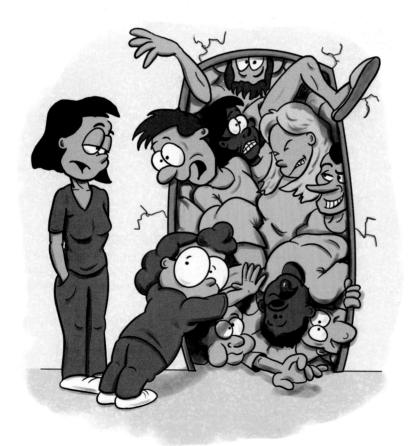

"Two things: First, it's two people to a room, not two hundred. Second, that's the closet."

admitting department of the room number. For example, the RN may determine that the adult patient being admitted is confused. In that case, the patient should be placed near the nurse's station for close observation because of the high risk for injury. Considering this information, the RN selects a room near the nurse's station. Figure 11-1 depicts a sample admission flowchart.

Problems that arise during the admission process that may affect the room assignment in a negative way include the following:

- No beds available on the desired unit
- Need to move or transfer another patient before an admission
- Lack of information from the referring agency
- Specialized staff required to be called in, or reassigned, to meet the patient's needs

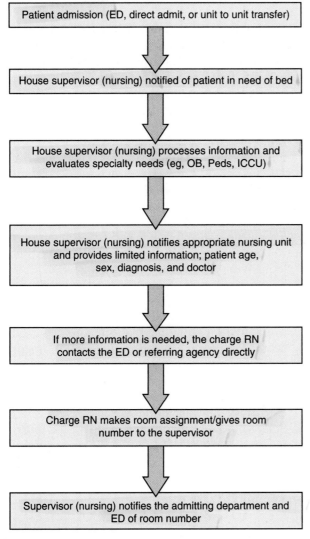

FIGURE 11-1
Admission flowchart.

Box 11-5 lists factors to consider when assigning rooms to patients. Box 11-6 depicts the room assignment process as it relates to the steps of the nursing process.

PITFALLS IN NURSING JUDGMENT

The failure to use sound nursing judgment in the clinical setting has a negative impact on patient care decisions. The nurse's inability to gather data or weigh the significance of each piece of data can lead to errors in the process. Factors that contribute to faulty judgments include:

- Knowledge gaps
- Ineffective problem solving
- Inadequate decision making
- Inappropriate prioritization
- Incompetent application of cognitive skills
- Failure to identify impact of action/inaction on the outcome

Box 11-6 Assigning Patient Rooms Using the Steps of the Nursing Process

ROOM ASSIGNMENT PROCESS

ASSESSMENT
1. Gather available data using medical diagnosis and pertinent history.
2. Determine whether patient needs require placement close to nurses' station.
3. Determine need for isolation or special precautions.
4. Identify rooms available.
5. Gather information about current patients and circumstances in rooms available.

ANALYSIS
1. Analyze the disease processes of the newly admitted patient.
2. Evaluate physical layout of the room being considered for the new patient.
3. Compare the needs of new and current patients to room availability.

OUTCOME IDENTIFICATION
1. Identify who the roommate of the new patient will be.
2. Evaluate the expected effects for new and current patient.

PLAN
1. Determine what room placement would be best for the patient, based on his/her functional status.

IMPLEMENTATION
1. Place patient in assigned room.

EVALUATION
1. Continue to monitor, evaluate and reevaluate patient's status based on changes in laboratory data, further diagnostic test findings, and changes in patient's condition.
2. New room reassignment may need to be made. For example, diagnostic tests indicate the need for isolation or occurrence of confusion indicates the need to move patient close to nurse's station for more careful observation.

It is imperative that the quality of patient care not be compromised by the nurse's inadequacies. Failure to apply critical thinking or a lack of skill and competency for the situation can result in faulty nursing judgments.

SUMMARY

Critical thinking is essential in the development of the ability to make comparisons that result in decisions affecting care delivery. Managing care requires identifying the needs of multiple patients requiring varied nursing expertise. Evaluating the individual care needs and comparing the competencies and skills of available health care personnel to determine the best choice involve nursing judgment.

The nurse must possess sound clinical judgment to make appropriate decisions about unit-specific patient care. Multiple factors must be considered, including the strengths and weaknesses possessed by nurses in varied caregiving situations. Additionally, the specific needs of individual patients must be taken into consideration when making patient room assignments. Recognition of the effects is essential to enhance clinical nursing judgment.

KEY POINTS

- Making decisions regarding the care of multiple patients requires nursing judgment.
- Nursing judgment is the ability to analyze and interpret the individual needs of a group, evaluate the significance of each circumstance, compare the effect on the outcome of each action or alternative, and draw conclusions to make a decision that achieves the best outcome for everyone affected.
- The following factors should be considered when making decisions regarding care of multiple patients: physical status and stability of each patient, implications of delaying care, priorities of care for each patient, expertise and experience of available personnel, and the needs of each patient.
- Competent nurses use analytical thinking in making clinical judgments.
- The first step in comparing patient needs is to gather information about each patient. Next, the problems of each patient should be identified and a list formulated. Expected outcomes need to be determined for each patient problem.
- The patient's condition is considered when identifying the priority of patient needs.
- Nursing judgment is required in the proper assignment of float nurses. Guidelines for float nurses have been established that can be used to ensure that patient care is not compromised.
- When floating to an unfamiliar environment, each nurse has strengths and weaknesses related to experience and specialty. Assignments can be made to the float nurse that take advantage of the nurse's strengths.
- Selecting the best room assignment for multiple patients requires application of nursing judgment.

REFERENCES

Benner, P. (1982). Issues in competency-based testing. *Nursing Outlook, 30*(5), 303–309.

Burckhardt, J. A., Irwin, B. J., & Phillips-Arikian, V. (2001). *Kaplan NCLEX-RN*. New York: Simon & Schuster.

Deloughery, G. (1998). *Issues and trends in nursing.* St. Louis: Mosby.

Facione, N. C. (1995). *Critical thinking and clinical judgment.* Presented at Goals 2000 conference in San Diego.

Foundation for Critical Thinking (1997). *Critical thinking: Basic theory and instructional structures.* Santa Rosa, CA: Author.

Guido, G. W. (2001). *Legal and ethical issues in nursing.* Upper Saddle River, NJ: Prentice Hall.

Hall, J. K. (1996). *Nursing ethics and law.* Philadelphia: W. B. Saunders

Hansten, R. I., & Washburn, M. J. (1998). *Clinical delegation skills: A handbook for professional practice.* Gaithersburg, MD: Aspen.

Harrington, N., Smith, N. E., & Spratt, W. E. (1996). *LPN to RN transitions.* Philadelphia: Lippincott-Raven.

Kidner, M. A. (1999). How to keep float nurses from sinking. *RN, 62*(9), 35–39.

Marquis, B. L., & Huston, C. J. (2003). *Leadership roles and management functions in nursing.* Philadelphia: Lippincott Williams & Wilkins.

McCloskey, J. C., & Grace, H. K. (1997). *Current issues in nursing.* St. Louis: Mosby.

Potter, P., & Perry, A. (2001). *Fundamentals of nursing.* St. Louis: Mosby.

Ringsven, M. K., & Bond, D. (1997). *Gerontology and leadership skills for nurses.* Albany: Delmar.

Wojner, A. W. (2001). *Outcomes management: Applications to clinical practice.* St. Louis: Mosby.

Zerwekh, J., & Claborn, J. C. (2000). *Nursing today: Transitions and trends.* Philadelphia: W. B. Saunders.

Student Worksheets

 SKILL SHEET: APPLYING NURSING JUDGMENT IN CLINICAL SETTINGS

Purpose

To enable the student to develop and demonstrate the ability to use sound judgment when making decisions about care for multiple patients.

Objective

To apply an organized process that facilitates appropriate judgment and reasoning skill in making decisions for groups of patients.

Steps: Applying Nursing Judgment in Clinical Settings

ASSESSMENT
1. Identify the problems of each patient.
2. Describe them clearly and precisely.
3. Evaluate all data for actual problems, potential problems, and collaborative problems.

ANALYSIS
1. Evaluate the identified problems of the patients.
2. Determine the degree of threat to life or safety for each.
3. Rank the priority problems using Maslow's Hierarchy of Needs.
4. Analyze the needs of the group for an entire shift.

OUTCOME IDENTIFICATION
1. Compare patients.
2. Determine which problems are most urgent on the basis of needs, changing or unstable status, and problem complexity.
3. Develop plan of care outcomes for each patient.
4. Establish options that best correlate with priorities and that demonstrate the least undesirable side effects.

PLAN
1. Consider scheduled nursing activities first.
2. Focus on nonscheduled activities second.
3. Anticipate the time it will take to attend to priority problems.
4. Decide how to combine activities to allow resolution of more than one problem at a time.
5. Consider how to involve the patient as a decision maker to participate in care.
6. Develop a working plan for the entire shift based on priorities to achieve the desired outcome.

IMPLEMENTATION
1. Implement nursing interventions and actions for patients with high-priority needs first.
2. Implement nursing interventions and actions for medium-priority problems that are not life threatening next (e.g., problems that do not threaten health or coping).
3. Implement nursing interventions and actions for low-priority needs last.
4. Delegate interventions and actions as indicated.

5. Ensure appropriate accountability.
6. Supervise performance of tasks, as indicated.
7. Identify problems not within the scope of nursing; refer them for treatment to the appropriate health team member.

EVALUATION

1. Continuously evaluate and reevaluate problems and needs after initial assessment, adjust ranking of problems as indicated.
2. Monitor responses of patients to strategies.
3. Adjust priorities based on the critical or urgent basis of needs, patient's changing status, and complexity of care involved.
4. Modify parts of the plan that are not working.
5. Reassign delegated activities and interventions as patient's situation or condition changes.

COMPETENCY VALIDATION: APPLYING NURSING JUDGMENT IN CLINICAL SETTINGS

COMPETENCY STATEMENT

The student will demonstrate the ability to identify and define problems, needs, and priorities and to develop strategies to resolve multiple problems to produce desired outcomes.
The student demonstrated the ability to do the following:

1. Identify problems of each patient.
2. Compare patients and determine which problems were most urgent on the basis of basic needs, changing or unstable status, and problem complexity.
3. Anticipate the time it will take to attend to priority problems.
4. Decide how to combine activities to resolve more than one problem at a time.
5. Identify how to involve the patient as a decision maker to participate in care.

COMPETENT

- Understands reason for task and is able to perform task independently
- Understands reason for task but needs supervision
- Understands reason for task and is able to perform task with assistance

NOT COMPETENT

- Understands reason for task but performs task at provisional level
- Is unable to state reason for task and performs task at a dependent level

SKILL CHECKLIST: APPLYING NURSING JUDGMENT IN CLINICAL SETTINGS

DECISION MAKING IN GROUPS	SATISFACTORY	UNSATISFACTORY	NI/COMMENTS
ASSESSMENT			
1. Gather information about each patient in the group.			
2. Assess the acuity level and stability of each patient.			
3. Assess the skills and competencies of the staff.			
4. Clarify the data and fill the data gaps.			
ANALYSIS			
1. Analyze the patients by disease process.			
2. Identify the most urgent needs.			
3. Compare the acuity level, needs, and stability of each patient in the group.			
4. Compare the urgency of the needs to the effect of delay in treatment.			
5. Compare the needs of the patients to the staff available.			
OUTCOME IDENTIFICATION			
1. Identify the expected outcomes.			
2. Evaluate the effect of delay in treatment for each patient.			
3. Compare the expected outcomes.			
PLAN			
1. Identify the expected effects of specific interventions on the desired outcomes.			
2. Identify the priorities and circumstances of the situation.			
3. Choose the plan that best correlates with priorities and that demonstrates the least undesirable side effects.			
4. Develop a plan for the shift (hospital stay) early.			
5. Delegate tasks as indicated.			
IMPLEMENTATION			
1. Initiate the plan.			
2. Involve the patient in the care when appropriate.			
3. Combine activities to resolve more than one problem at a time.			

DECISION MAKING IN GROUPS	SATISFACTORY	UNSATISFACTORY	NI/COMMENTS
EVALUATION 1. Determine success of plan.			
2. Establish whether the desired outcome was achieved.			
3. Take responsibility for decisions.			
4. Evaluate and reevaluate effect of decision and make adjustments accordingly.			

 SCENARIOS TO ACCOMPANY STUDENT WORKSHEETS

Consider the following patient scenarios on the nursing unit. The setting is a medical-surgical unit with a staff of two RNs, one LPN/LVN, and one UAP. Tonight, one of the regular RNs called in sick, and Central Staffing just called with a replacement nurse from the obstetric unit. Using a primary care delivery system, plan the work assignment with the staff members available.

Room 101: An 83-year-old woman, 7 days after colectomy. The incision has staples, and the dressing has been removed. The patient is to be discharged tomorrow. The day shift reports a new rash on her back.

Room 102: A 77-year-old woman admitted for a 23-hour observation. She has a history of leukemia with hemoglobin of 6.2 g/dL and a hematocrit of 23.4%. Medical orders include: infuse 2 units packed red blood cells (PRBC) through the port-A-Cath and repeat hemoglobin and hematocrit (H&H) 2 hours after blood infusion.

Room 103: A 35-year-old woman 2 days after mastectomy. She is very happy that all the lymph nodes tested negative and is anxious for discharge.

Room 104: A 73-year-old man admitted with a prolapsed hemorrhoid. He is scheduled for surgery, has normal saline infusing at 100 mL/hr, is on nothing by mouth (NPO) except medication, and needs preoperative teaching.

Room 105: An 83-year-old woman, 1 day after left total-knee replacement. Medical orders include: morphine sulfate (MS) by PCA pump for pain, continuous passive motion (CPM) machine at 0 to 45 degrees, oxygen (O_2) at 2 L per nasal cannula, IV fluids—lactated Ringer's infusing at 25 mL/hr, and a Foley catheter to straight drainage.

Room 106: An 82-year-old man is admitted to telemetry. He arrived on the unit during report, needs admitted, and is scheduled for the catheterization in early morning.

Room 107: A 72-year-old woman admitted with type 1 diabetes mellitus, left leg neuropathy, and peptic ulcer disease. Her medical orders include: sliding scale insulin, no weight bearing on left leg, ambulate with walker, and occupational therapy (OT) and physical therapy (PT) evaluation.

Room 108: A 27-year-old man admitted 5 days ago following a ruptured appendix. Medical orders include intravenous antibiotics (IVAB) and a saline lock for intermittent infusion. The intravenous site has signs of phlebitis present.

Room 109: A 67-year-old woman who had a sigmoidoscopy with polypectomy for rectal hemorrhage. She is on 23-hour observation with a saline lock for intermittent infusion of IVAB.

Room 110: A 79-year-old man admitted 3 days ago for a new-onset cerebral vascular accident (CVA) with left facial droop. He has a history of type 1 diabetes mellitus and hypertension. Medical order includes a saline lock for intermittent infusion, sliding scale insulin, and rehabilitation evaluation.

Room 111: A 44-year-old woman, 1 day after mastectomy. Her prognosis is poor. Medical orders include 5% dextrose in normal saline (D-5 NS) infusing at 100 mL/hr, morphine sulfate (MS) by PCA pump, and a wound drainage device. She vomited three times on day shift.

Room 112: A 64-year-old man admitted 4 days ago for a possible bowel obstruction. He is scheduled for upper gastrointestinal (UGI) radiography with a small bowel follow through (SMFT) in the morning. Medical orders include 5% dextrose in 0.45 normal saline (D-5 ½ NS) infusing at 100 mL/hr and IVAB.

Using the Checklist as a guideline for decisions, consider the skills and competencies of the staff members to select the assignment that achieves the most desirable outcomes for all patients involved. Use the table below to assign duties to available staff members.

RN:
OB FLOAT NURSE:
LPN/LVN:
UAP:

See the Answer Key in Appendix A for sample answers for this exercise.

PRACTICE EXERCISES: APPLYING NURSING JUDGMENT IN CLINICAL SETTINGS

 ## SCENARIOS: MAKING ROOM ASSIGNMENTS

SCENARIO 1

A 4-year-old girl was admitted to your pediatric unit from the ER. The ER nurse reports the patient's primary diagnosis is positive respiratory syncytial virus (RSV) she also has a rash that appears to be measles. The patient will be arriving on the nursing unit with her mother, father, and grandmother. All family members would like to stay with the child overnight. The patient's medical history is unremarkable. The child cries often but is easily comforted by her mother.

The situation on your unit: 3 double rooms, no private rooms. Room 214 beds A and B are occupied by boys with the same diagnosis, postoperative hernia repair. Room 215 bed A is empty; bed B is occupied by a girl with measles and fever. Room 216 bed A is occupied by an overflow adult patient to be discharged in the morning, with a diagnosis of abdominal pain of unknown origin.

Hospital census is low.

Questions to consider:

1. What transmission precautions does your patient require?

_____

_____

_____

2. What is required for this type of precaution?

_____

_____

_____

3. Where would you put the patient?

_____

_____

_____

SCENARIO 2

The admitting office calls with an admission from Dr. Joe's office, a pediatrician. You know from experience that Dr. Joe does not like his patients to share the same room. The patient is a 10-year-old boy with a diagnosis of viral meningitis. The patient's mother and father will be bringing him to the hospital and have requested a private room. The patient is an only child. No remarkable history.

The situation on your unit: 4 double rooms, 1 private room. Room 302 bed A is occupied by a 12-year-old boy, diagnosis ankle fracture caused by a motor vehicle accident (MVA). Bed B is empty. Room 304 bed A is occupied by a 10-year-old girl, diagnosis concussion. Bed B is empty. There is a 6-year-old girl in the private room, diagnosis rule out (R/O) Lyme disease. Room 305 bed B is empty. Room 305 bed A is occupied by a 6-month-old girl with severe burns to her upper chest.

Hospital census is high.

Questions to consider:

1. What transmission precautions does your patient require?

_____

_____

_____

2. What is required for this type of precaution?

_____

_____

_____

3. Where would you put the patient?

_____

_____

_____

Scenario 3

You are working on an adult medical-surgical unit. A nurse from the ER calls with an admission. The patient is a 72-year-old man with cardiac arrhythmias and possible tuberculosis (TB). The patient has a history of lung cancer. The patient's wife, 5 children, and 3 grandchildren are in the waiting room. The patient is stable and does not require ICCU placement at this time.

The situation on your unit: 14 double bed rooms, 4 private rooms. All of the rooms on the unit have negative air pressure. All double beds are occupied except for 2 male beds. In Room 306 bed A is a 68-year-old English professor, diagnosis R/O myocardial infarction. Bed B is empty. In Room 307 bed A is a 36-year-old man, retired city mayor admitted with angina. Bed B is empty.

Hospital census is low.

Questions to consider:

1. What transmission precautions does you patient require?

_____

_____

_____

2. What is required for this type of precaution?

_____

_____

_____

3. Where would you put the patient?

_____

_____

_____

SCENARIO 4

A 24-year-old man was admitted to your medical unit from the ER. The ER nurse reports the patient's primary diagnosis is colitis. He is also diabetic. The patient will be arriving on the unit with his wife, mother, and sister. The patient is stable.

The situation on your unit: 16 double rooms; 2 private rooms with negative air pressure. All double beds are occupied except for 2 male beds. In one room is a 26-year-old male salesman, diagnosis *Campylobacter* gastroenteritis. In the other double room is a 44-year-old male electrician, diagnosis postoperative arthroscopy.

Both negative air pressure rooms are occupied, one by a 50-year-old housewife with vancomycin-resistant *Enterococcus* (VRE), the other by a 42-year-old banker who is postoperative tonsillectomy and adenoidectomy (T&A).

Hospital census is low.

Questions to consider:

1. What transmission precautions does you patient require?

_____

_____

_____

2. What is required for this type of precaution?

_____

_____

3. Where would you put this patient?

_____

_____

_____

SCENARIO 5

A 7-year-old boy was admitted to your pediatric unit from the ER. The ER nurse reports the patient's primary diagnosis is sickle cell crisis. He also has a rash that appears to be impetigo. The patient will arrive on the unit with his mother, sister, and grandmother. All family members would like to stay with the child overnight. The patient is stable.

The situation on your unit: 4 double rooms, 2 private rooms with negative air pressure.

Room 213 A is occupied by a 12-year-old boy with a fractured femur, who is in skeletal traction. Bed B is occupied by a 6-year-old boy with nephrotic syndrome. Room 214 bed A is occupied by a 70-year-old man with a major infected decubitus. Bed B is empty. Room 215 bed A is occupied by a 6-year-old child, postoperative T&A. Bed B is occupied by a 16-year-old child, postoperative appendectomy. Room 216 bed A is empty, and bed B is occupied by an 8-year-old girl with a new diagnosis of diabetes. There is a 3-year-old girl in one private room with sedation for magnetic resonance imaging (MRI) to R/O brain tumor. The other private room is occupied by a 15-year-old girl with a diagnosis of TB.

Hospital census is high.

Questions to consider:

1. What transmission precautions does your patient require?

_____

_____

_____

2. What is required for this type of precaution?

_____

_____

_____

3. Where would you put the patient?

_____

_____

_____

CRITICAL THINKING EXERCISES

1. Which of the following patients should the nurse assign to a UAP?
   A. A 45-year-old with an open wound to the right upper leg, which cultured positive for methicillin-resistant *Staphylococcus aureus* (MRSA). The wound requires a dressing change.
   B. A 26-year-old, 2 days after splenectomy. The patient has orders to increase activity.
   C. A 46-year-old woman after mastectomy. She needs discharge teaching related to emptying wound drainage device.
   D. A 75-year-old man who is in traction and requires a bed bath.
2. Which of the following patients should the nurse assign to a UAP?
   A. Injection of meperidine (Demerol) to a patient complaining of pain.
   B. Administration of a bolus gastrointestinal tube (G-tube) feeding to a 4-year-old.
   C. A 14-year-old admitted 2 days ago with tibial fracture who has external fixation. The patient requires pin care.
   D. A 21-year-old 1 day after appendectomy, with a fever during the night. The patient needs to be ambulated this evening.
3. Which of the following patients should the nurse assign to an experienced UAP?
   A. A 45-year-old with a fracture of the left leg who rings his call light because he needs to use the urinal.
   B. A 52-year-old man admitted for gastroenteritis. He has antiemetic medications ordered.
   C. A 42-year-old woman experiencing abdominal discomfort. Her abdomen is distended. She has had only 50 mL of urine output in the past 24 hours.
   D. A patient, with a chest tube, who is ambulating in the hall.
4. Which of the following patients should the nurse assign to an experienced UAP?
   A. A 33-year-old man who was involved in a MVA 2 days ago. He has a cast with an external fixator to his left wrist.
   B. An 80-year-old man admitted for dehydration. He has a stage III decubitus to the coccyx. The wound requires medicated dressing changes twice a day.
   C. A 67-year-old woman with a G-tube for feeding. Her diagnosis is congestive heart failure (CHF) and debilitating arthritis.
   D. A 24-year-old, 2 days after appendectomy, who needs vital signs taken.
5. Which of the following patients should the nurse assign to an LPN/LVN?
   A. An 11-year-old diabetic patient who is severely dehydrated, with blood sugar readings in the 800s.
   B. An 85-year-old man, 2 days after G-tube placement. He has a pressure ulcer to his coccyx that cultured positive for MRSA.
   C. An 89-year-old woman with a diagnosis of dementia who is bladder incontinent and requires hygienic care.
   D. A 62-year-old male patient with suspected gastrointestinal bleed who require a stool specimen for occult blood.

6. Which of the following patients should the nurse assign to an LPN/LVN?
   A. A 36-year-old woman, 2 days after appendectomy, who requires ambulation.
   B. A 78-year-old patient, admitted with a fractured hip, postoperative day 4. The wound requires a sterile dressing change daily.
   C. A new colostomy patient, who requires fitting of the drainage appliance and the first irrigation procedure.
   D. An 82-year-old woman, 2 days after above-the-knee amputation. She is receiving peritoneal dialysis.

7. Which of the following patients should the nurse assign to an LPN/LVN?
   A. A 57-year-old man hospitalized with dehydration. He is receiving nasogastric (NG) tube feedings around the clock. He is stable and having no signs of pain or discomfort. Vital signs: blood pressure, 132/88 mm Hg; pulse, 88 beats/min; respirations, 20 breaths/min; temperature, 99.4°F (37.4°C). His family is at the bedside.
   B. A 49-year-old woman admitted for a cardiac catheterization today. She needs the consent form completed, labs drawn, preprocedure teaching, and preprocedure medications administered.
   C. A 63-year-old patient with a cerebral vascular accident (CVA) and right-side deficit. He requires assistance with feeding.
   D. A 24-year-old man admitted for altered level of conscious (LOC) and R/O increased intracranial pressure following a MVA. He has a NG tube set to low, intermittent suction, and a Foley catheter for gravity drainage.

8. Which of the following patients should the nurse assign to an LPN/LVN?
   A. A 46-year-old patient with new-onset diabetes, who is being discharged home today.
   B. A 96-year-old man, 3 days postoperative, with a daily sterile dressing change.
   C. A patient 2 days after a right total-knee replacement who needs intake and output measured.
   D. A 37-year-old woman who needs blood glucose measured before meals and at bedtime.

9. Which of the following patients should the RN assign to another RN, or retain personal responsibility for?
   A. A 27-year-old man with hepatitis C, urine positive for illegal drugs, and threatening to leave against medical advice (AMA) if he "doesn't get pain medications now."
   B. A 22-year-old with an overdose of unknown substance: blood pressure, 70/49 mm Hg; pulse, 142 beats/min; respirations, 12 breaths/min, shallow and labored. Responds minimally to painful stimuli.
   C. A 33-year-old woman, 3 days after open reduction internal fixation (ORIF). Physician orders read: discontinue catheter today.
   D. A 38-year-old long-time diabetic patient with stasis ulcers of lower legs. Wounds require dressing changes twice a day.

10. Which of the following patients should the RN assign to another RN, or retain personal responsibility for?
    A. A 6-year-old who is 1 day postoperative. A unit of blood is ordered for today.
    B. A 25-year-old, 9 hours after cesarean section. She has petechiae and ecchymoses of the skin and had uncontrolled hemorrhage during surgery. Platelet count is decreased (50,000 mm³).
    C. A 7-year-old admitted with pneumonia who is in an oxygen tent and requires handheld nebulizer (HHN) every 4 hours.
    D. A 7-year-old girl admitted for a T&A this morning. Preoperative teaching was done, and she is awaiting transport to the operating room.

11. Which of the following patients should the RN assign to another RN, or personally retain responsibility for?
    A. A 3-year-old girl admitted yesterday with laryngotracheobronchitis who has a tracheostomy.
    B. A 5-year-old girl admitted after gastric lavage for Tylenol ingestion.
    C. A 52-year-old man who had transurethral resection of the prostate (TURP) earlier this morning. He has a continuous bladder irrigation (CBI), which is draining pink urine with small clots.
    D. A 62-year-old woman who had a left below-the-knee amputation (BKA) yesterday. She has been diabetic for more than 30 years.

12. Which of the following patients should the RN assign to another RN, or retain personal responsibility for?
    A. An 80-year-old woman with a diagnosis of acute myocardial infarction (MI). She has a Nitroglycerin drip to be titrated (adjusted to pain level).
    B. A 23-year-old postmastectomy patient with a low hemoglobin level. She needs 2 units of blood to be transfused.
    C. A 43-year-old, 2 days after an open cholecystectomy with wound drainage device. The patient requires a sterile abdominal dressing change daily.
    D. A 72-year-old with a history of chronic obstructive pulmonary disease (COPD) and insulin-dependent diabetes mellitus (IDDM), admitted with pneumonia. He is stable and needs to be ambulated in hall.

13. Which of the following patients should the nurse see first?
    A. A 40-year-old 7-day postpartum female with bright red vaginal bleeding and a hemoglobin level of 7.0 g/dL.
    B. A diabetic patient with a blood sugar of 400 mg/dL and no orders for insulin coverage.
    C. A 46-year-old end-stage renal disease patient who had an arteriovenous (AV) fistula placement 2 days ago. No thrill or bruit noted.
    D. A 50-year-old woman, 2 days after knee replacement. She refuses to use CPM machine due to pain.

14. You have just returned from lunch. As you step off the elevator, all of these patients are ringing their call bells. Which one should you see first?
    A. A 22-year-old woman newly admitted with a diagnosis of intestinal obstruction, vomiting fecal emesis. She has a doctor's order of NG tube insertion and administration of meperidine (Demerol), 25 mg, and Phenergan, 25 mg, by intravenous push (IVP).
    B. A 17-year-old motorcycle rider who was hit by a truck. He was brought to the ER by ambulance. He has an obvious compound fracture of the femur. He was alert and oriented upon arrival, but is now confused.
    C. A 28-year-old woman with acute psychosis. She is on suicide precautions. PCU is unavailable. The patient is crying, stating that she thinks she is going to die. Vital signs are: blood pressure, 196/128 mm Hg; pulse, 138 beats/min and regular; respiration, 31 breaths/min; temperature, 96.9°F (36°C).
    D. A 24-year-old woman, post cesarean section, who is exhibiting a gradually decreasing blood pressure and an increase in pulse. No excessive vaginal bleeding is noted. She states that she has a taste of blood in the back of her throat.

15. The nurse receives change-of-shift report and has been assigned each of these patients. Which one should be assessed first?
    A. A 17-year-old patient, 2 days after casting for a radial fracture. He is complaining of severe pain in his arm, his fingers are edematous, and pulses are weak.
    B. A 16-year-old boy who is scheduled for a colonoscopy in the morning and has not had his bowel prep.
    C. A 49-year-old woman with a history of COPD, admitted for deep vein thrombosis (DVT). She is experiencing chest discomfort and dyspnea.
    D. A 72-year-old man who is scheduled for total hip replacement in need of preparation for surgery and has not signed the consent form.

16. You have just returned from lunch and as you get off the elevator, all of these patients ring their call bell. Which one should you answer first?
    A. A 36-year-old patient with terminal lung cancer being transferred to hospice home care.
    B. A 32-year-old patient refusing chemotherapy to treat cancer of the stomach.
    C. A 22-year-old patient admitted for diabetic ketoacidosis with an insulin drip. He has normal saline (0.9% NS) infusing at 100 mL/hr and an order for an immediate (STAT) sodium bicarbonate IVP.
    D. A 25-year-old patient admitted in acute sickle cell crisis with acute joint pain and dehydration.

17. You have just returned from lunch, and as you get off the elevator, all of these patients ring their call bell. Which one should you answer first?
    A. A 37-year-old woman who is supposed to have a fasting blood sugar in morning but has been allowed to eat breakfast before the procedure.
    B. A 78-year-old man who has bronchopneumonia and has not had an HHN treatment this morning.
    C. A 20-year-old woman involved in a car accident, with no visual injuries admitted during the night. She is slow to respond to verbal command and has an odor of alcohol.
    D. A 55-year old woman admitted with diarrhea and vomiting and a current potassium level of 2.5 mEq/L.
18. You are the charge nurse on a medical-surgical unit tonight. Central staffing has informed you that an oncology nurse will be floated to your unit as a replacement for the call-in. Which of the following patients would be the best assignment?
    A. A 40-year-old man, 3 days after right total-knee replacement. He is stable and tolerates CPM at 0 to 90 degrees well. Constavac was removed today.
    B. A 32-year-old woman, 1 day after total-knee replacement. Her partial thromboplastin time (PTT) is 110 seconds, and a heparin drip is infusing at 900 units per hour.
    C. A 74-year-old man, 1 hour after cardiac catheterization, who is anticipating discharge in 6 hours.
    D. A 42-year-old woman admitted yesterday for cirrhosis of the liver. She has a Port-A-Cath accessed for IVAB.
19. You are the charge nurse on an ICCU tonight. Central staffing has informed you that a medical-surgical nurse will be floated to your unit to replace the nurse who called in. Which of the following patients would be the best assignment?
    A. A 23-year-old woman, diagnosis cocaine addiction, with abdominal cramps and vaginal bleeding.
    B. A 55-year-old man admitted with an abdominal aortic aneurysm who is scheduled for dissection repair as soon as possible.
    C. A 33-year-old man admitted with a subarachnoid hematoma. The patient is unconscious and requires assistance with breathing.
    D. A 45-year-old man admitted to the hospital with a laceration of the spleen and minor cuts and bruises acquired due to an altercation. He is scheduled for exploratory surgery.
20. You are the charge nurse in an emergency unit tonight. Central staffing has informed you that a pediatric nurse will be floated to your unit as a replacement for the call-in. Which of the following patients would be the best assignment?
    A. A 60-year-old patient transported by ambulance from home with shortness of breath (SOB), labored respirations, nonproductive cough, and congested lung sounds. He is very lethargic and has circumoral pallor.
    B. A 90-year-old man who is brought into the ER by his daughter. His chief complaint is nausea and vomiting of coffee-ground emesis for 2 days. His daughter has power of attorney.
    C. A 30-year-old patient with cerebral palsy. He has difficulty voicing his chief complaint.
    D. An 18-year-old woman admitted with head trauma following a MVA. Respirations are labored. She has an altered LOC. Blood pressure is 180/105 mm Hg. Pupils are pinpoint.
21. You are the charge nurse on a pediatric unit tonight. Central staffing has informed you that an ICCU nurse will be floated to your unit as a replacement for the call-in. Which of the following patients would be the best assignment?
    A. Siamese twins, 9 months old, who are joined at the hip. The babies were born at 29 weeks' gestational age (GTA). The patients are in the ER awaiting an empty bed in pediatrics. They are being admitted for treatment of severe chicken pox. The babies are crying. They need IV hydration. The mother is a nurse and states that her babies always require a peripherally inserted central catheter (PICC) line when ill.
    B. A 15-month-old boy admitted for bronchiolitis. He is in an oxygen tent, has an IV of dextrose in 0.45 normal saline (D-5 ½ NS) infusing at 60 mL/hr. His mother is at the bedside.
    C. A 7-year-old boy who needs discharge instructions for home use of an HHN, medications, and other home care.
    D. A 9-year-old boy admitted with possible sepsis. He has a rapid, irregular pulse, temperature of 103.2°F (39.6°C) and blood pressure of 80/50 mm Hg. His mother is in the way. She is crying, repeatedly saying, "Please don't let my baby die." She is causing a disturbance on the unit.

22. You are the charge nurse on an obstetric unit tonight. Central staffing has informed you that a medical-surgical nurse will be floated to your unit as a replacement for a call-in. Which of the following patients would be the best assignment?
    A. A 24-year-old woman, 2 days after a cesarean section with orders for wound care and ambulation.
    B. An 18-year-old woman in active labor who needs an IV placement initiated and vital signs taken every hour.
    C. A 23-year-old, 2 hours after vaginal delivery with a third-degree vaginal laceration. She has Menkes' disease.
    D. A 28-year-old woman who is 6 months' pregnant with a diagnosis of placenta previa. She has active bleeding.

23. You are the charge nurse on an oncology unit tonight. Central staffing has informed you that a psychiatric nurse will be floated to your unit as a replacement for a call-in. Which of the following patients would be the best assignment?
    A. A 43-year-old man with terminal cancer who is asking for an increase in dose of morphine being administered by a PCA pump.
    B. A 30-year-old woman who has just been diagnosed with cancer of the breast.
    C. A 66-year-old woman admitted for a chemotherapy treatment.
    D. A 70-year-old woman admitted with a hemoglobin level of 8.0 mg/dL and hematocrit of 32%. She needs an IV initiated and 2 units of blood transfused.

24. You are the charge nurse on a psychiatric unit tonight. Central staffing has informed you that an ER nurse will be floated to your unit as a replacement for a call-in. Which of the following patients would be the best assignment?
    A. A 19-year-old son of the hospital administrator, admitted for depression. He claims a history of sexual abuse.
    B. A 35-year-old woman with symptoms of withdrawal from cocaine abuse.
    C. A 36-year-old bipolar patient in a manic state. She was awake during the night throwing chairs in the lounge.
    D. A 76-year-old woman with cognitive impairment who is in need of one-to-one supervision.

25. You are the expert nurse and working with a new nurse. As you walk down the hall, you observe the new nurse doing all of the following. Which one of these actions would you tell the nurse to stop doing?
    A. While monitoring a patient receiving 1 unit of packed red blood cells with 5% dextrose in normal saline (D-5 0.9NS), the new nurse performs the assessment of a new patient admitted to the same room.
    B. The new nurse is initiating venipuncture with a 20-gauge Intracath on a postoperative cholecystectomy patient whose IV had infiltrated.
    C. The new nurse is following orders to begin reverse isolation on a 45-year-old woman who received chemotherapy last week. As the nurse enters the patient's room, the nurse is wearing only a facial mask.
    D. The new nurse prepares to give meperidine (Demerol), 8 mg IV. The nurse asks a fellow RN to witness his or her waste of 2 mg/2 mL out of a 10-mg/10-mL vial. The nurse wastes the 2 mL in a sink and washes out the sink. The nurse documents the waste and administers the medication.

26. You are the expert nurse and working with a new nurse. As you walk down the hall, you observe the new nurse doing all of the following. Which one of these actions would you tell the nurse to stop doing?
    A. After performing the morning assessment of a 28-year-old diabetic patient scheduled for an esophagogastroduodenoscopy (EGD) this morning, the nurse administers his morning intermediate-acting (NPH) insulin 20 units and regular insulin, 10 units subcutaneously, in the abdomen.
    B. The new nurse introduced herself, explained the procedure, gathered venipuncture supplies, and applied a tourniquet. Using sterile technique, the nurse inserted a 22-gauge catheter into the left distal cephalic.
    C. Before medication administration, the new nurse instilled 10 mL of air into a G-tube and auscultated for air sounds to ensure G-tube placement. Next, the nurse aspirated gastric contents and checked the acid alkaline level (pH) of aspirated contents to verify placement.
    D. The new nurse administered a subcutaneous injection of Lovenox without aspirating before or massaging the injection site after.

27. You are the expert nurse and working with a new nurse. As you walk down the hall, you observe the new nurse doing all of the following. Which one of these actions would you tell the nurse to stop doing?
    A. The nurse hangs a 1,000-mL bag of 5% dextrose in normal saline (D-5 0.9 NS) with 20 mEq of potassium chloride intravenously. The nurse documents in the chart that mucous membranes are dry, skin turgor is poor, and there has been no urine output since admission.
    B. The nurse administers a bolus feeding through a patient's G-tube by gravity, making sure not hold tubing more than 18 inches above patient.
    C. The nurse then assesses the circulation, pulse, movement, and sensation (CPMS) of a supine patient who has a cast to the left lower leg and foot.
    D. The new nurse is giving Lasix, 40 mg IVP. The nurse checked the medication order, identified the patient by name band, cleansed the saline lock with alcohol, and injected saline to flush the lock. The nurse then gave the Lasix slowly, followed by a saline flush.
28. The admitting office has just called your nursing unit to admit a 38-year-old man with a medical diagnosis of diabetes mellitus, out of control. The patient has a history of Addison's disease. Which one of the following patients would be the best roommate for the patient?
    A. A 38-year-old man admitted for diabetes, out of control. He has an open wound on the left heel, which cultured positive for MRSA.
    B. An 87-year-old man with a history of Alzheimer's and CHF, who is incontinent of urine and feces. He was admitted today with a diagnosis of urinary tract infection (UTI) and dehydration.
    C. A 70-year-old man with a history of lung cancer. He has been receiving chemotherapy and radiation for the past month. His white blood cell count is 2.3 mm³.
    D. A 74-year-old man with an old tracheostomy. His breathing is slightly labored. He has a productive cough with yellow sputum. He has a low-grade temperature.
29. The admitting office has just called to inform you of the admission of a 12-year old with a sickle cell crisis. Which of the following patients would be the best roommate?
    A. A 15-year-old patient admitted with a fever, malaise, night sweats, and a productive, dry cough.
    B. A 79-year-old patient admitted for acute exacerbation of asthma. He has a history of severe colitis.
    C. A 78-year-old patient admitted with an acute painful rash with vesicles on the trunk. He related that his grandchild has the chicken pox.
    D. An 18-year-old patient with an open wound fracture and contusion, resulting from an MVA. He is postoperative following orthopedic surgical repair. Culture of the wound drainage reveals positive MRSA. The incision is covered with a dressing.

ANSWER KEY

CHAPTER 1

Critical Thinking

SCENARIO TO ACCOMPANY STUDENT WORKSHEETS

Sample Answers

SITUATION	WHAT POSSIBLE INFERENCE CAN BE MADE?	WHAT ASSUMPTION LED TO THE INFERENCE?
The physician informed the patient that the lab data results are positive for cancer and that the disease has spread to the liver. The patient is very upset and crying.	The diagnosis of cancer caused the patient to feel sad.	All patients that learn they have a life-threatening disease are sad.
The physician told the patient that his WBC (white blood cell count) was abnormal and that it indicated an infection.	A variation in the WBC indicates an infection.	All patients with a variation in the WBC have an infection.
The patient rang the call light for pain medication. The nurse had gone to lunch, and a delay resulted in the patient experiencing extreme pain for an extended time.	The patient was in pain because the nurse attended to her own needs instead of the patient's needs.	All nurses cause patients to experience pain while attending to their own needs.
The hospital is operated by a managed care company that frequently short-staffs the patient care areas. As a result of the working conditions, many of the nurses have quit. The result of increased short-staffing is poor patient care and overworked nurses.	This managed care group has short-staffed the patient care areas.	All hospitals operated by managed care groups deliver poor patient care to the hospitalized patient.
The patient was admitted to the nursing unit at the beginning of the 12-hour shift. The nursing staff had nine primary care patients to attend to. The nurse assigned to the patient was so busy that she failed to write a plan of care for the patient. The nurse failed to monitor the intravenous fluids and urinary output. As a result of the nurse's neglect, the patient went into cardiac failure due to the fluid overload.	Failure to develop a plan of care caused injury to the patient.	Any time that a plan of care is not developed, injury results.

PRACTICE EXERCISES: CRITICAL THINKING

Scenario: Using Skills of Critical Thinking

Interpretation: Clarify what the behavior means.
An unsteady gait and ambulating to the bathroom without assistance and without an assistive device places the patient at greater risk for falls.

Analysis: During the assessment, what questions should the nurse ask to determine the best plan of care?
Is there a history of past falls?
Could side effects of current medications contribute to the risk?
What is the degree of confusion?
What can be done to increase the safety in the present environment?
What is the best plan of care?

Evaluation: What outcomes do you expect to achieve with your patient today?
The patient will remain free of injuries as a result of caregiver's actions to minimize risk factors that might precipitate falls. The staff will adjust the bed height and use safe transfer procedures. Safety behavior will be demonstrated by the patient in proper use of assistive devices and use of well-fitting shoes.

Inference: What conclusion (explanation for behavior) could the nurse make based on the analysis?
The confusion could be related to medication, environment, or use of equipment.
The Risk Assessment Score is increased.
The most appropriate nursing diagnosis would be High risk for injury related to falls.
Additional interventions may be beneficial for this patient.

Explanation: During implementation, how can the nurse justify the actions being initiated?
A confused patient has a greater risk for injury with certain medications, in an unsafe environment, with inappropriate use of, or lack of, appropriate assistive devices that contribute to increasing risk for falls.

Self-regulation: What issues should the nurse reexamine to correct or improve the nursing care?
Do I know all the facts?
Is there biased thinking here?
Have I made accurate assumptions and evaluated correctly?
What do I need to change to correct my thinking?

Quiz

1. *One hour. If you started at 5:00, your second would be at 5:30, and the final one at 6:00.*

2. *70, because 30 divided by one half equals 60 (30/0.5 = 60 + 10 = 70).*

3. *The match.*

4. *Two apples. Remember, <u>you</u> took the apples.*

5. *All of them.*

6. *White. The house has to be at the North Pole; therefore, the bear must be a polar bear.*

7. *None. Noah, not Moses, took the animals on the ark.*

8. *One hour. You had to wind up the clock. Therefore, it was a mechanical one—12-hour analog, not 24-hour digital.*

Adapted from Davies, R., & McDermott, D. (1996). *45 Activities for developing a learning organization*. Aldershot, UK: Gower Publishing Limited.

SCENARIO TO ACCOMPANY STUDENT WORKSHEETS

Sample Answers

Frank Fellow is a 72-year-old man who was admitted to the step-down unit from intensive coronary care 24 hours after cardioversion. Patient education is to include self-administration of heparin, 5,000 units subcutaneously twice a day. The patient has a visual impairment and is experiencing difficulty drawing the correct dosage of medication from the vial. He can administer the injection independently.

During the evening while you are teaching the patient and his wife, the patient complains of left-sided chest pain rated at 5 on a 0 to 10 scale. He is moderately short of breath. Upon hearing his complaints of shortness of breath, his spouse becomes frantic and tearful.

1. Underline the problems in the scenario:

2. Identify the alternatives. What should the nurse do?
   Delegate the emotional support of the frantic wife to a co-worker.
   Perform an assessment of the patient, gathering physical data as well as asking the patient for input. Assessment reveals topical burns on his chest with dressing covering them. These are a result of the cardioversion. A review of the medication record reveals that pain medication was given within the hour. Key point: Reassure the patient. He is probably anxious and stressed about self-injections. Gaining patient cooperation by addressing his concerns (and those of the wife) is essential. Identify alternative interventions for pain management.

PRACTICE EXERCISES: PROBLEM SOLVING

Scenarios: Identifying Problem-Solving Methods

SCENARIO 1
   What problem-solving method was used?
   Do it yourself
   What other problem-solving methods could have been included?
   Combine knowledge

SCENARIO 2
   What problem-solving method was used?
   Assign someone
   What other problem-solving methods could have been included?
   Do it yourself or combine knowledge

SCENARIO 3
   What problem-solving method was used?
   Influence others
   What other problem-solving methods could have been included?
   Combine knowledge

Scenarios: Detecting Errors in the Problem-Solving Process

SCENARIO 4
   What error in the problem-solving process is Jane making?
   Failure to identify actual problem

What is the actual problem?
Excessive concern with punctuality and poor coping mechanisms

SCENARIO 5

What error in the problem-solving process is the nurse making?
Failure to identify all possible scenarios
What would be a strategy to remedy this error?
Take time to consider all options

SCENARIO 6

What error in the problem-solving process is Dante making?
Failure to monitor implementation
What would be a strategy to remedy this error?
Follow up on solutions and monitor progress

FUN EXERCISES

1. *Sandbox*
2. *Man overboard*
3. *I understand*
4. *Reading between the lines*
5. *Long underwear*
6. *Crossroads*
7. *Tricycle*
8. *Downtown*
9. *Split level*
10. *Neon light*
11. *Life after death*
12. *Backward glance*
13. *Three degrees below zero*
14. *Circles under the eyes*
15. *Paradise (pair of dice)*
16. *High chair*
17. *Touchdown*
18. *Six feet underground*
19. *Mind over matter*
20. *He's beside himself*
21. *Scrambled eggs*
22. *Onside kick (as in football)*

DEMONSTRATION OF THE PROBLEM-SOLVING PROCESS

SAMPLE ANSWERS

ASSESSMENT

Recognize that problem exists: the paper is due in 1 week, and the group has made no progress. Make a list of needs.
Need passing grade to continue in program. Need for family approval.
Collect, compile, organize data.
Due date, requirements, strengths and weaknesses of group members.

ANALYSIS

Define problem clearly.
Need well-written paper submitted in 1 week.
Establish priorities.
High priority because need passing grade.
Develop list of strategies: include do paper self, divide evenly and hope for best, schedule group meeting to discuss progress, complain to instructor, threaten team members.

OUTCOME IDENTIFICATION

Likelihood of each occurring
For each strategy ask: Do you really think that is going to happen?
Establish desired outcome.
Good paper without alienating classmates.

STRATEGY	NEGATIVE EFFECT	POSITIVE EFFECT
Do paper self	Lack of trust from group, Less time to study for test.	Paper will be done to your standards.
Divide evenly, hope for best	Paper may not get finished or may be poorly done.	Will not require as much time.
Complain to instructor	May reflect poorly on ability to work with groups.	Instructor may intervene with group members.
Threaten team members	Team members may respond negatively to confrontation.	May not be selected to be in team with these members again.
Schedule group meeting to discuss progress	May not all attend.	Can openly discuss expectations and division of labor.

PLAN

Choose alternative with best chance of success.
Group meeting to discuss lack of progress
List of resources
Instructor, textbook on group dynamics
List of desired actions
Schedule time and place for meeting.
Time schedule
Needs to be done quickly because of rapidly approaching due date
Assignments
Establish tentative plan for division of labor

IMPLEMENTATION

Have group meeting. Assign duties.
Directions to personnel
Give dates for submission of parts of paper. Discuss desired font, etc. Volunteer to proof final draft.

EVALUATION

Monitor response.
Remind of due dates. Request sections as they become due.

SCENARIO TO ACCOMPANY STUDENT WORKSHEETS

SAMPLE ANSWERS

Options to consider:

- *Collaborate with the physician for alternative medication that is prepackaged so that patient is not required to draw up the dosage. As an example, Lovenox is a prepackaged unit dose so that self-injection is all that is required.*
- *Teach the wife to draw up and administer the injections.*
- *Continue to teach the patient how to draw up and administer the drug as best as he can.*

PRACTICE EXERCISES: DECISION MAKING

SCENARIOS: USING DECISION-MAKING SKILLS

SCENARIO 1

Based on the scenario, identify the problem that would require a decision.
If you were Jean, how could you pass the test and still attend the party?
Identify solutions:

- Call in sick for work, attend the party, and cram before and after the party.
  Pro: Will be able to attend party and study.
  Con: Boss will be angry and may fire you.
- Attend the party, go to work, and just hope for the best on the test.
  Pro: Will be able to attend party, and boss won't be angry.
  Con: Probably will fail out of nursing school.
- Call in sick, stay home from the party, and study very hard.
  Pro: Will pass the exam and stay in nursing program.
  Con: Won't get to attend the party, and boss will be angry.

Identify the outcome you wanted to achieve with the decision you made.
To pass the exam and be able to continue in the nursing program and become a nurse in May.
Place an asterisk (*) beside the selected alternative that achieves the desired outcome. (Answers may vary. Have a group discussion with your instructor to determine the best outcome.)
What if Jean's goal were different? What if the goal were to make money to pay the rent and buy groceries because her mother lost her job and has been ill the past 3 weeks? Would your choice be different?

SCENARIO 2

Based on the scenario, identify the problem that would require a decision.
How should time be allocated to allow for studying?
Identify two solutions.

- Study when she first gets home, without stopping for supper and chores until studying is done.
  Pro: Will get studying done while not being so tired from housework.
  Con: Will be hungry and in a messy house.
- Leave studying until after supper and chores are done.
  Pro: Anxiety will be decreased about messy house and husband being hungry.
  Con: Will be too tired to study, stressed from being tired and not being finished with studying.

- Ask husband to do supper and help with the chores.
  Pro: Will get studying done.
  Con: Will have distractions with husband cooking; will feel inadequate for not being all things to all people.

Identify the outcome you wanted to achieve with the decision you made.
To make good grades.
Place an asterisk (*) beside the selected alternative that achieves the desired outcome. (Answers may vary. Have a group discussion with your instructor to determine the best outcome.)

SCENARIO 3

Identify a problem that required you to make a decision.
Should Joel attend nursing school in the fall?
Identify solutions:

- Go to school and work part-time too.
  Pro: Will get an education for a better job and eventually make more money.
  Con: Will be stressed, interrupt family routine, and make grades lower than desired owing to job and family demands.
- Go to school and quit job.
  Pro: Will get an education for a better job and have fewer disruptions with family. Also, will have more time to study.
  Con: Will have less money to spend while going to school.
- Don't start school, and keep on working as a UAP.
  Pro: Life will be uninterrupted.
  Con: Will have a job with poor pay and little chance for advancement.

Identify the outcome you wanted to achieve with the decision you made.
To go to school and have time to devote to studies to ensure doing well on boards.
Place an asterisk (*) beside the selected alternative that achieves the desired outcome. (Answers may vary. Have a group discussion with your instructor to determine the best outcome.)

SCENARIO 4

Based on the scenario, identify a problem that would require a decision.
Michelle's son will be upset if his mom does not attend his Christmas program.
Identify solutions:

- Call in sick for that day.
  Pro: Will be able to attend son's program.
  Con: May be suspended for requesting time off and then calling in sick.
- Trade shifts with someone else.
  Pro: Will be able to attend son's program.
  Con: Will have to work on day off to replace regular shift.
- Go to work and miss program.
  Pro: Boss won't be angry.
  Con: Son will be upset because Mom missed the Christmas program.

Identify the outcome you wanted to achieve with the decision you made.
To have the day off and attend the program.
Place an asterisk (*) beside the option that correlates with the priorities and demonstrates the least undesirable side effects. (Answers may vary. Have a group discussion with your instructor to determine the best outcome.)

SCENARIO 5

Identify a problem that requires you to make a decision.
The patient is in pain before the time she can have another pill, and another painful procedure is about to occur.

Identify solutions:

- Give the pain pill early this time.
  Pro: Patient will be pain free and more likely to comply with therapy.
  Con: Face being chastised for not following the doctor's orders and risking possible legal issues.
- Call the doctor and report the pain.
  Pro: Be absolutely within legal limits.
  Con: Doctor will be interrupted and probably angry.
- Ask the patient to wait the 30 minutes.
  Pro: Nurse will not have to decide.
  Con: Patient who is already in pain will have a procedure that will increase her pain (violation of the Patient Care Partnership).
- Give pain medication as written and get patient up in chair without it.
  Pro: Nurse will not have to decide.
  Con: Patient's pain will be increased.

Identify the outcome you want to achieve.
To have patient participate in prescribed therapy without undue pain.
Place an asterisk (*) beside the selected alternative that achieves the desired outcome. (Answers may vary. Have a group discussion with your instructor to determine the best outcome.)

SCENARIO 6

Identify a problem that requires you to make a decision.
Whether or not to put the IV needle back in.
Identify solutions:

- Restart the IV.
  Pro: Patient will continue to get IV fluids and antibiotics.
  Con: Temporary discomfort of the needle stick.
- Leave the needle out.
  Pro: Patient can move more freely without discomfort.
  Con: Patient will not get the antibiotics needed for treatment of his disease.
- Ignore the situation and let someone else deal with it.
  Pro: Nurse will not be bothered with the procedure.
  Con: Fluids will continue to leak, and patient will not get needed treatment.

Identify the outcome you wanted to achieve with the decision you made.
For the patient to get the necessary treatment to resolve the pneumonia on my shift.
Place an asterisk (*) beside the option that correlates with priorities and demonstrates the least undesirable side effects. (Answers may vary. Have a group discussion with your instructor to determine the best outcome.)

SCENARIO 7

Identify a problem that required you to make a decision.
Whether or not to get her up this morning.
Identify solutions:

- Get her up per doctor's order.
  Pro: Promotes mobility, and early mobility reduces chance for blood clots.
  Con: She may still be under the effect of anesthetic and injure herself.
- Leave her in bed until this afternoon.
  Pro: Patient can better assist in the transfer and minimize risk for injury. Also promotes rest.
  Con: Bed rest increases risk for skin breakdown and promotes blood clots.

Identify the outcome you want to achieve with the decision you make.
Minimize risk for injury and promote rest to facilitate healing.
Place an asterisk (*) beside the option that correlates with priorities and demonstrates the least undesirable side effects. (Answers may vary. Have a group discussion with your instructor to determine the best outcome.)

SCENARIO TO ACCOMPANY STUDENT WORKSHEETS

Sample Answers

DATA CLUSTER	DATA CLUSTER
Patient is 73 years old, lives with 55-year-old developmentally disabled son	1+ pitting edema in lower extremities
Recent diagnosis of congestive heart failure	Fine crackles in bases bilaterally
Anticipated need for digitalis preparation and ongoing diuretic therapy	Occasional dry, nonproductive cough
	Alert and oriented
	Respirations 24 breaths/min at rest

1. List the priority nursing diagnoses (review NANDA list and place in order of priority).
   Activity intolerance related to diminished cardiac output as evidenced by 1+ pitting edema, fine crackles, nonproductive cough, respirations 24 breath/min at rest.
   Deficient knowledge related to disease process, precautions, and side effects of diuretic and digitalis therapy as evidenced by patient saying she has never taken medication for anything like this.

2. Identify interventions in order of priority to assess at the beginning of your shift.
   Measure respiratory rate and oxygen saturation to determine oxygenation.
   Establish baseline vitals to evaluate effectiveness of medication.
   Assess urinary output to evaluate diuretic therapy.
   Assess the serum electrolyte data.

PRACTICE EXERCISES: PRIORITY SETTING

Setting Priorities of Nursing Diagnoses

Use Maslow's Hierarchy of Needs to identify the level of needs of the nursing diagnoses in the column 1, and place the corresponding number in the blank beside column 2.

1. Physiologic
2. Safety and security
3. Love and belonging
4. Self-esteem
5. Self-actualization

COLUMN 1	COLUMN 2
Activity intolerance	1
Imbalanced nutrition: Less than body requirements	1
Anxiety	2
Social isolation	3
Ineffective role performance	3
Ineffective airway clearance	1
Chronic confusion	2
Impaired tissue integrity	1
Constipation	1
Acute pain	1
Disturbed sleep pattern	1
Deficient fluid volume	1

Scenario: Identifying Priority Nursing Diagnoses

COLUMN 1	COLUMN 2
Situational low self-esteem related to fear of prolonged disability and threat to job	4
Ineffective breathing pattern related to effects of anesthesia and history of smoking	1
High risk for ineffective coping related to effects of acute illness, lack of support system	3
High risk for infection related to hazards of invasive lines and contamination of peritoneum with gastric juices	2
Acute pain related to surgical incision and irritation of gastric juice during bleed	1

Scenarios: Prioritizing Nursing Activities

SCENARIO 1

List the five top-priority nursing activities at this time.

1. *Replace oxygen.*
2. *Raise bed to high Fowler's position.*
3. *Encourage patient to deep breathe and cough.*
4. *Assess for fluid overload (crackles and increased blood pressure).*
5. *Assess pulse quality and check for edema (Is pulse bounding?).*

SCENARIO 2

What is your initial action at this time and why?

1. *Apply pressure with gauze pad to stop bleeding.*

2. *Assess respirations, breath sounds, and chest sounds (May have pneumothorax; however, this is a potential problem, and the actual problem of bleeding is the priority under these circumstances.)*
3. *Call physician or report to nurse.*

SCENARIO 3

What is your first priority?
These are all indicators of ketoacidosis without respiratory distress.

1. *Determine whether the patient took his morning dose of insulin.*
2. *Call the emergency department and determine whether insulin was given and the dosage.*
3. *Recheck Glucoscan.*
4. *Call the physician.*

SCENARIO 4

All of these are appropriate to this patient; which one is the priority at this time?

Deficient knowledge related to procedure
Anxiety related to procedure
Acute pain related to the disease process
Risk for imbalanced nutrition related to disease

Based on this decision select the priority nursing activity at this time.

Administer intramuscular (IM) pain medication
Sit and talk with patient
Call the physician
Offer to call a family member

SCENARIO 5

All of the following need to be completed. In what order would you perform them?

4	*Complete assessment*
7	*Teach patient about complications of diabetes and circulation*
6	*Perform morning care and grooming*
2	*Administer morning insulin injection*
3	*Take vital signs*
1	*Perform finger stick for blood glucose monitoring*
5	*Assist with breakfast tray*

SCENARIO 6

Which nursing activity is the priority? Identify in order of priority as numbers 1 through 5, with number 1 being top priority.

2	*Make sure the paracentesis equipment is available.*
3	*Perform a body system assessment*
5	*Ensure that the patient voids to empty the bladder*
4	*Take vital signs*
1	*Get patient signature on informed consent*

TIME MANAGEMENT

EVALUATING USE OF TIME

Review the following Daily Time Log. Under the comments, note what you would do differently to be more efficient and to provide better care. (Not every entry needs a comment.)

TIME	ACTIVITIES	EVALUATION OF TIME USE
7:00–7:30	Received shift report; checked medication administration record (MAR); delegated vitals for stable patients	
7:30–8:00	Shared "horror stories of yesterday" with nurse who had day off; check labs	Postpone stories for break; make unit rounds
8:00–8:30	Assessed patients, served meal trays, helped nursing assistant (NA), cleaned up spills on carpet	Delegate tray pass; call housekeeper for spills
8:30–9:00	Evaluated Mrs. Green's shortness of breath; finished picking up trays; started treatments	Delegate picking up trays and start medications pass
9:00–9:30	Started medication pass; took two phone calls from patient's families	Return calls after medications pass, then do treatments
9:30–10:00	Rechecked Mrs. Green; break, 9:30–9:45; finished treatments; finished 9:00 AM medications	
10:00–10:30	Documented treatments; documented Mrs. Green's shortness of breath episode	Chart at time of distress
10:30–11:00	Made rounds; took pharmacy calls and called lab	
11:00–11:30	Postponed NA's performance appraisal; evaluated Mrs. Green's chest pain; called doctor	Distressed patient is the priority
11:30–12:00	Lunch break	
12:00–12:30	Prepared lunch trays; assisted with distribution and feeding	Could delegate
12:30–1:00	Delegated noon vitals to NA; doctor to see Mrs. Green; transcribed new orders	Delegate vitals earlier
1:00–1:30	Began afternoon treatments	
1:30–2:00	Started 1:00 PM medications; completed NA performance appraisal; interrupted twice for phone calls	Start medications earlier; have unit secretary take messages
2:00–2:30	Made rounds on patients; transcribed orders—did not finish	
2:30–3:00	Completed afternoon charting	Chart at time of care
3:00–3:30	Reported off to evening shift; 10 minutes late for report	Start on time now; next nurse sitting

Adapted from Ringsven, M. K., & Bond, D. (1991). *Gerontology and leadership skills for nurses*. Boston: Delmar. Copyright 1997. Reprinted with permission of Delmar Learning, a division of Thomson Learning: www.thomsonrights.com (fax, 800-730-2215).

SCENARIO: EVALUATING USE OF TIME

DAILY TIME LOG

TIME	ACTIVITIES	EVALUATION OF TIME USE
7:00–7:30	Receive shift report; check MAR; review morning Glucoscan	
7:30–8:00	Check MAR; give insulin; perform head-to-toe assessment, including vital signs	
8:00–8:30	Call physician; call lab for blood draw; call Radiography; perform chart assessment and process orders	
8:30–9:00	Delegate compression device and Aqua K-pad; initiate heparin therapy; delegate serving breakfast	
9:00–9:30	Administer meds; review labs; delegate tray removal and recording input and output	
9:30–10:00	Assist Radiography with portable chest radiograph; break, 9:30–9:45	
10:00–10:30	Perform patient teaching; maintain bed rest until results are back and physician arrives to assess them	
10:30–11:00	Reassess patient; delegate Glucoscan; doctor here to assess; process new orders	
11:00–11:30	Document interventions	
11:30–12:00	Take and record vital signs; give insulin SS	
12:00–12:30	Lunch break, 12:00–12:30; delegate serving lunch	
12:30–1:00	Review plan of care and revise	
1:00–1:30	Administer medications	
1:30–2:00	Perform patient teaching	
2:00–2:30	Document evaluation of care	
2:30–3:00	Record input and output totals, clear intravenous pump; check follow-up PTT for heparin drip	
3:00–3:30	Give report	

Adapted from Ringsven, M. K., & Bond, D. (1991). *Gerontology and leadership skills for nurses.* Boston: Delmar. Copyright 1997. Reprinted with permission of Delmar Learning, a division of Thomson Learning: www.thomsonrights.com (fax, 800-730-2215).

SCENARIOS TO ACCOMPANY STUDENT WORKSHEETS

Identifying and Clustering Cues

SCENARIO 1

A 72-year-old woman was admitted following a motor vehicle accident. In the emergency department (ED), an x-ray revealed that the head of the left femur was fractured. She is scheduled for an open reduction and internal fixation (ORIF) later today. At present, she rates the pain at 8 on a 1 to 10 scale. The son mentioned during the assessment that his mother is sometimes forgetful.

Vital signs include the following: blood pressure, 168/92 mm Hg, temperature, 98°F (36.7°C); pulse, 102 beats/min and irregular; respirations, 26 breaths/min. Breath sounds are clear bilaterally, respirations even and unlabored, and peripheral pulses present and palpable at 2+ except left foot. The left pedal pulse is weak and barely palpable and capillary refill response is 5 seconds. The patient is alert and oriented, is able to move all extremities except the left leg, and verbalizes appropriate responses to all questioning. She relates allergies to sulfa and ampicillin.

During the assessment, the patient is very anxious and states that she has never been in the hospital before. She did confide that she had spent a lot of time at the hospital when her husband died from cancer last year. Significant medical history includes high blood pressure controlled with medication.

1. Underline all of the cues and problems in the above scenario.
2. Sort and cluster the relevant data using Diagnostic-Related Groups.

Circulation:
Hypertension controlled with medication
Current blood pressure of 168/92 mm Hg (probable response to pain)
Pulse, 102 beats/min (irregular heartbeat)
Pedal pulse diminished in left foot
Delayed capillary refill time in left foot

Activity/Rest:
Gait and mobility impairment resulting from fracture of left leg

Neurosensory:
Movement impaired in left leg
Weakness and loss of function in left leg

Pain/Discomfort:
Pain rated at 8

Safety:
Allergy to sulfa and ampicillin
Forgetful at times

Ego Integrity:
She is very anxious.
Fear of hospitalization

Teaching/Learning:
Scheduled for ORIF, needs pre-operative teaching
Need for informed consent due to impending surgery
No previous exposure for self as patient in hospital

SCENARIO 2

A 68-year-old man presented in the ED with an <u>acute epistaxis</u> (nosebleed) 2 hours earlier. At the time the bleeding started, he also experienced <u>blurred vision,</u> which he stated had never happened before. Upon questioning, the patient related that he had been experiencing early-morning <u>headaches for the past 3 to 4 months.</u> The initial <u>blood pressure of 198/116 mm Hg</u> was treated with medication in the ED, and the epistaxis subsequently stopped without specific intervention. The patient was admitted for further diagnostic tests and follow-up care.

On arrival to the medical-surgical unit, the following vital signs were obtained: blood pressure, 142/88 mm Hg; temperature, 98.2°F (36.8°C); pulse, 98 beats/min; respirations, 28 breaths/min. The patient verbalizes <u>weakness and fatigue</u> gradually increasing during the past 4 months. He ambulates with a steady gait, and muscle strength and hand grasp are equal and strong bilaterally. He also relates feeling "<u>palpitations</u>" and <u>shortness of breath on exertion.</u> He attributes his symptoms to working a lot of overtime and being <u>stressed because of his wife's illness.</u> He states he <u>did not seek medical attention because he thought he was just tired.</u> Current <u>body weight is 328 pounds; height is 5 feet, 10 inches.</u> On the lab draw, his blood <u>sugar was 228 mg/dL</u> (he states he had not eaten this morning before arriving in the ED). He has a <u>history of smoking</u> since the age of 23 years, and he <u>always adds salt</u> to his food at the table.

1. Underline all of the cues and problems in the above scenario.
2. Sort and cluster the relevant data using the Diagnostic-Related Groups.

Ego Integrity:
Wife's illness
Stress factors resulting from work and financial concerns
Denial of own illness

Food/Fluid:
Food preferences include high sodium
Obesity (weight, 328 pounds)
Blood sugar (228 mg/dL fasting)

Neurosensory:
Headaches during past 3 to 4 months
Episode of epistaxis with visual blurring

Pain/Discomfort:
Headaches noted above

Respirations:
Exertional dyspnea
History of smoking

Circulation:
Elevated blood pressure
Palpitations
Fatigue and weakness

Teaching/Learning:
Needs teaching for self-monitoring blood pressure
Needs dietary modifications for carbohydrates and salt specifically
Needs weight reduction strategies
Physiologic effects of cigarettes

PRACTICE EXERCISES: ADVANCED NURSING PROCESS APPLICATIONS

Identifying and Clustering Cues Practice Exercises

SCENARIO 1

A 53-year-old woman was admitted on a 23-hour observation for a laparoscopic cholecystectomy. On the admission database, she verbalized frequent episodes of nausea, belching, and heartburn when eating fatty foods. Immediately before admission, the severity of the epigastric distress and right upper abdominal pain had increased. The patient has a saline lock in the left hand; Steri-Strips to the four puncture wound sites on the abdomen, and pain management with oral medication. She is scheduled for discharge today.

1. Underline all of the cues and problems in the above scenario.
2. Select the appropriate Diagnostic-Related Groups. Sort and cluster the relevant data into the groupings.
   Teaching/Learning: Assistance with wound care, self care, and discharge needs
   Dietary teaching

3. Identify the priority nursing diagnosis.
   Deficient knowledge R/T home management of postoperative status secondary to cholecystectomy AEB verbalized questions about follow-up care and dietary prescription.

4. What is the expected outcome?
   Before discharge, patient will verbalize knowledge about self-care, indicators to report to primary health care provider, components of a low-fat diet with gradual introduction of fats over 4 to 6 months, and follow-up care.

SCENARIO 2

A 28-year-old woman was admitted with a diagnosis of recurrent inflammatory bowel disease. She has been on prednisone for 10 years and experienced a gradual weight loss of 30 pounds in the past year. Symptoms include 5 to 10 loose stools per day, nausea, and frequent intermittent pain.

During the physical assessment, the patient described patterns of fatigue with normal daily chores and sleep patterns being disturbed at night as a result of the frequent episodes of diarrhea. Anxiously, she reported recently quitting her job because of inability to cope with all of the problems the disease causes at work. Her current body weight is 106 pounds, and her height is 5 feet, 7 inches. She has poor muscle tone, pale mucous membranes, and poor skin turgor. There are visible hemorrhoids and a fissure noted in the anal area, and she verbalizes noting small amounts of red blood during bowel movements.

1. Underline all of the cues and problems in the above scenario.
2. Identify the appropriate diagnostic groups. Sort and cluster the relevant data using the groupings.

Activity/Rest:
Fatigue
Sleep disturbed due to diarrhea

Ego Integrity:
Anxiety and emotional upset
Loss of job and income related to disease
Withdrawal from normal activities as a result of illness

Elimination:
Frequent (5 to 10) stools per day
Red blood during bowel movements (indicates rectal bleeding)
Hemorrhoids and rectal fissure

Food/Fluid:
Gradual weight loss (30 pounds in 1 year)
Current body weight: 106 pounds; height, 5 feet, 7 inches

Nausea and anorexia
Weakness, poor muscle tone
Poor skin turgor
Pale mucous membranes

Pain/Discomfort:
Frequent intermittent pain

Safety:
Prednisone for 10 years (predisposed to osteoporosis)

3. Based on these clusters, identify the priority nursing diagnoses and place in order of priority.
   1. *Diarrhea*
   2. *Deficient fluid volume*
   3. *Deficient nutrition*
   4. *Skin breakdown*
   5. *Chronic pain*
   6. *Individual ineffective coping*
   7. *Fatigue*

   (When the first two diagnoses are treated, the other problems will diminish without planned interventions. Diarrhea is the most urgent because it can lead to life-threatening electrolyte disturbance; deficient fluid volume can also be life threatening.)

4. What are the expected outcomes for the two priority nursing diagnoses?
   Within 2 days of admission, the patient will report decreased frequency of stools and more normal consistency.
   Within 24 hours of admission, the patient will stabilize fluid volume as evidenced by balanced intake and output, urinary output of more than 30 mL/hour, vital signs within baseline range, stable blood pressure with position change, good skin turgor, capillary refill time of less than 3 seconds, moist mucous membranes, and diarrhea controlled.

SCENARIO 3

Marie Kelly, who is 53 years old, was admitted from the emergency room with <u>chronic renal failure</u> has a long <u>history of diabetes mellitus</u> and <u>hypertension</u> and is on hemodialysis. Her symptoms include <u>extreme fatigue, general malaise,</u> and <u>occasional confusion</u> from the chronic uremia. She has no known allergies. Physical assessment reveals <u>generalized tissue and pitting edema of feet and legs, pallor, and bronze-gray, yellow skin.</u> She verbalizes that urine output is normally <u>anuric</u> and that <u>constipation</u> is always a problem. Her skin has numerous <u>crusted areas</u> on both arms, and she is <u>scratching</u> during the assessment. She complains of frequent <u>nausea and vomiting</u> and an <u>unpleasant metallic taste</u> in her mouth.

1. Underline all of the cues and problems in the above scenario.
2. After identification of the cues (defining characteristics), sort them into appropriate data clusters.

Activity/Rest:
Extreme fatigue
General malaise

Circulation:
History of hypertension
Generalized tissue and pitting edema
Pallor: bronze-gray, yellow skin

Food/Fluid:
History of diabetes
Generalized tissue and pitting edema
Complains of frequent nausea and vomiting and unpleasant metallic taste

Elimination:
Chronic renal failure
Constipation
Anuric

Neurosensory:
Occasional confusion

Safety:
Itching skin, frequent scratching
Crusting and scratch marks on arms
No known allergies

3. Identify two priority nursing diagnoses (write in three-part format) and list in order of urgency.
   Excess fluid volume R/T inability of kidneys to excrete fluid AEB generalized tissue and pitting edema of feet and legs, anuria
   Impaired skin integrity R/T scratching skin secondary to accumulation of toxins in skin and edema causing alterations in skin turgor AEB generalized tissue edema, crusts, and scratching on arms

4. What are the expected outcomes for the nursing diagnoses?
   After dialysis, the patient will have normal fluid volume evidenced by stable weight, adequate skin turgor, vital signs within baseline normal values, and decreasing edema in tissue.
   Patient will identify effective measures to maintain skin integrity as evidenced by verbalization and demonstration of behaviors and techniques to promote healing of crusts and to prevent further skin breakdown.

SCENARIO 4

Ronald Johnson, a 73-year-old man, was seen in the emergency room for the following symptoms: right-sided hemiparesis, expressive aphasia, and dysphagia. He is drowsy and demonstrates slurred speech and altered mental status. The wife states, "I found him in the hallway outside the bathroom." She also requests a laxative because he has been constipated all morning. A computed tomography (CT) scan and angiogram completed in the emergency ED revealed a blockage in the middle cerebral artery.

1. Underline all of the cues and problems in the above scenario.
2. After identification of the cues (defining characteristics), sort them into appropriate data clusters.

Circulation:
Blockage in middle cerebral artery

Food/Fluid:
Dysphagia

Neurosensory:
Altered mental status
Expressive aphasia
Drowsy
Slurred speech

Activity/Rest:
Right side hemiparesis

Elimination:
Constipation

3. Identify three priority nursing diagnoses (write in three-part format) and list in order of urgency.
   Ineffective tissue perfusion (cerebral) R/T interruption of arterial blood blow AEB altered mental status, expressive aphasia, drowsiness, and slurred speech
   Impaired physical mobility R/T right-sided hemiparesis, weakness, and cognitive impairment AEB inability to move purposefully the left side of body and decreased muscle strength and control

Risk for ineffective airway clearance R/T loss of cough reflex, loss of gag reflex, dysphagia, and cognitive impairment

4. Use your critical thinking skills to develop another nursing diagnosis that is implied in the above scenario. This one will only have two parts because it is a "risk for" diagnosis and no cues are present.
   High risk for injury R/T increase in intracranial pressure

5. What are the expected outcomes for the two identified priority nursing diagnoses?
   Patient will demonstrate improved cerebral tissue perfusion as evidenced by improved mental status and reduction of speech impairment and visual disturbance.
   Before hospital discharge, patient will demonstrate appropriate transfer and ambulation techniques.

Advanced Applications: Using the Nursing Process

SCENARIO

1. Identify the cues (defining characteristics) for the nursing diagnosis and place into data clusters.

   Food/Fluid:
   Verbalized that he stopped drinking fluids due to pain on urination
   Dizziness and low output
   Temperature, 99.2°F; pulse, 98 beats/min; blood pressure, 98/60 mm Hg sitting
   Skin turgor is flaccid, mucous membranes dry, and musculature is weak
   Elimination
   Abdominal pain rated at 10
   Past history of cancer of the prostate
   30 mL dark-brown urine without visible signs of bleeding upon catheter insertion
   Foley in place at present
   Pain on elimination

   Teaching/Learning:
   Intentional failure to drink fluid after chemotherapy when catheter was removed
   Patient's failure to recognize symptoms of urinary tract infection

ANALYSIS (DIAGNOSIS)

2. Identify the two priority nursing diagnoses (based on NANDA and written in three-part format).
   Deficient fluid volume R/T lack of knowledge regarding therapeutic regimen for disease AEB low fluid intake
   Lack of knowledge R/T therapeutic regimen for disease treatment AEB inability to follow treatment regimen at home

3. Which data definitely need further discussion with the patient?
   The Teaching/Learning cluster: The patient is dehydrated because of intentional inadequate intake. This must be corrected because of potential harm to the kidney tissue. Chemotherapy and antibiotics can damage the kidney tissue without adequate fluid to flush them through.

OUTCOME IDENTIFICATION

4. Identify the outcome desired and the indicators (based on NOC) that the outcomes have been achieved.
   Maintain fluid volume balance AEB:
   Normal skin turgor, moist mucous membranes, stable weight, blood pressure and pulse within normal range for patient and stable with position change, capillary refill time less than 3 seconds, usual mental status, and blood urea nitrogen and hematocrit within normal range.

PLAN

5. Develop a nursing plan of care based on this patient's current health care needs.

IMPLEMENTATION

Initiate the interventions as outlined in the plan of care.

EVALUATION

Monitor the patient for the following responses to interventions.

- *Maintains urine output >1,300 mL/day*
- *Maintains normal blood pressure, pulse, and body temperature*
- *Maintains elastic skin turgor; moist tongue and mucous membranes; and orientation to person, place and time.*
- *Describes symptoms that indicate the need to consult with health care provider.*

Lippincott's Interactive Care Plan Creator

Name: Student
Client Initials: JL
ID: 123
Admission Date: 09/14/03
Course: Cognitive Skills in Nursing
Age: 61
Sex: M
Instructor: Saundra
Date: 07/02/2002

MEDICAL DIAGNOSES	NURSING DIAGNOSES	PATIENT OUTCOMES/GOALS	NURSING ACTIVITIES	RATIONALE	EVALUATIONS
Dehydration	**Fluid Volume Deficit**				
	DEFINING CHARACTERISTICS:				
	Fluid intake, inadequate	Maintain fluid volume balance within 24 hours of admission	Fluid, oral, increasing intake of, teach about	The oral route is preferred for maintaining fluid balance.	Fluid balance (NOC 0601) 24-hour intake and output balanced Serum electrolytes WNL Hematocrit WNL Urine specific gravity WNL
	Mucous membrane, dryness		Intake and output, measure	A urine output of < 30 mL/hr is insufficient for normal renal function and indicates hypovolemia or onset of renal damage.	Skin hydration Moist mucous membranes Body weight stable
	Skin, turgor, decreased		Intake and output, teach about		Peripheral pulses palpable Orthostatic hypotension not present
	Urine output, decreased		Blood pressure, measurement of, perform	Observe for decreased pulse pressure first, then hypotension. A decreased pulse pressure is an earlier indicator of shock that is the systolic blood pressure. Decreased intravascular volume results in hypotension and decreased tissue oxygenation.	
	Weakness		Intravenous infusion, equipment or site, check	Isotonic IV fluids such as 0.9%, N/S or lactated Ringer's allow replacement of intravascular volume.	
	Blood pressure, decreased Temperature, body, increased Dizziness Pulse, increased		Postural blood pressure, assess	A 15-mm HG drop when upright or an increase of 15 beats/min in the pulse rate are seen with deficit fluid volume.	

SCENARIOS TO ACCOMPANY STUDENT WORKSHEETS

Sample Answers

PATIENT	OUTCOMES	TASK/PROCESS	WHO WILL PERFORM IT?
Room 101	Within 24 hours of discharge, the patient will be free of symptoms of bleeding AEB labs and physical data.	Monitor for changes in vitals and active signs of bleeding or change in lab data.	RN: assess and interpret data and lab values LPN/LVN: collect data and report UAP: obtain routine vitals, intake and output and report
	Before the EGD, the patient will verbalize understanding of the procedure, complications, and follow-up care before signing the informed consent.	Perform patient teaching and evaluate the informed consent.	RN: teach and evaluate consent
	No hospital-acquired injuries.	Provide for safety needs.	All staff to monitor for safety.
Room 102	Within 24 hours of discharge, the patient will verbalize pain reduction to less than 3 on a 1 to 10 scale, with oral pain medications.	Manage pain control with PCA pump. Monitor fluid volume status.	RN: pain management for PCA LPN/LVN: data gathering and reporting UAP: obtain intake and output and report
	Within 24 hours of discharge, patient verbalizes knowledge about disease process, home care of drains, medication, care of the surgical incision, and potential complications.	Perform patient teaching and discharge planning. Evaluate emotional status and coping mechanisms Collaborate with Reach for Recovery (breast cancer support group).	RN: teaching plan RN: evaluation and nursing judgment RN: collaborate with support group
Room 103		Assess vital signs, monitor tissue perfusion and quality of output.	RN: assessment and interpretation of data LPN/LVN: data gathering and reporting UAP: comfort measures and report of progress
		Monitor fluid volume status and fluid restrictions.	RN: evaluate the fluid volume status LPN/LVN: collect data and report UAP: obtain intake and output and report
		Manage diabetes control with Glucoscan and sliding scale insulin. Perform patient teaching and obtain informed consent.	LPN/LVN: perform Glucoscan and give sliding scale insulin RN: evaluation and nursing judgment

(continued)

PATIENT	OUTCOMES	TASK/PROCESS	WHO WILL PERFORM IT?
Room 104	Within 24 hours of discharge, patient will have vital signs WNL and other signs of stable fluid volume. No signs of infection will be present on discharge.	Assess vital signs, monitor fluid volume status (intake = output) and quality of output.	RN: assessment, interpretation of data, evaluation of fluid volume status LPN/LVN: data gathering and reporting UAP: obtain intake and output and report
		Take initial baseline vital signs and monitor labs.	RN: assessment and interpretation of data
		Perform patient teaching and informed consent.	RN: evaluation and nursing judgment
Room 105	By discharge, the patient will demonstrate effective coping strategies AEB diminished anxiety with the transfer.	Evaluate emotional status and coping strategies.	RN: evaluation and nursing judgment
		Perform patient teaching and discharge planning.	RN: evaluation and nursing judgment
		Coordinate transfer with the nursing home staff.	RN: collaborate with nursing home staff and assess patient needs to complete transfer papers
Room 106		Monitor fluid volume status and interpret lab data.	RN: evaluate the fluid volume status and interpretation of data LPN/LVN: collect data and report UAP: obtain intake and output and report
		Take initial baseline vital signs and monitor labs.	RN: assessment and interpretation of data

Adapted from Zerwekh, J., & Claborn, J. C. (2000). *Nursing today: Transitions and trends.* Philadelphia: W. B. Saunders.

The final step in the process involves a written assignment sheet. Who can perform each task?

RN:

All initial assessments
All IVs and IV medications (101, 102, 103, 104, 105, 106)
Discharge planning (101, 102, 104, 105, 106)
Collaborate with the nursing home (105)
Collaborate with Reach for Recovery (breast cancer support group) (102)
Evaluate procedure preparation (103, 104)
Evaluate preoperative/preprocedure teaching and informed consent (101,103)
Collaborate with family (102, 105)
Collaborate with social service (102)
Collaborate with dialysis nurse (103)
Monitor labs (104, 106)
Infuse blood (106)
Plan work assignments for oncoming shift

LPN/LVN:

All medications except IVs
Prepare for surgery (103)
Glucoscans (103)
Stool specimens (104)
Hemoccult stool (106)
Monitor, empty, and record drain (102)
Assist UAP with hygienic care all patients
Assist with turns

UAP:

Turn patient every 2 hours (101, 105)
Obtain vital signs and intake and output for all patients
Hygienic care all patients
Assist with admissions, discharge, and transfers
Foley catheter care (101)
Feeding (105)

Special Notes

*All staff assist with answering call lights
All staff monitor for safety needs (101, 105)
NPO (101, 103, 104)

PRACTICE EXERCISES: DELEGATION

Scenarios: Delegating Tasks

SCENARIO 1

1. Identify the tasks for the new admission that could be delegated to the UAP.
   Initial greeting and vital signs

The following tasks need to be completed during your shift in addition to other tasks of assessing patients, passing medications, completing documentation, processing physician's orders, and performing discharge planning.
A. Teach a patient to give own insulin
B. Assist the physician with a paracentesis
C. Write the plan of care for a newly admitted patient
D. Perform wound assessment and photo-documentation
E. Perform blood glucose tests for three patients
F. Phone report of labs to the physician
G. Insert Foley catheter
H. Collect intake and output data
I. Evaluate patient response to pain medication

2. Identify those tasks that you as the RN could not delegate and explain why.
Assessment, evaluation, and nursing judgment cannot be delegated. These include A, B, C, D, F, and I.

3. Identify those tasks that you could delegate to an experienced LPN/LVN who has demonstrated competent skills.
A competent, experienced LPN/LVN could assist in teaching the insulin injection, but the RN must assess the patient's knowledge and understanding. The LPN/LVN would possess the skills necessary to assist with a sterile procedure, contribute data for the care plan development, take photo of pressure wound, and evaluate pain response to medication; however, the RN must write the care plan and perform the wound assessment.

4. The RN delegates the vital signs, baths, and intake and output for eight patients to the UAP. What is the RN's accountability for the delegated work?
The RN must define patient parameters to the UAP that must be reported to the RN.

5. Describe the directions and communication you would use in defining the patient parameters to be reported by the UAP.
The nurse should identify the tasks and communicate performance expectations. Parameters should be established so that the UAP understands to report significant vital signs, fluid imbalances, and changes in status. The UAP should be instructed to ask for assistance and support. The UAP should understand from whom to seek assistance.

SCENARIO 2

1. Identify the tasks for the new admission that could be delegated to the UAP.
Initial greetings and vital signs. Apply oxygen setup, obtain oxygen saturation, and report to RN.

The following tasks need to be completed during your shift in addition to other tasks of assessing patients, passing medications, documentation, processing physician's orders, and discharge planning.
A. Incentive spirometry every 4 hours for postoperative patients
B. Pain management for postoperative patients
C. Remove IV from painful IV site
D. Restart IV
E. Apply oxygen setup for new admission
F. Obtain oxygen saturation level on new admission
G. Perform admission assessment on new admission
H. Develop plan of care for new admission
I. Perform blood glucose tests for two patients
J. Administer tube feeding every 4 hours for geriatric patient
K. Perform wound reassessment and dressing changes for decubitus sores

2. Identify those tasks that you as the RN could not delegate and explain why.
A, B, D, G, and H. D, G, and H all require higher-level skills as well as assessment., evaluation, and nursing judgment. B could be a shared responsibility with the LPN/LVN. Although the

LPN/LVN could administer pain medication, it is still the RN's evaluation skills that determine whether the expected outcome has been achieved.

3. Identify those tasks that you could delegate to the LPN/LVN.
   A, B, C, I, J, K. C, J, and K are tasks clearly within the LPN/LVN's scope of practice. B is a shared responsibility with the RN. See note above. For item A, the LPN/LVN can have the patient use the device, but the RN should do evaluation and interpretation of the patient status. On item I, covering blood sugar with sliding scale insulin is within the LPN/LVN's realm.

4. Identify those tasks that you would delegate to the UAP.
   E, F, and I. If I is on the UAP's competency list, performing blood glucose checks is acceptable as long as the patient is stable.

Evaluating Skills and Competencies of the Caregiver

1. An 11-year-old female diabetic patient running a blood sugar of 800 is severely dehydrated.
   RN

2. A 67-year-old female patient with a gastrointestinal tube for feeding with a diagnosis of congestive heart failure and debilitating arthritis
   LPN/LVN

3. An 89-year-old female patient with bladder incontinence and a diagnosis of dementia who needs hygienic care
   UAP

4. A 52-year-old female patient experiencing abdominal discomfort and abdominal distention, who has had 50 mL urine output in past 24 hours
   RN

5. A 14-year-old patient admitted 2 days ago with a tibial fracture and an external fixator that requires pin site care
   LPN/LVN

6. An 85-year-old patient, 2 days after gastrointestinal tube placement, with a methicillin-resistant *Staphylococcus aureus* (MRSA)–positive culture, who needs a dressing change to a pressure ulcer to the coccyx
   LPN/LVN

7. A 36-year-old female patient, 2 days after appendectomy, who needs to be ambulated
   UAP

8. A 78-year-old patient, admitted with a fractured hip, 4 days after surgery, who requires a sterile dressing change
   LPN/LVN

9. A new colostomy patient who requires fitting of the appliance and the first irrigation procedure
   RN

10. A 38-year-old patient, 2 days after an above-the-knee amputation, who is receiving peritoneal dialysis
    RN

11. A 29-year-old female patient admitted for a cardiac catheterization today, in need of an informed consent, lab work to be drawn, and patient teaching
    RN

12. A patient with a right-sided cerebral vascular accident who requires assistance with feeding
    UAP

13. A 46-year-old new-onset diabetes patient being discharged today
    RN

14. A 37-year-old female patient in need of a blood glucose test before meals (ac) and at bedtime (hs)
    UAP

15. A 29-year-old patient, 2 days after a right total-knee operation, in need of having intake and output recorded
    UAP

16. A 33-year-old female patient, 3 days after an open-reduction, internal-fixation right leg operation, who needs the catheter discontinued today
    LPN/LVN

17. A 27-year-old male patient positive for hepatitis C, with urine positive for illegal drugs, who is threatening to leave against medical advice if he "doesn't get pain medication now"
    RN

18. An 89-year-old female patient admitted with dementia and urinary incontinence needing hygienic care
    UAP

19. A 24-year-old patient, 2 days after appendectomy, who needs vital signs taken
    UAP

20. A 21-year-old patient, 2 days after appendectomy, who ran a fever last night and needs to be ambulated today
    UAP

Chapter 7 COMMUNICATION

SCENARIO TO ACCOMPANY STUDENT WORKSHEETS: GIVING REPORT

SAMPLE ANSWERS

1. What information do you need to gather before report?
   Assessment information: auscultation of chest, degree of peripheral edema, blood sugar results, vital signs, condition of needle site, activity toleration, current condition
   Kardex information: treatment plan with nursing diagnose
   Reports or worksheets from team members—intake and output.
   Information received in report
   Changes in condition during the shift
   Tests performed and results received
   Patient education performed

2. Should all the information obtained with an assessment be communicated during report?
   No, only information that is appropriate and relevant

3. In giving report, what things should be included?
   See list in skill sheet under Implementation

4. After giving report, you think of items that you forgot. At times, you must call the unit after arriving home with additional information. What strategies could be used to decrease the incidence of this?
   Organize information on a report sheet
   Recheck to make sure all information is gathered before starting
   Rehearse report
   Ask that socialization among staff decrease during report. This can be distracting and result in disorganized, fragmented report.

SCENARIO TO ACCOMPANY STUDENT WORKSHEETS: CALLING THE PHYSICIAN

Sample Answers

1. What are the steps in notifying the doctor?
   See skills checklist under Implementation

2. What would you tell the doctor?
   The transfer sheet indicates vomiting of bright red blood.
   Vital signs
   Tender abdomen with hyperactive bowel sounds
   Current medications
   Reddened area on coccyx
   Mental status
   History of CVA with expressive aphasia and Alzheimer's disease

3. What orders might you receive?
   IV fluids, x-rays and other diagnostic tests, lab work including a CBC and electrolytes, turn every 2 hours, discontinue medications at this time

4. What would you do if unable to contact the physician?
   Attempt to contact at available numbers and page
   Document attempts to contact
   Check on routine or standing orders
   Keep patient NPO
   Other options depend on institution—may contact physician's service, house staff, or nursing supervisor.

PRACTICE EXERCISES: COMMUNICATION

Calling the Physician: Sample Answers

1. You are a staff nurse on a surgical unit. A patient has returned from knee replacement surgery 2 hours ago. The patient is complaining of incisional pain. Should you call the doctor?
   This is normally not necessary. Pain is expected following this surgery, and the physician has most likely written orders in anticipation of this. Check the postoperative order sheet for the pain medication ordered by the physician.

2. You are a staff nurse at a long-term care facility. A new resident has been admitted to your wing. What should you do before contacting the physician?
   Assess the patient first. Obtain a thorough history including allergies. List current medications. Analyze the data for significance and note abnormal findings.

3. What orders would you expect to receive from the call?
   Orders for: activity, diet and fluids, medications, therapies (physical, occupational, speech, etc.), treatments (such as wound care), and lab and diagnostic tests.

PRACTICE EXERCISES: PATIENT TEACHING

Writing Objectives: Sample Answers

1. Mr. Smith has been newly diagnosed with diabetes mellitus. Write an additional objective for the teaching plan. (There are many possibilities for answers)
   At the end of the hour session and given a list of dietary exchanges and dietary requirements, Mr. Smith will correctly compose a sample food plan for one entire day.

2. How would you evaluate successful attainment of this objective?
   Compare Mr. Smith's written plan to his established dietary guidelines.

CHAPTER 9 Applying Clinical Reasoning to Various Practice Settings

SCENARIO TO ACCOMPANY STUDENT WORKSHEETS: USING CLINICAL REASONING SKILLS

Sample Answers

PHYSICAL ASSESSMENT DATA

1. What would you need to do about these findings?
   Call the doctor with the lab results to obtain IV fluid orders. Also, need to monitor electrolytes closely. When rehydration begins, the potassium will drop, which can cause some rhythm disturbance. May need to have order for telemetry.

2. Is the current intravenous (IV) therapy consistent with the lab data and medical diagnosis?
   No. The patient should have fluids, either 0.9% NS or lactated Ringer's solution.

   Unlike the nursing process, cognitive skills (critical thinking) can occur in any sequence. The nurse must decide when to apply these skills in clinical practice. Apply the skills to the following example:
   While reviewing the chart to gather data, the nurse notes that the patient was given 500 mg of amoxicillin, and the doctor's order sheet was for 250 mg of amoxicillin three times daily.
   Use your critical thinking skills to analyze this finding.

3. Use interpretation to describe what this means.
   A medication error has occurred because the wrong dose of medication was given.

4. Use analysis to determine the cause of the problem.
   How would this affect the patient?
   Why did the medication error occur?
   Was the medication given according to the five rights?
   Was the order for 500 mg?
   Should the next dose be held?
   Could the patient develop toxicity?

5. Identify what questions need to be answered to contribute data regarding the situation.
   Does the nurse need to call the primary care provider to get a blood level drawn?
   Was the nursing unit short-staffed, or was the nurse working an extra shift?

Was the writing of the doctor understandable?
Was the order transcribed and checked according to protocol?

6. Evaluation: Identify the outcome expected from the administration of the drug and determine whether progress was made toward the outcome.
   An antibiotic should destroy microbes; however, and overmedication can cause a toxic reaction as a result of damage to renal blood flow, causing harm to the patient.

7. Inferences: What conclusions can be drawn from the situation that will affect the nurse's decision?
   The nurse should monitor the patient's condition.
   A violation of the five rights has occurred.
   Fatigue and overwork may contribute to errors.
   Illegible handwriting may contribute to errors.
   Failure to follow standard protocol for processing orders may contribute to errors.

8. Explanation: Describe what to do. Why?
   The physician must be informed and an occurrence report made to identify ways to avoid this incident in the future.

9. Self-regulation: Describe what the nurse should do differently the next time to improve delivery of care (medication administration).
   Have no further medication error occur.

PRACTICE EXERCISES: CLINICAL REASONING IN VARIOUS PRACTICE SETTINGS

SCENARIO 1: MENTAL STATUS EXAMINATION

ASSESSMENT

1. To further assess the patient's mental status, what should the nurse do?
   Perform a Mini-Mental Status Examination.

2. Demonstrate application of the cognitive skills to the care needs related to Mr. Bender.
   Interpretation:
   The patient suffers from altered mental status.

   Analysis:
   What is the degree of confusion?
   What is the Risk Assessment Score?
   Has the patient fallen previously?
   Does the patient use assistive devices for mobility?
   What are the side effects of the medication being taken?
   How can we best keep the environment safe for this situation?
   Will the precautions to protect the patient from accidents and injury interfere with the patient's autonomy?

   Evaluation:
   Is the patient receiving care safely and effectively in the hospital environment?
   Is the patient able to meet his care needs with restrictions necessitated by hospitalization?
   Has the patient sustained any hospital-acquired injuries related to falls during this hospitalization?
   Inference:
   Altered mental status can cause the patient to be at increased risk for injury in an unfamiliar environment.
   The nurse should monitor the patient for behavior indicative of altered mental status during ongoing care.

Explanation:

Altered mental status contributes to the inability to interpret visual and auditory stimuli and impairs one's ability to find one's way around the environment.

Implementing full precautions can prevent injury.

Self-regulation:

"Do I know all the facts?"

"Is my thinking biased?"

"Am I making accurate assumptions?"

ANALYSIS

1. Which cue needs further discussion with the patient's wife other and why?

   The patient's wife states that the patient has a poor short-term memory but recalls things that happened in his childhood. The wife has expressed that "lately it is becoming an increasing concern." The wife may no longer feel able to take care of him in the home environment.

2. Based on this information, the nurse should suspect what condition?

   Alzheimer's disease

3. Identify the priority nursing diagnosis for this patient at this time.

   High risk for injury

OUTCOME IDENTIFICATION

1. Identify the goals appropriate to this patient's care.

   The patient will have no accidents or injuries related to hospitalization.

2. Which of these goals should receive priority in the care of the patient?

   Placement of barriers to prevent falls

3. List the indicators that should be recorded to indicate the goal has been met.

   NOC (1913) Safety Status: Physical Injury
   Skin abrasions
   Bruises
   Fractures
   To perform at level 5 (to have none)
   NOC (1909) Safety Behavior: Fall Prevention
   Placement of barriers to prevent falls
   Correct use of assistive devices
   Provision of personal assistance
   To perform at level 5

PLAN

1. Identify interventions appropriate for the hospital environment to prevent injuries.

   NIC (6460) Dementia Management
   Determine type and extent of cognitive impairment (using standardized tool).
   Include the wife in planning, providing, and evaluating care.
   Provide low-stimulation environment.
   Identify and remove potential dangers.
   Introduce self when initiating contact.
   Give simple directions, one at a time.
   Use distraction to manage behavior, rather than confrontation.
   Monitor nutrition and weight.
   Provide reality orientation cues.
   Monitor carefully for physiologic causes of increased confusion (especially low blood sugar secondary to hypoglycemia).
   Avoid use of physical restraints.

IMPLEMENTATION

1. Because the patient has altered mental status, how would instructions be different for a procedure?

    The altered mental status will affect the patient's ability to comply with instructions. Individuals performing procedures and tests should be aware of the cognitive impairment. For procedures requiring informed consent, the wife (or power of attorney [POA] for health care) should be consulted when obtaining consent.

EVALUATION

1. Describe the effectiveness in progressing toward the desired outcome.

    The patient will be able to meet his physical and emotional care needs during hospitalization safely. The patient will have no hospital-acquired injuries.

SCENARIO 2: CRITICAL CARE SETTING

1. What is the primary problem or issue?

    The patient is saying, "I want to know about the procedure before I sign." The issue is about informed consent, not about refusing to sign. The patient should be informed about risks and benefits. Additionally, he should be told what alternatives exist, including not having the proposed intervention.

2. What alternatives does the nurse have in planning interventions?

    A. Voice his or her opinion based on past experiences to convince the patient to sign the permit.

    B. Ask the nursing supervisor to intervene on the patient's behalf with the physician to work out a plan to protect the patient's right to make an informed choice.

    *C. **Best option.** Help the patient to write down his questions, call the physician back and ask him or her to communicate the desired information on the telephone to the patient.*

SCENARIO 3: CRITICAL CARE SETTING

1. What should the nurse do now?

    Make sure the patient understands the risks and benefits of blood administration. Call the physician and inform him or her about the variation; also inform the nursing supervisor. After conferring with all involved, if the physician makes the determination to proceed with the procedure, then cross out the Blood Consent section and have the patient sign only the surgical consent. Call the operating room and alert them before sending the patient. Clearly document what was discussed with the patient and the understanding that he expressed about the risks and benefits.

2. After surgery, the patient returns to his room on a ventilator and is very drowsy. Postoperative orders include:

    Type and cross-match 4 units of packed red blood cells (PRBCs) and transfuse 2 units when available.

    Give 2 units fresh frozen plasma (FFP) when available.

    The hemoglobin and hematocrit values are 4.9 mg/dL and 15.3%, respectively. What should the nurse do?

    Call the physician who ordered the blood products and explain the patient's choice. If the physician is uncomfortable with the patient's decision, he or she may consult the hospital ethics committee.

3. The surgeon cancels the order for the PRBCs and the FFP and talks to the patient's daughter about the situation and prognosis. An hour after the surgeon leaves, the patient's daughter, who is not a Jehovah's Witness, approaches the nurse and says she wants her father to have the blood. She further states that "if it is given while he is asleep, he will never know he got it." What should the nurse do now?

    A paternalistic approach to the patient's rights is almost never acceptable. The nurse is accountable to the patient in this circumstance, not the daughter. Who will know? The nurse will know. The damage to the nurse's opinion of himself or herself will be irreparable.

SCENARIO 4: CRITICAL CARE SETTING

1. The nurse starts to give the Lasix, when the patient states, "I do not want that shot!" The nurse asks, "Why?" The patient states, "It makes me urinate so much, and I have such a hard time when I use the bedpan or commode." She further elaborates, "I get leg cramps that hurt so bad!" What alternative courses of action does the nurse have?

    A. **Best option.** *Patient teaching. If there is not an order for a bedside commode, get one. Discuss leg cramps and diagnosis. Call the physician to obtain a medication order to relieve the discomfort.*

    B. *Call the physician and obtain an order for Foley catheter insertion before administration of the Lasix.*

SCENARIO 5: CRITICAL CARE SETTING

1. What should the nurse do now?

    Call the physician and the cardiac catheter lab. The initial preparation in the physician's office should have included an explanation of the procedure. When the patient arrives at the unit, the nurse should explain the procedure to the patient. Early intervention almost always produces a better result.

SCENARIO 6: OBSTETRIC AND PEDIATRIC CARE SETTING

1. As her nurse, what will you do to help her with the present situation? Why?

    Catheterize the patient. A full bladder hinders the baby's descent into the birth canal.

SCENARIO 7: OBSTETRIC AND PEDIATRIC CARE SETTING

1. What is the correct action to take at this time? Why?

    Place the baby under the heat lamp to elevate the temperature to at least 98.6°F (38.8°C). Explain to the mother the reason for this and tell her you will bring her baby to her as soon as the temperature reaches an acceptable range.

SCENARIO 8: OBSTETRIC AND PEDIATRIC CARE SETTING

1. As her nurse, what would you do to help Debra remain positive about her ability to breast-feed her baby?

    Possible interventions:

    Tell Debra to get some rest and try again when she is not so exhausted.

    Show Debra some videos on breast-feeding.

    Help Debra position the baby so that they both are comfortable.

    Teach Debra to express some milk onto the nipple to entice the baby to suck.

SCENARIO 9: ACUTE CARE SETTING

1. What should the nurse do about the labs?

    Given his circumstance, these are expected results of a renal patient.

    Consult with the dialysis nurse to establish the treatment schedule. Calling the physician is unnecessary as long as the dialysis routine is continued. Administer the sliding scale insulin.

SCENARIO 10: ACUTE CARE SETTING

1. What should the nurse do first?

    Assess vital signs (include orthostatic blood pressure with head of bed elevated).

    Call the physician with vitals and hematocrit and hemoglobin results.

    Prepare to initiate blood transfusion when available.

SCENARIO 11: ACUTE CARE SETTING

1. What alternatives should the nurse consider?

    A confused 92-year-old is a safety risk and was placed there to prevent injury. In addition, this is an ethical issue. There are limited alternatives. The bed on the pediatric unit should be the room of choice if the daughter continues to demand a private room for her mother.

2. After all of the alternatives are explored, the nurse determines that Mrs. Blue must be placed in a semiprivate room. How should the nurse proceed?
   Kindly but gently tell the daughter this is the only option available. Contact the hospital's patient representative to support the daughter.

SCENARIO 12: ACUTE CARE SETTING

1. What are some alternatives the nurse can consider in providing for the care needs of this patient?
   Critical care beds should be used for those that will gain the most benefit from the level of care provided. Explore alternatives such as family members staying, obtaining a sitter, and adjusting assignments for additional support of the team assigned to Mrs. Blue.

SCENARIO 13: HOME CARE SETTING

1. Outline the care needs of each patient. Identify what the nurse should do first.
   Patient 1:
   This is a clean wound, and there is a premature baby to consider.

   Patient 2:
   This is an immunosuppressed patient with HIV.

   Patient 3:
   This is an immunosuppressed patient with CRF.

   Patient 4:
   This is a dirty, lengthy, complex visit. The home care nurse needs to check with the charge nurse and have Patient 4 transferred to someone else. He needs to be replaced in this nurse's work assignment with a clean case to avoid contamination to other patients.

SCENARIO 14: HOME CARE SETTING

1. What is the primary problem or issue here?
   Medication compliance is probably the biggest issue with home care. The patient may not have enough money to buy all of her medications, such as the Coumadin.

SCENARIO 15: HOME CARE SETTING

1. What should the nurse do?
   This hospice patient is heavily medicated with narcotics (side effect, constipation) and is dehydrated (dark urine and constipation). Her assessment should be thorough and her care palliative. A trip to the emergency room would potentially cause her more discomfort. Assess recent stool history. Routinely, hospice patients have protocols in place related to constipation. Check for impaction, and evacuate it. This setting demands a great deal of autonomy and independent thinking from the nurse.

SCENARIO 16: PSYCHIATRIC CARE SETTING

1. What would be the first action of the nurse?
   Consult medication administration record (MAR) for previous administration of psychotropic medications.

2. What might the nurse interpret as the cause of any abnormal symptom?
   Neuroleptic malignant syndrome

3. Write an appropriate nursing diagnosis for the patient need.
   Ineffective breathing pattern R/T inadequate ventilation AEB tachypnea and neuromuscular rigidity.

4. Write an outcome statement that the nurse could use with this diagnosis.
   Respiratory rate will be maintained within normal limits.

5. Following the initial assessment and action in question 1, what would be the appropriate nursing plan of care?
   Call the physician. If appropriate, arrange transfer to the intensive care unit.

SCENARIO 17: PSYCHIATRIC CARE SETTING

1. Analyze each option for the risks and benefits of choosing it.
    A. *Call for help from unit staff.*
       Benefit: immediate response, less chance of injury with better-trained individuals
       Rick: other employees may be injured
       Other employees may not hear request or may not be able to leave current activity, resulting in delay.
    B. *Call for hospital security.*
       Benefit: may obtain added assistance from increased number of individuals
       Risk: may require more time to summon this help

    C. *Enter lounge alone and attempt to quiet patient.*
       Benefit: can remove other patients quickly; agitated patient may respond if a relationship exists with caregiver
       Risk: event may escalate, with injury to employee and other patients; may delay obtaining assistance

    D. *Go to supply room for restraining devices.*
       Benefit: devices would be handy if needed
       Risk: not least restrictive measure; seclusion would be more appropriate
       Requires strict documentation; other patients may be injured while nurse is in supply room

SCENARIO 18: PSYCHIATRIC CARE SETTING

1. What should Ashley do?
    The co-worker's responsibility regarding the impaired nurse is clearly addressed in the ANA Standards.
    The Nurse Practice Act dictates that the impaired nurse must be reported. Policy within the institution delineates who will be notified. Routinely, it is the nursing supervisor or charge nurse.

Chapter 10 **Ethical Decision Making**

SCENARIO TO ACCOMPANY STUDENT WORKSHEETS

Sample Answers

PLAN

1. *Confer with the nursing supervisor.*
2. *Consult the Ethics Committee.*
3. *Do nothing. The physician is aware of the issues and will select the best option for the circumstances.*

IMPLEMENTATION

Because of the urgency of the situation, consult with the nursing supervisor for now. The patient has a right to advance directives, and respect demands that health care personnel listen. The best option is to consult the Ethics Committee, but because of the instability of the patient, asking the nursing supervisor to intervene is better for now. At a later time, an Ethics Committee meeting should address the issue and educate the physician further on this subject. Doing nothing may cause the patient and family to be pressured into doing something they do not want.

EVALUATION

The nurse should continue to monitor the patient and family to ensure that their requests are honored and that they have the information necessary to continue making decisions.
    See the Answer Key in Appendix A for sample answers for this exercise.

PRACTICE EXERCISES: ETHICAL DECISION MAKING

Scenarios: Using the ANA Code of Ethics

Use the ANA Code of Ethics to determine what the patient could reasonably expect from the nurse in the following situations.

1. *Treat all patients with respect and dignity. ANA Standard 1.*
   As soon as the charge nurse detects a problem, she should remove the patient from the situation to protect him. Doing nothing will cause psychological harm. If possible, reassign the patient or assume responsibility for his care and confront the nurse about the situation.

2. *The nurse's primary duty is to the patient. ANA Standard 2.*
   The nurse is accountable to act as a patient advocate. The family is not the party for which the nurse is accountable. The problem is that the nurse is searching for the best way to assist the patient to receive the treatment that she really wants. Share the daughter's concerns with the patient and encourage the patient to communicate her wishes to the daughter.

3. *The nurse should protect the patient from harm. ANA Standard 5.*
   The patient has a reasonable expectation that the nurse will act in a manner that will not harm him or her. Listen to the concerns of the patient and family, acknowledge the mistake, and do it in a manner that the patient and others know of your sorrow. Second, counsel the new nurse to understand why the incident occurred and determine the best course of action to prevent the mistake from occurring in the future.

4. *The nurse is responsible for personal professional conduct in the work environment consistent with the values of nursing. ANA Standard 6.*
   Remove the nurse from the situation to protect the patients from potential danger and then confront the employee. Refer the employee to the employee assistance department, or follow the institutional protocol for dealing with an impaired nurse.

5. *Collaborate with other health care providers to meet the patient's total health needs. ANA Standard 8.*
   Discuss the problem with the nurse to identify the exact problem and contributing factors. Review the agency's reporting procedure for accuracy and clarity.

6. *The nurse is responsible and accountable for appropriate delegation. ANA Standard 4.*
   First, treat the patient emergency with appropriate interventions and mediation such as Narcan, assessing oxygen saturation, obtaining vital signs, and administering oxygen. If you do not have treatment orders already in place, call the physician and obtain orders. Second, this is inappropriate delegation. The patient care assignment is the responsibility of the RN. Each skill level can be determined by the associated job description, and workers in the skill level are accountable and responsible to know their job boundaries. Having a discussion with the nurse and UAP to determine the facts and dealing with the situation based on the facts are imperative to achieving safe care for all patients.

7. *The nurse is responsible for maintaining integrity in practice and profession. ANA Standard 9.*
   This is unacceptable, and the nurse will be prosecuted for murder. The nurse–patient relationship is built on trust. The patient should be able to expect respect as a person.

8. *The nurse has a duty to participate in knowledge development. ANA Standard 7.*
   The nurse should contribute data and input into the knowledge base by completing the occurrence report for faulty equipment and other documentation requested for trial studies. This provides data to protect future patients from harm.

9. *Delegate appropriately to ensure administration of optimum patient care. ANA Standard 4.*
   By refusing to delegate, the nurse has more to do than is humanly possible for one person. The nurse should ask a more experienced nurse for assistance with delegation to resolve the immediate situation. Second, the nurse should request information on delegation principles. As a result of increased knowledge and learning how to delegate safely, patient care will improve.

10. *The nurse's primary duty is to the patient. ANA Standard 2.*

The nurse is accountable to act as a patient advocate. The family is not the party for which the nurse is accountable. If the patient has indicated in some way that she did not want to know, the moral duty to tell has been resolved. The problem here is the nurse is searching for the best way to assist the patient to receive the treatment that she really wants. Share the husband's concerns with the patient and encourage the patient to communicate her wishes to the husband.

11. *The nurse has a responsibility to protect the patient's rights, that is, confidentiality. ANA Standard 3.*

Personal information the patient gives to the nurse and information obtained from the medical records during delivery of care should be held in confidence. "The patient has a right to expect that all communications and records pertaining to his care be treated as confidential" (American Hospital Association, 1992). The nurse should tell the caller that all patient information is confidential.

12. *Treat all patients with respect, dignity and as unique individuals. ANA Standard 1.*

As soon as the charge nurse detects a problem, it is important to remove the patient from the situation to protect him. Doing nothing will cause psychological harm. If possible, reassign the patient or assume responsibility for the care, and confront the nurse about the situation.

Scenarios: Making Ethical Decisions

SCENARIO 1

Options
1. *Ethics consult is the only viable option. This will facilitate discussion of quality of life and gather input from family, physician, and other experienced professionals.*
2. Do nothing. Respect family's opinion because they are now the decision makers. This leaves everybody in crisis.

SCENARIO 2

Options
1. Do nothing and just accept the physician's order.
2. Call the physician back and get reprimanded.
3. *Review the chart to determine whether there is another physician that can be called.*
4. Notify the nursing supervisor.

SCENARIO 3

Options
1. Do nothing. Leaves everybody in crisis.
2. *Ethics consult is an option for all to express views and come to an understanding and agreement. If the patient clearly lacks decision-making capacity, and the family can't agree after the consult, the Healthcare Surrogate Act compels that someone be appointed. This requires time to have a court-appointed decision maker thoroughly assess the patient's situation.*
3. Obtain social services consultation to discuss power of attorney (POA) and advance directives with the patient.

SCENARIO 4

Options
1. Do nothing about the concern. Give the drug.
2. *Call the nursing supervisor and ask him or her to intervene. Do not give the drug because this is an invalid order.*

SCENARIO 5

Options

1. Do nothing. The patient has already signed an informed consent. Proceed with the procedure because further delay may cause harm to the patient.
2. Call the nursing supervisor and ask him or her to intervene.
3. *Assess the patient's reason for refusal. It may be a misunderstanding or anxiety. The nurse is the patient advocate. Clarify with the patient his understanding of a pacemaker. A patient has a right to informed consent and may rescind that consent at any time. He has a right to refuse treatment options as long as he fully understands the risks involved and is willing to accept the consequences. The health care provider's role involves helping the individual with life decisions. Call the physician out of the OR and ask him or her to discuss this issue further.*

SCENARIO 6

Options

1. Indirect intervention. Use distraction, determine whether family can come sit or whether a sitter is available to stay.
2. *Assess the patient for mentation; assess the physician's order and the chart to determine the reason for the device. If the restraints have been placed because of staffing issues, remove them. Put the bed in low position and explore the use of a lap tray with a chair while observing behavior. Consult with the nurse manager to discuss staffing issues. Complete an occurrence report to avoid further incidents.*
3. Do nothing. Leave restraints on and assume that she needs them because you have an order.

SCENARIO 7

Options

1. Do nothing. This violates the patient's right to appropriate pain management.
2. *Call the physician for breakthrough pain medication that does not affect the respiratory system. Assess the description of the pain. Discuss with Irene the level of pain that is acceptable to her. Review the medication sheet to determine whether there are other supplemental drugs that might cover the breakthrough pain episodes. Consult with the pharmacist or other hospice nurses for options that have been effective in similar situations with other patients. Discuss the risks and benefits of various pain management drugs with the patient and family members. Determine an acceptable pain management regimen with the patient, taking into consideration the risks and benefits.*

SCENARIO 8

Answer

The nurse should assess the home situation and support system for the patient. When the home environment is unsafe or the patient does not have the necessary skill to function in the home setting, social services must be called.

What options should the nurse consider?

Options

1. Refuse to discharge the patient until she is able to perform skills for diabetic management independently.
   Outcome: Reimbursement issues for the hospital and a delay does not change the fact that the patient does not have the resources to buy supplies and medication.
2. Do nothing. Discharge the patient.
   Outcome: The nurse has failed to protect the patient from harm. This is an unsafe discharge. The diabetic patient must have insulin, syringes, and supplies to control the blood sugar and maintain diabetic control.

3. *Collaborate with social services and ask for an ethics consult. The patient has a right to a transition plan, and this is an unsafe discharge.*
   Outcome: Delaying the discharge until appropriate arrangements can be made through social services to help the patient find resources to obtain needed medical care and home care to arrange further patient teaching to ensure that she is able to perform needed skills independently are essential for this patient to have a safe discharge.

SCENARIO 9

ANSWER

Do nothing. There is no other choice except to perform the code unless the physician decides to write a no code order against the wishes of the two family members, and this is a rare occurrence. Continue to collaborate with social services and pastoral care to work with family members.

SCENARIO 10

OPTIONS

1. Do nothing. Abide by the patient wishes. Patient will most likely continue to deteriorate.
2. *Call an ethics consult to ensure that family can be involved. This will ensure that everyone understands that the patient could be ambulatory if the surgical intervention were successful. If the patient continues to refuse, the patient's choice must be honored.*
3. Patient teaching. Evaluate her understanding of surgery risks and benefits. After 4 years, it is unlikely that this will be effective, but it is important to at least try.

SCENARIO 11

OPTIONS

1. *There are no options for active treatment. Palliative treatment is the only alternative. Call social services and work with the patient to gain some insight and develop realistic expectations. The focus should be redirected to quality time and putting affairs in order.*
2. A psychiatric consult may be indicated if the situation continues, and the nurse should also ask the physician to explain the side effects of the drugs further.
3. Do nothing. Leaves everybody in a crisis.

SCENARIO 12

OPTIONS

1. *Encourage the patient to discuss these issues with his wife. Educate him about the consequences of his behavior to the unborn child and wife. Encourage him to disclose this information to his wife so that testing can be performed and treatment if indicated. Confidentiality prevents telling. Consult with social services to discuss these issues with the patient.*
2. Do nothing. This maintains confidentiality but denies wife and unborn child treatment if indicated.

SCENARIO TO ACCOMPANY STUDENT WORKSHEETS

Sample Answers

Using the Checklist as a guideline for decisions, consider the skills and competencies of the staff members to select the assignment that achieves the most desirable outcomes for all patients involved. Use the table below to assign duties to available staff members.

RN: This nurse would be best suited for unit-specific needs and situations with unpredictable outcomes, or potential for adverse affects.

Room 102: Blood infusion, manage central line care and interpret laboratory data

Room 105: Manage PCA pump for pain control, unit-specific equipment (CPM), neurovascular assessments, and postoperative care of the orthopedic patient

Room 106: Unit-specific care needs for teaching, informed consent, interpretation of labs and telemetry strips; develop plan of care for new admission (disease-specific plan)

Room 111: Manage PCA pump for pain control, emotional needs with death and dying, unit-specific care

Discharge Planning

Collaborate with Reach for Recovery (breast cancer support group)

Evaluate procedure preparation

Evaluate preoperative/preprocedure teaching and informed consent

Monitor labs

Infuse blood

Plan work assignments for oncoming shift

OB FLOAT NURSE:

This nurse would be best suited for care of the abdominal surgery patient (experience with cesarean sections), perirectal and vaginal care, parenteral therapy and antibiotics, monitoring for hemorrhage, and patients who do not have unit-specific care and teaching needs.

Room 101: Abdominal incision and postoperative needs

Room 104: Perineal care, pain management, preoperative preparation, and preoperative teaching

Room 108: Abdominal incision, parenteral therapy, and initiate venipuncture

Room 109: Peri-care and monitor for hemorrhage or further bleeding

IV medications for LPN (share pair)

Cover IVs and IV medications for patients in Rooms 101, 102, 103, 107, 108, 109, 110, 112

LPN/LVN:

This nurse is best suited for stable patients with predictable outcomes, routine care assignments, and cases requiring the technical skills of the LPN/LVN.

Room 103: Stable patient with predictable outcome

Room 107: Stable patient with predictable outcome

Room 110: Stable patient with predictable outcome

Room 112: Stable patient with predictable outcome

Routine and oral medications for float nurse (share pair)

All medications except IVs for patients in Rooms 101, 102, 103, 107, 108, 109, 110, 112

PRACTICE EXERCISES: APPLYING NURSING JUDGMENT IN CLINICAL SETTINGS

Scenarios: Making Room Assignments

SCENARIO 1

1. What transmission precautions does your patient require?
   Respiratory isolation

2. What is required for this type of precaution?
   Private room

3. Where would you put the patient?
   Move the adult patient to another floor and place the new patient in Room 216 bed A.

SCENARIO 2

1. What transmission precautions does your patient require?
   Contact isolation

2. What is required for this type of precaution?
   Private room

3. Where would you put the patient?
   Move the 6-year-old patient with Lyme disease in with the 10-year-old patient with a concussion and place the new patient in Room 305.

SCENARIO 3

1. What transmission precautions does you patient require?
   Respiratory isolation

2. What is required for this type of precaution?
   Negative airflow room

3. Where would you put the patient?
   Move the 36-year-old mayor with angina from the private room. Place the new patient in the negative airflow room.

SCENARIO 4

1. What transmission precautions does you patient require?
   Standard precautions

2. What is required for this type of precaution?
   Universal precautions

3. Where would you put this patient?
   Place the new patient with the 44-year-old electrician, diagnosis postoperative arthroscopy.

SCENARIO 5

1. What transmission precautions does your patient require?
   Contact precautions

2. What is required for this type of precaution?
   Private room

3. Where would you put the patient?
   Move the 3-year-old with MRI sedation in with the 8-year-old diabetic patient. Place the new patient in the private room.

Critical Thinking Exercises

1. D. *Routine care needs*
2. D. *Routine care needs*
3. A. *Routine care needs*
4. D. *Routine care needs*
5. B. *Dressing change to wound*
6. B. *Requires dressing change*
7. A. *Stable patient*
8. B. *Sterile dressing change*
9. B. *Threat to ABCs related to physiologic needs (option A is urgent, but psychosocial needs and pain do not supersede the evaluation, assessment, and judgment required for option B)*
10. B. *Threat for spontaneous bleed related to platelet count.*
11. B. *Physiologic threat for cell death related to Tylenol ingestion (option A has tracheostomy; thus, threat to airway is stabilized)*
12. A. *Requires high level of evaluation, assessment, and judgment*
13. A. *Active bleed is most urgent*
14. D. *Symptoms of shock already present*
15. C. *Symptoms of pulmonary embolus (common complications of DVT) threaten airway*
16. C. *Acidosis is life threatening*
17. D. *Potassium level of 2.5 mEq/L is life threatening*
18. D. *The oncology nurse has high level of expertise with PAC*
19. D. *Surgical preparation is familiar procedure to medical-surgical nurse*
20. C. *Nonverbal patients are familiar to pediatric nurse*
21. D. *Maintaining cardiovascular stability and emotional support are aspects of care familiar to the ICCU nurse*
22. A. *Abdominal wounds and surgical care patients are familiar to the medical-surgical nurse*
23. B. *High need for emotional support and someone to listen*
24. B. *High level of confidentiality is critical for ER nurse*
25. A. *Dextrose clots the blood*
26. A. *Do not give regular insulin when patient is NPO for a procedure without clarification*
27. A. *Do not give potassium in IV fluids when there is no urinary output*
28. B. *Addison's disease patient must be protected from infection*
29. B. *Sickle cell disease patient must be protected from infection*

North American Nursing Diagnosis Association (NANDA) Accepted Nursing Diagnoses

Activity intolerance
Activity intolerance, risk for
Adaptive capacity, decreased: Intracranial
Adjustment, impaired
Airway clearance, ineffective
Anxiety
Anxiety, death
Aspiration, risk for
Bed mobility, impaired
Body image, disturbed
Body temperature, risk for imbalanced
Breast-feeding, effective
Breast-feeding, ineffective
Breast-feeding, interrupted
Breathing pattern, ineffective
Cardiac output, decreased
Caregiver role strain
Caregiver role strain, risk for
Communication, impaired verbal
Confusion, acute
Confusion, chronic
Constipation
Constipation, perceived
Constipation, risk for
Coping, community: Readiness for enhanced
Coping, defensive
Coping, family: Compromised
Coping, family: Disabled
Coping, family: Readiness for enhanced
Coping, ineffective
Coping, ineffective community
Decisional conflict
Denial, ineffective
Dentition, altered
Development, risk for delayed

Diarrhea
Disuse syndrome, risk for
Diversional activity, deficient
Dysreflexia
Dysreflexia, risk for
Energy field disturbance
Environmental interpretation syndrome, impaired
Failure to thrive, adult
Falls, risk for
Family processes, dysfunctional: Alcoholism
Family processes, interrupted
Fatigue
Fear
Fluid volume, deficient
Fluid volume, deficient, risk for
Fluid volume, excess
Fluid volume, imbalanced, risk for
Gas exchange, impaired
Grieving, anticipatory
Grieving, dysfunctional
Growth and development, delayed
Growth, risk for disproportionate
Health maintenance, ineffective
Home maintenance, impaired
Hopelessness
Hyperthermia
Hypothermia
Incontinence, bowel
Incontinence, functional urinary
Incontinence, reflex urinary
Incontinence, stress urinary
Incontinence, total urinary
Incontinence, urge urinary
Incontinence, urge urinary, risk for
Infant behavior, disorganized
Infant behavior, readiness for enhanced organized
Infant feeding pattern, ineffective
Infection, risk for
Injury, risk for perioperative positioning
Injury, risk for
Intracranial adaptive capacity, decreased
Knowledge, deficient
Latex allergy response
Latex allergy response, risk for
Loneliness, risk for
Memory, impaired
Nausea
Noncompliance
Nutrition, imbalanced: Less than body requirements
Nutrition, imbalanced: more than body requirements
Nutrition, imbalanced, risk for: More than body requirements
Oral mucous membrane, impaired
Pain, acute
Pain, chronic
Parental role conflict
Parent–infant/child attachment, risk for impaired

Parenting, impaired
Parenting, impaired, risk for
Peripheral neurovascular dysfunction, risk for
Personal identity, disturbed
Physical mobility, impaired
Poisoning, risk for
Post-trauma syndrome
Post-trauma syndrome, risk for
Powerlessness
Powerlessness, risk for
Protection, ineffective
Rape trauma syndrome
Rape trauma syndrome: Compound reaction
Rape trauma syndrome: Silent reaction
Relocation stress syndrome
Relocation stress syndrome, risk for
Role performance, ineffective
Self-care deficit, bathing/hygiene
Self-care deficit, dressing/grooming
Self-care deficit, feeding
Self-care deficit, toileting
Self-esteem, chronic low
Self-esteem, low
Self-esteem, situational low
Self-esteem, situational low, risk for
Self-mutilation
Self-mutilation, risk for
Sensory perception, disturbed
Sexual dysfunction
Sexuality patterns, ineffective
Skin integrity, impaired
Skin integrity, impaired, risk for
Sleep deprivation
Sleep pattern, disturbed
Social interaction, impaired
Social isolation
Sorrow, chronic
Spiritual distress
Spiritual distress, risk for
Spiritual well-being, readiness for enhanced
Suffocation, risk for
Suicide, risk for
Surgical recovery, delayed
Swallowing, impaired
Therapeutic regimen management, effective
Therapeutic regimen management, ineffective
Therapeutic regimen management, ineffective community
Therapeutic regimen management, ineffective family
Thermoregulation, ineffective
Thought processes, disturbed
Tissue integrity, impaired
Tissue perfusion, ineffective
Toileting self-care deficit
Transfer ability, impaired
Trauma, risk for
Unilateral neglect

Urinary elimination, impaired
Urinary retention
Ventilation, impaired spontaneous
Ventilatory weaning response, dysfunctional
Violence, other-directed, risk for
Violence, self-directed, risk for
Walking, impaired
Wandering
Wheelchair mobility, impaired

INDEX

Note: Page numbers followed by f indicate figures; those followed by t indicate tables, and those followed by b indicate boxed material.

U

Understaffing, 203, 265
  ethical aspects of, 240–241
Unlicensed assistive personnel
  delegation to, 123–125. *See also* Delegation
  scope of practice for, 123b

V

Values
  clarification of, 229–230, 237, 237b
  in decision making, 38
  ethics and, 229
Veracity, 232
Verbal orders, 154–156, 156b

W

Walking rounds, 151
Working plan, development of, 261
Workload, excessive, 203, 240–241, 265